Advanced Endoscopic Sinus Surgery

Advanced Endoscopic Sinus Surgery

Editor
James A. Stankiewicz, M.D.
Professor and Vice Chairman
Department of Otolaryngology - Head and Neck Surgery
Loyola University at Chicago Medical Center
Maywood, Illinois

with 234 illustrations

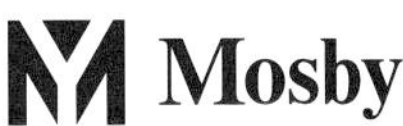

St. Louis Baltimore Berlin Boston Carlsbad Chicago London Madrid
Naples New York Philadelphia Sydney Tokyo Toronto

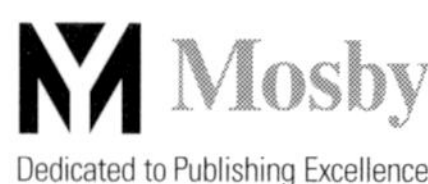

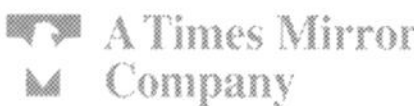

Publisher: Anne Patterson
Editor: Robert Hurley
Developmental Editor: Lauranne Billus
Project Manager: Christopher J. Baumle
Production Editor: David Orzechowski
Designer: Nancy McDonald
Manufacturing Supervisor: Karen Lewis

First Edition

Printed in the United States of America
Composition by Carlisle Communications, Ltd.
Printing/binding by Walsworth Publishing Company

Cover: From Cerebrospinal Fluid Fistula and Endoscopic Sinus Surgery, *Laryngoscope* 101:250–256, 1991.

Mosby–Year Book, Inc.
11830 Westline Industrial Drive
St. Louis, Missouri 63146

Library of Congress Cataloging-in-Publication Data

Advanced endoscopic sinus surgery / James A. Stankiewicz. -- 1st ed.
p. cm.
Includes bibliographical references and index.
ISBN 0-8151-7944-8 (alk. paper)
1. Paranasal sinuses—Endoscopic surgery. I. Stankiewicz, James A.
[DNLM: 1. Paranasal Sinuses—surgery. 2. Endoscopy. WV 340 A244 1944]
RF421.A28 1994
617.5'23—dc20
DNLM/DLC
for Library of Congress

94-23525
CIP

95 96 97 / 9 8 7 6 5 4 3 2

Contributors

Jack B. Anon, M.D., F.A.C.S.
Clinical Assistant Professor
University of Pittsburgh School of Medicine
Department of Otolaryngology
Pittsburgh, Pennsylvania

John P. Bent, III, M.D.
Department of Otolaryngology
University of Iowa Hospital and Clinics
Iowa City, Iowa

David W. Chambers, M.D.
Division of Otolaryngology
University of Missouri School of Medicine
Columbia, Missouri

James M. Chow, M.D.
Associate Professor
Department of Otolaryngology—Head and Neck Surgery
Loyola University Medical Center
Maywood, Illinois

James A. Duncavage, M.D.
Associate Professor and Vice Chairman
Department of Otolaryngology
Vanderbilt University Medical Center
Nashville, Tennessee

David H. Henick, M.D.
Fellow
Department of Otolaryngology
University of Pennsylvania
Philadelphia, Pennsylvania

Alfredo Herrara V., M.D.
Hospital Clinica San Rafael
Departmento de Otorrinolaringologia
Y Carugia De Cabeza Y Cuello
Bogota, COLOMBIA

Roger Jankowski, M.D.
Associate Professor
Department of Otolaryngology
Head and Neck Surgery
Hospital Central
Nancy Cedex
FRANCE

Jordan S. Josephson, M.D., F.A.C.S.
Director, Nasal and Sinus Center
New York, New York;
Consultant Staff
National Institutes of Health
Bethesda, Maryland;
Attending Physician
Manhattan Eye, Ear, and Throat Hospital
New York, New York

David W. Kennedy, M.D.
Professor and Chairman
Department of Otolaryngology
University of Pennsylvania Medical Center
Philadelphia, Pennsylvania

Frederick A. Kuhn, M.D.
Professor
Division of Otolaryngology
The Medical College of Georgia
Augusta, Georgia

Rodney Lusk, M.D.
Associate Professor
Washington University
St. Louis Children's Hospital
St. Louis, Missouri

Mark May, M.D., F.A.C.S.
Shadyside Hospital
Facial Paralysis and Sinus Surgery Center
Pittsburgh, Pennsylvania

Ralph B. Metson, M.D., F.A.C.S.
Assistant Professor
Harvard University
Otolaryngology—Head and Neck Surgery
Private Practice
Boston, Massachusetts

David S. Parsons, M.D., F.A.A.P., F.A.C.S.
Professor of Surgery and Pediatrics
Division of Otolaryngology
University of Missouri School of Medicine
Columbia, Missouri

Barry Schaitkin, M.D.
Shadyside Hospital
Facial Paralysis and Sinus Surgery Center
Pittsburgh, Pennsylvania

Reuben C. Setliff, III, M.D.
Private Practice in
Otolaryngology
North Platte, Nebraska

Seth J. Silberman, M.D.
The Sinus Center
Cleveland, Ohio

James A. Stankiewicz, M.D.
Professor and Vice Chairman
Department of Otolaryngology—Head and Neck Surgery
Loyola University Medical Center
Maywood, Illinois

Leonard H. Wurman, M.D., F.A.C.S.
Division of Otolaryngology—Head and Neck Surgery
Ear, Nose, and Throat Associates of Wausau, S.C.
Wausau Hospital Center
Wausau, Wisconsin

S. James Zinreich, M.D.
Associate Professor
The Johns Hopkins Medical Institutions
Department of Radiology
Baltimore, Maryland

To Joanne, my wife, for continuing patience and love despite much lost time.
To my children—Jim, Damien, Mara, Justin—the lights of my life!
To my parents, Adam and Mildred: Thank you! Time is short but my love is forever.

Preface

Since 1985, endoscopic diagnosis and surgery have moved from their beginnings in the United States to advanced diagnostic and treatment alternatives for numerous pathologic problems affecting the nose and sinuses. Therefore, it is appropriate that this textbook—the first dealing with advanced endoscopic sinus surgery—be written. Although other textbooks have dealt with the viewpoints of one or two authors regarding selected advanced topics in endoscopic sinus surgery, this book presents a wide variety of advanced topics in this area. These topics are discussed by the investigators who have pioneered and refined the endoscopic treatment for these problems. The book is written in an easy-to-read format and features numerous illustrations and short chapters for the advanced practitioner. Each chapter is filled with pearls of knowledge from the experts. Some of the techniques, such as Dr. Setliff's chapter on the microdebrider or "Hummer," are described for the first time. Dr. Lusk and Dr. Parsons, the foremost pediatric sinus surgeons in the United States, present their up-to-date viewpoints of the best way to handle revision and primary endoscopic sinus surgery (including the "Hummer" technique) in children. Dr. Fred Kuhn, who has the most experience in frontal sinus endoscopy, discusses his surgical approaches to the frontal sinuses. Dr. David Kennedy, the acknowledged leader and pioneer in endoscopic sinus diagnosis and surgery in the United States, provides his expert insight into fungal sinusitis and orbital decompression. Dr. Mark May, perhaps the best teacher in endoscopic sinus diagnosis and surgery, and his associate, Dr. Barry Schaitkin, describe their experiences with the troublesome revision sinus patient.

I hope this book

- provides information that will assist practitioners in their preparation and performance of advanced sinus surgery;
- provides wise counsel about techniques for performing safe surgery and avoiding complications; and
- acts as a handy reference that will be used over and over again.

As one peruses the table of contents, I feel the scope and potential usefulness of this textbook will be readily apparent.

I would like to thank all of the authors for their outstanding efforts to make this book an excellent reference for advanced endoscopic sinus surgery.

Acknowledgements

To my secretary, Susan Whelton, for her skill and valuable assistance; to Joanne Zichmiller for helping me locate and order materials; to Sandra Cello Lang and her staff for their excellent medical media work; to Lauranne Billus for coordinating the project; to David Orzechowski for his editing expertise; to Dr. Gregory Matz and the Department of Otolaryngology for their advice and support; and to Wendy Miller, R.N., M.S.N., for her help and support. Without these people, no book would be possible.

Contents

Advanced Endoscopic Sinus Surgery

1

Revision Endoscopic Sinus Surgery

Barry Schaitkin and Mark May

Revision endoscopic sinus surgery challenges the surgeon's skill and experience because the usual anatomic reference points are altered by previous surgery and scarring, as well as disease. In this presentation we review indications for revision surgery in our patients. We also describe the anatomic landmarks we rely upon to perform revision surgery effectively and nearly without complications.

Common Reasons for Revision Surgery

THE MIDDLE TURBINATE

The most common reason for failure of endoscopic sinus surgery in our patients followed up for 2 years or longer has been lateralization and adhesions of the middle turbinate with obstructed drainage of the frontal, maxillary, or anterior ethmoid sinuses (Fig. 1–1). Adhesions occur when the mucosa from the lateral aspect of the middle turbinate is denuded during endonasal endoscopic surgery.[1–3] We have eliminated this cause of failure by removing the lateral aspect of the middle turbinate (when the middle meatus is narrowed by a concha bullosa) or its anterior two-thirds (when the middle turbinate is polypoid, lateralized, or floppy) (Fig. 1–2).

NATURAL OSTIUM

Presence of a normal, active mucociliary system as described by Messerklinger[4] is associated with drainage of the maxillary sinus through the natural ostium. Thus, the patient's symptoms are usually not relieved, and suppurative sinusitis persists when drainage tracts are made in the inferior meatus (a nasoantral window) or the posterior fontanelle rather than through the natural ostium. This is often the problem when patients continue to have symptoms or develop new symptoms of maxillary ostium obstruction after endoscopic sinus surgery. We have found this to occur primarily within the first 6 months after surgery and, as discovered during revision surgery, it results from not connecting the natural ostium to a middle meatal antrostomy. Symptoms were relieved by revision surgery in which obstruction of the ostium was corrected by removing the middle turbinate, by removing recurrent polyps blocking the natural ostium, or by reopening a stenotic ostium.

ANTERIOR ETHMOID AND FRONTAL SINUS

Persistent disease in the anterior ethmoid system leading to frontal sinus obstruction was another cause of endoscopic sinus surgery failure in our series. The anatomy of the nasofrontal area was well described by Von Alyea,[5] and more recently by Kuhn et al.,[6] who focused on aspects of anatomy in this area from the perspective of endoscopic sinus surgery.

The path that frontal sinus drainage takes into the nasofrontal recess varies depending upon how the uncinate process attaches; most often this process attaches to the orbit, and the frontal sinus drains medial to the infundibulum. Although this area was previously difficult to treat surgically, new instruments introduced by Bolger and Kuhn[4] make operations in this space easier.

Patients with extensive scarring due to previous surgery and recurrent polyposis that obstructs the nasofrontal isthmus can now be treated by revision endonasal endoscopic surgery. Previously, revision surgery was performed via an external approach, but now we use a frontal sinus ostioplasty technique that was originally described by Wolfgang Draf[7] and was modified by May.[8]

SPHENOID

Postoperative problems in the sphenoid sinus led to failure of endoscopic sinus surgery for a small number of patients treated early in our series. In

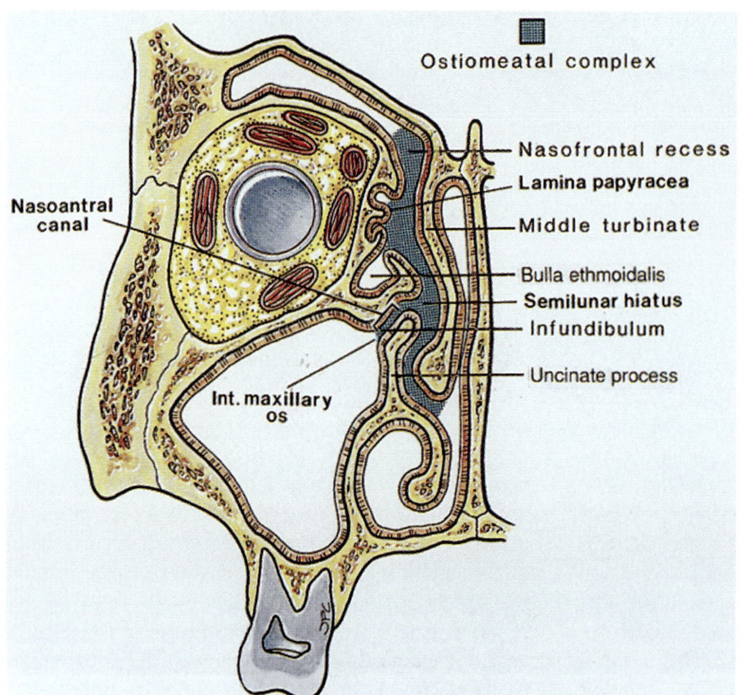

Fig. 1–1. Coronal section demonstrating anatomic basis for middle turbinate adhesions to obstruct maxillary, anterior ethmoid, and frontal sinus drainage. (From: Levine HL, and May M. Endoscopic Sinus Surgery. New York: Thieme Medical Publishers, 1993. By permission.)

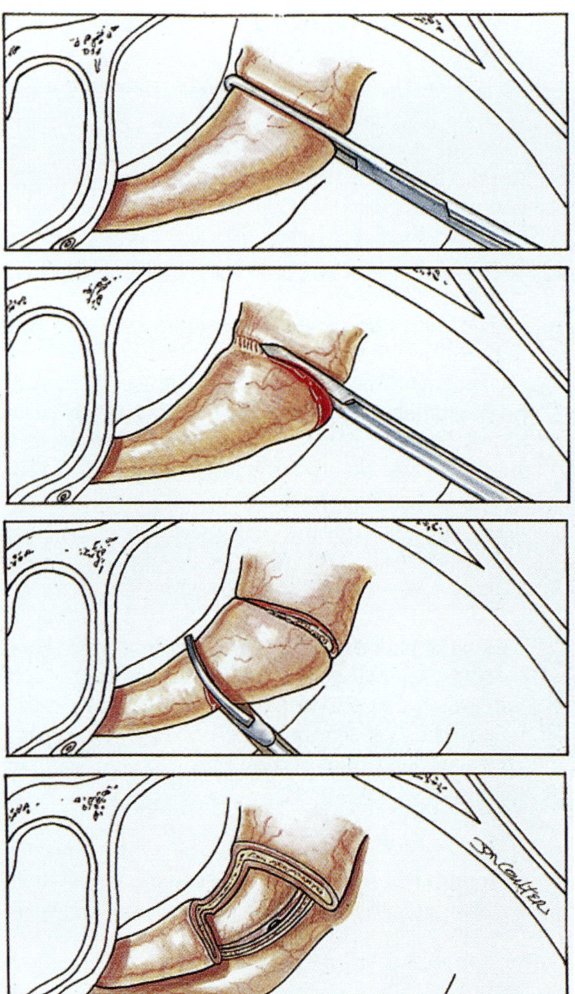

Fig. 1–2. Step by step approach for resecting anterior two-thirds of middle turbinate. (From: Levine HL, and May M. Endoscopic Sinus Surgery. New York: Thieme Medical Publishers, 1993. By permission.)

most cases, sphenoid sinus opacification was evident on preoperative radiologic images, but the sinus was not opened during the original surgical procedure. Instead, the surgeon believed he had opened the sphenoid when in fact he was in the posterior ethmoid. Later in this presentation, we discuss how to avoid making this error.

RECURRENT POLYPOSIS

Recurrence of polyps is a common reason to perform revision surgery. Complete removal of polyps and the use of topical or parenteral steroid therapy are effective in achieving prolonged palliation. In spite of this, recurrent polyps may require revision surgery. The surgical technique presented provides a safe approach to revision surgery for any problem, including recurrent polyposis.

Surgical Technique

The surgical technique we use for revision procedures is designed to keep the surgeon oriented to sinus anatomy and to avoid complications. When using the following six anatomic reference points,[9] our incidence of complications after revision surgery was no greater than after initial surgery. The landmarks, in the order in which we commonly look for them during the procedure, are as follows:

THE ANTERIOR ARCH

The first reference point is the arch formed between the posterior superior aspect of the lacrimal bone and the anterior superior attachment of the middle turbinate (Fig. 1–3). This bony arch is present even when the middle turbinate has been resected. The arch defines the anterior border and the entrance into the ethmoid complex. This keeps the surgeon from venturing medial to the lateral lamella of the cribiform plate where, lacking a cap from the frontal bone, the bone is one-tenth the thickness.[10] Staying laterally along the lamina papyracea decreases the risk of penetration of the ethmoid roof.

THE MAXILLARY SINUS ANTROSTOMY

If the maxillary sinus ostium has been obscured by scarring or polypoid disease, the ostium can be located in two ways. Pushing on the posterior fontanelle can force an air bubble through a patent but hidden sinus ostium. The place where the bubble arises can then be used as the focus of a wide maxillary sinus antrostomy, which is often necessary in revision surgery.

Alternatively, the posterior fontanelle can be located safely by identifying the soft mobile membrane that lies just superior to the inferior turbinate. Once entered, the sinus can be opened widely from the lacrimal bone anteriorly to the palatine bone posteriorly to include the natural ostium. The location of the natural ostium may be confirmed by visualizing it through an angled telescope or, in more difficult cases, directly via maxillary sinus sinoscopy through a canine fossa puncture.

Opening the maxillary antrum widely allows the surgeon to identify the next two landmarks—the lamina papyracea and "the ridge."

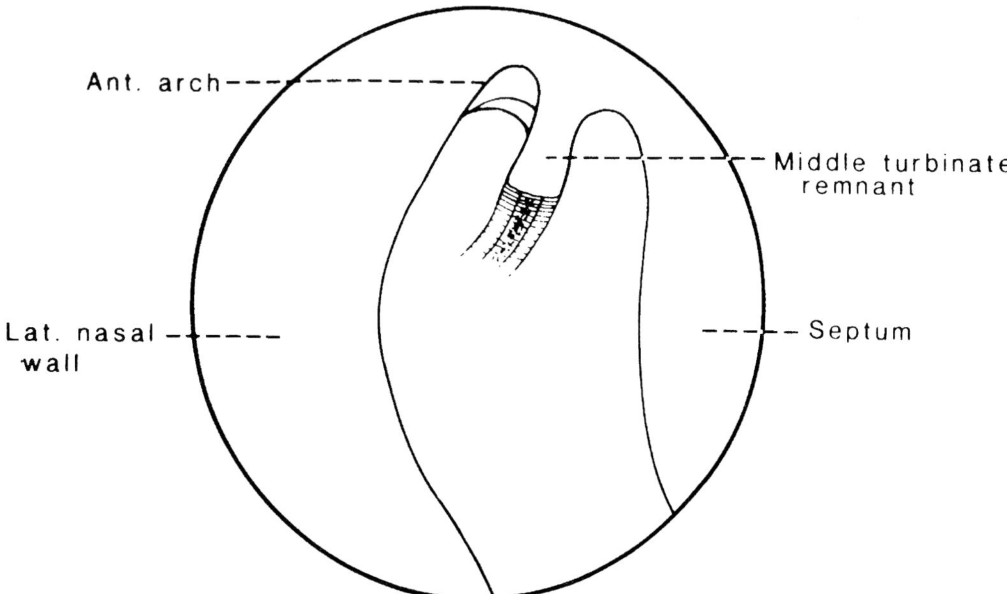

Fig. 1–3. Endoscopic view of right anterior arch in patient with middle turbinate resected and stump remaining. (From: May M, Schaitkin B, Kay SL: Revision endoscopic sinus surgery: six friendly surgical landmarks. *Laryngoscope* 104:766–767, 1994. By permission.)

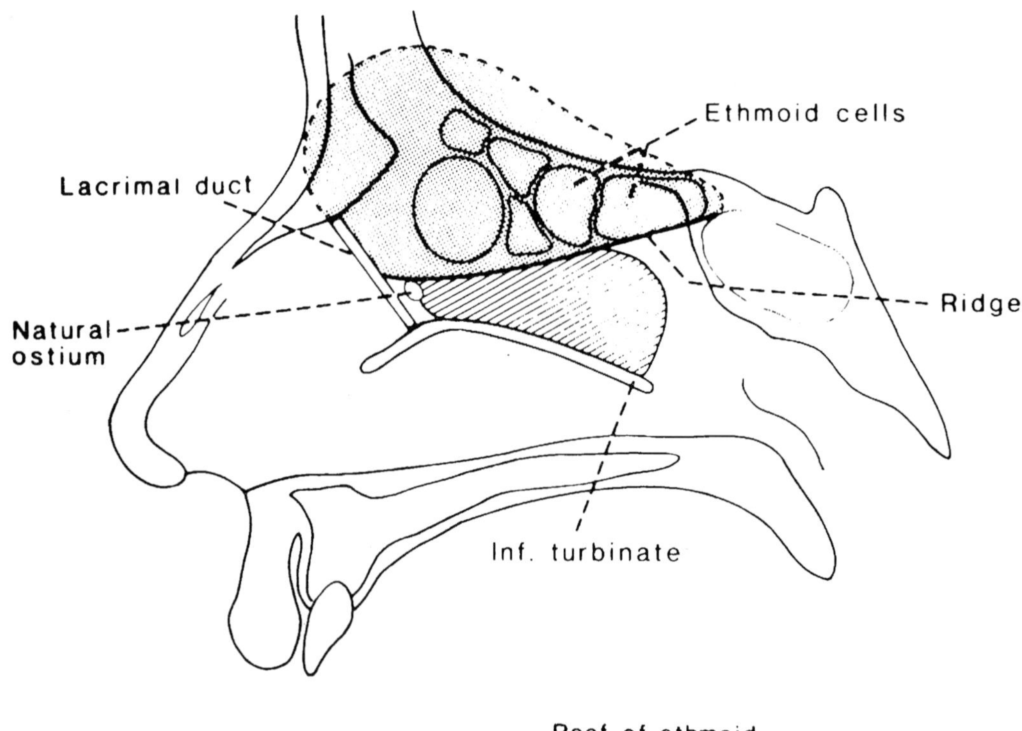

A

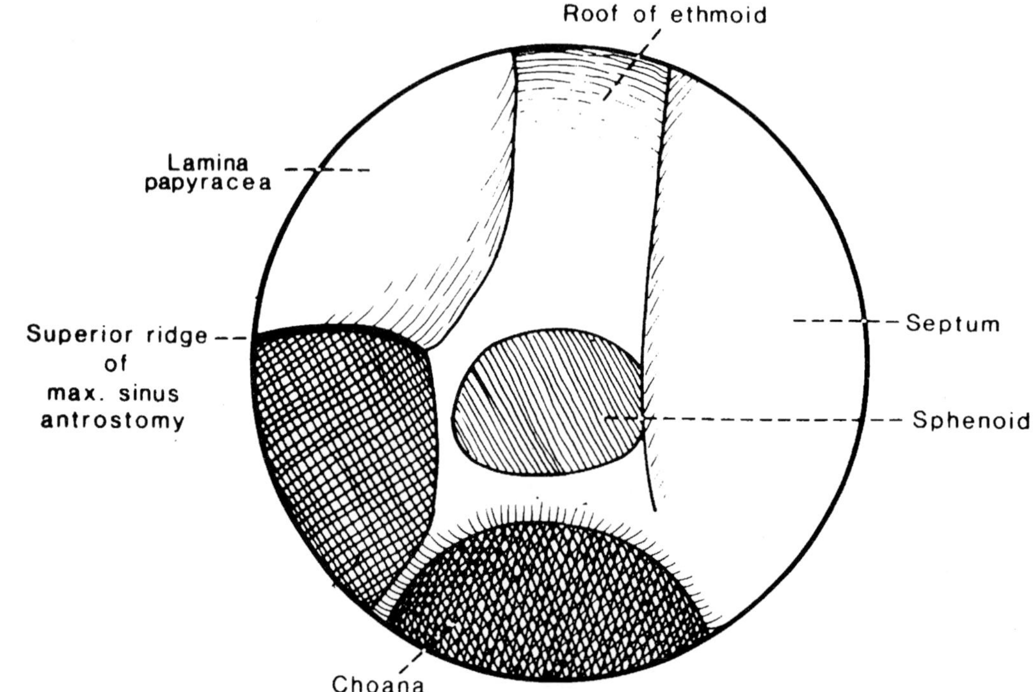

B

Fig. 1–4. **A,** Sagittal view demonstrating the ridge with ethmoid cells above and sphenoid sinus below. **B,** Endoscopic view right posterior choanal depicts the ridge forming roof of antrostomy and level of an opened sphenoid sinus. (From: May M, Schaitkin B, Kay SL: Revision endoscopic sinus surgery: six friendly surgical landmarks. *Larynoscope* 104:766–767, 1994. By permission.)

THE LAMINA PAPYRACEA

The patient's recent CT scans should be reviewed to identify any violation of the lamina papyracea by disease or previous surgery. The lamina is located just superior to the maxillary antrostomy and can be appreciated by following the floor of the orbit medially. As the surgeon advances the endoscope through the antrostomy, the lamina appears as a flat plate of bone that often looks yellow because of the orbital fat that lies behind it. The roof of the ethmoid sinus is approached by moving along the lamina papyracea so as to remain where the bone is thickest because it is covered by the frontal bone.

THE RIDGE

The ridge is the bony extension of the orbital floor between the maxillary antrostomy inferiorly and the lamina papyracea superiorly. Viewed endoscopically, the posterior ethmoid complex will be above this ridge and the sphenoid sinus below. Thus, the ridge and the antrostomy itself are useful landmarks to assure that one has entered the sphenoid sinus and is not in a posterior ethmoid cell (Fig. 1–4).

THE POSTERIOR CHOANAL ARCH

Identifying the posterior choanal arch helps the surgeon safely locate the anterior face of the sphenoid sinus during any endoscopic sinus surgery, but is especially helpful during revision surgery or when the natural ostium of the sphenoid is difficult to visualize because of extensive disease in the sphenoethmoid recess. After locating the posterior choanal arch and posterior aspect of the nasal septum, the surgeon grasps the mucosa over the front face of the sphenoid and dissects it inferiorly to displace branches of the sphenopalatine artery. The exposed bone near the nasal septum and 1 cm above the arch is cracked with a closed straight sinus forceps and the opening to the sphenoid sinus is enlarged inferiorly with Kerrison forceps. This medial inferior portion is the safest part of the sphenoid sinus to enter. The sphenoid sinus is then enlarged superiorly and laterally, following the details of sinus size and the relationships of the carotid artery and optic nerve provided on axial and coronal CT scans. The front face of the sphenoid sinus is opened to its roof, thus including the natural ostium of the sphenoid sinus.

THE SPHENOID SINUS ROOF

The ethmoid and sphenoid sinuses have a common roof, which is easily appreciated by examining sagittal images (Fig. 1–5). Using the roof of the sphenoid sinus as a guide to the roof of the ethmoid sinus, the surgeon can complete the revision surgery, work-

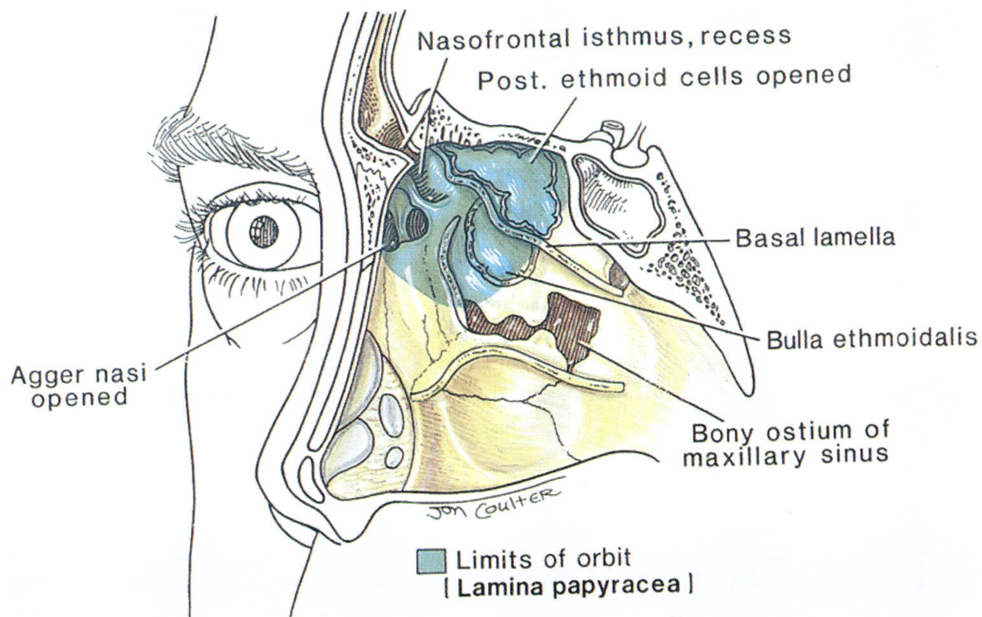

Fig. 1–5. Sagittal representation shows the common roof shared by ethmoid and sphenoid sinus. (From: Levine HL, and May M. Endoscopic Sinus Surgery. New York: Thieme Medical Publishers, 1993. By permission.)

ing from posterior to anterior. The lateral portion of the surgical area is addressed first, moving along the lamina papyracea for the reasons mentioned previously.

During revision surgery, *the skull base* is exposed last, after identification of all six of the landmarks. This helps prevent penetration of the skull base and potential complications. To expose all of the ethmoid sinus roof requires removal of remnants of lamella connecting the lamina papyracea to the middle turbinate and superior turbinate (when present). This exposure is necessary to remove all residual disease.

REFERENCES

1. Schaefer SD, Manning S, Close LG. Endoscopic paranasal sinus surgery: Indications and considerations. *Laryngoscope* 1989;99:1–5.
2. Lazar RH, Younis RT, Long TE, et al. Revision functional endonasal sinus surgery. *Ear Nose Thorat J* 1992;71:131–133.
3. Stankiewicz JA. Complications in endoscopic intranasal ethmoidectomy: An update. *Laryngoscope* 1989;99:686–690.
4. Messerklinger W. Nasendoskopie: Der mittlere Nasengang und seine unspezifischen Entzundungen. *HNO* 1972;20:212–215.
5. Van Alyea OF. Frontal sinus drainage. *Ann Otol Rhinol Laryngol* 1946;55:267.
6. Kuhn FA, Bolger WE, Tisdal RG. The agger nasi cell in frontal recess obstruction: An anatomic, rheologic and clinical correlation. *Op Tech Otolaryngol Head Neck Surg* 1991;2:226–231.
7. Draf W. Endonasal microendoscopic frontal sinus surgery, the Fulda concept. *Op Tech Otolaryngol Head Neck Surg* 1991;2:234–240.
8. May M. Frontal sinus surgery: Endonasal endoscopic ostioplasty rather than external osteoplasty. *Op Tech Otolaryngol Head Neck Surg* 1991;2:247–256.
9. May M, Schaitkin B, Kay SL. Revision endoscopic sinus surgery: Six friendly surgical landmarks. *Laryngoscope* 1994. In press.
10. Kaintz J, Stammberger H. The roof of the anterior ethmoid: The place of least resistance in the skull base. *Am J Rhinol* 1989;3:191–199.

2

Maxillary Sinus Revision Surgery

James A. Duncavage

The maxillary sinus must constantly clear its mucociliary blanket directly out the maxillary ostium. The maxillary sinus ostium has been examined anatomically in the past. According to Lang, the maxillary ostium is an elliptical cleft with a long sagittal axis.[1] The ostium has been measured to be between 2 to 6 mm wide and 7 to 11 mm long. The ostia varies greatly in both width and length, ranging in diameter from 3 to 19 mm and in length from 1 to 20 mm. The ostium should be thought of as a three-dimensional space with width, height, and length. The anatomic studies of the maxillary ostium have shown a marked variability in size and in the location of the ostium within the infundibulum. This high variability in size and location of the maxillary ostium should be kept in mind as you read this chapter on maxillary sinus revision surgery.

Physiology

Ciliary movement within the maxillary sinus carries the mucous blanket in all directions toward the ostium. The ciliary beats have been measured to be 250 to 300 beats per minute with the effective forward beat about one-quarter of the return beat. Remember, the maxillary sinus must clear itself against gravity. Many factors can affect the ciliary clearance. The chemical mediators of allergy change the mucous blanket and may have an effect on the cilia. Infection causes loss of cilia and resulting mucous stagnation. The changes from environmental pollution are probably similar to those of infection and allergy. Also, unidentified chemical mediators of asthma may adversely affect the maxillary mucociliary clearance.

Previous Maxillary Sinus Surgery

The Caldwell-Luc operation may have been used to treat maxillary sinus disease in the patient you are now seeing for persistent maxillary sinusitis. I have found that it is not possible to remove completely all maxillary sinus mucosa. The remaining mucociliary blanket will continue to clear the mucous via the natural ostium.

The patient may have had an inferior meatus antrostomy previous to your consultation. I examine the inferior meatus by inserting a 30° and 70° endoscope. Many times I see purulent material coming out the inferior meatus antrostomy. On internal maxillary sinoscopy, I often find purulent secretions on the medial maxillary wall.

Many patients have a middle turbinate that was preserved during ethmoid surgery. I have found in some patients that the middle turbinate has lateralized due to scarring of the middle turbinate to the lateral wall. An obstruction to the mucociliary clearance of the maxillary sinus can then occur. Even if a middle meatus antrostomy has been used, if the middle turbinate scars over the opening, a blockage to mucociliary flow can occur.

A widely patent middle meatus antrostomy with persistent maxillary sinus disease is often observed in my practice. A close endoscopic exam with a 30° and 70° endoscope may reveal an uncinate remnant or scarring of the remaining infundibulum. The uncinate remnant or the scarred infundibulum will obstruct the area of the natural maxillary ostium.

Another finding I have observed with a widely patent middle meatus antrostomy is circular flow. If the maxillary ostium is not continuous with the middle meatus antrostomy, then the maxillary sinus will still clear the mucociliary blanket via the natural ostium. Some of the mucous coming out the natural ostium will then flow back into the surgical antrostomy and be again cleared by the maxillary mucociliary clearance via the natural ostium. There will be incomplete clearance if some of the mucous is constantly recycled. I have observed this recycled mucous to become overgrown with bacteria, usually *Staphylococcus* or *Pseudomonas* spp. I have also found the natural maxillary ostium and an accessory ostium to be involved occasionally with this circular flow of mucous.

Evaluation of the Patient

The patient who presents with continued maxillary sinus infection after medical and surgical treatment should be approached in a systematic way. A complete nasal and sinus history is obtained. I inquire about any relief experienced with antibiotics. If antibiotics help but the infection returns, then I suspect a mechanical problem such as obstruction. I also review what surgical procedure has been used to treat the maxillary sinusitis. I note whether the patient has inhalant allergies or asthma. These two conditions will have an effect on mucociliary clearance. I have noted that the diabetic patient in my practice has an especially difficult time with both bacterial and fungal infections. I also ask about the types of antibiotics used and the duration of their use.

The next step is the physical exam. The nasal speculum is used to examine the general health of the nasal lining. Then a 30° endoscope is passed. The inferior meatus is examined. If an inferior meatus antrostomy is present it is inspected, as is the maxillary sinus. The inferior turbinate is then inspected. I observe if it has been reduced in size surgically.

The middle meatus is now examined. I observe for an antrostomy, for circular flow, for scarring and for purulent drainage. I then rotate the endoscope 90° and observe the nasofrontal recess. Purulent drainage from the frontal sinus can be a source of chronic maxillary infection. I culture all purulent drainage with a small wire cotton tipped swab bent 90° on the end. I culture for aerobes and fungus and adjust the antibiotics based on the sensitivities.

The CT scan can be helpful, but it must be interpreted in conjunction with medical management and physical exam. If the patient is on steroids and antibiotics at the time of the CT scan, the CT scan may be normal.

I will obtain a CT scan when the patient's course of antibiotics and steroids is completed. I usually wait at least 2 weeks. I also have found the CT helpful when I am trying to decide if scarring of the infundibulum has occurred. The coronal CT may show residual uncinate present. This may not be apparent on exam.

Revision Surgery

I will now go through each different problem I have seen and describe how I revised the maxillary sinus.

1. I have found that the patient with purulent maxillary sinusitis and inferior meatus antrostomy continues to have maxillary sinusitis due to maxillary ostium occlusion. I treat this with an endoscopically placed middle meatus antrostomy. I use the technique as described by Kennedy (Fig. 2–1).[2]
2. A scarred middle turbinate obstructing the middle meatus is managed by partial middle turbinectomy. If an antrostomy in the middle meatus is present, I check it at the time of

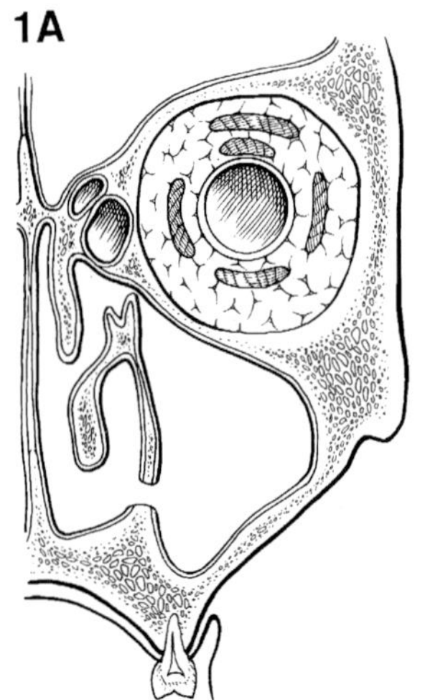

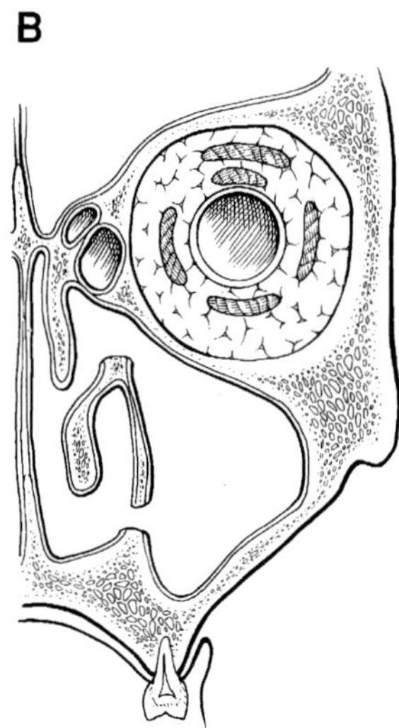

Fig. 2–1. **A,** Previous inferior meatus antrostomy with an obstructed middle meatus. **B,** An endoscopically placed middle meatus antrostomy.

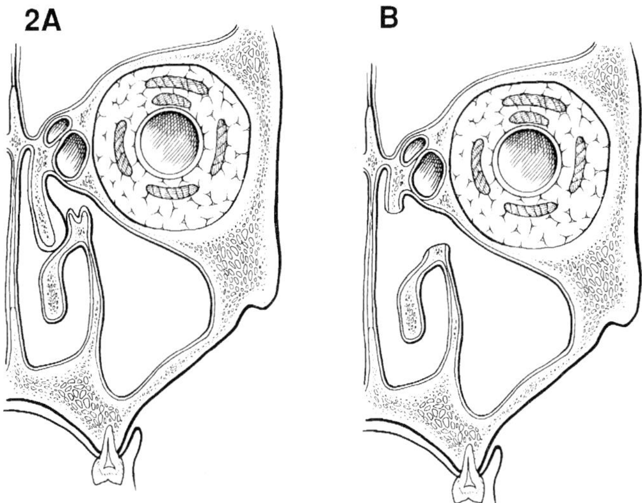

Fig. 2–2. **A,** A middle turbinate is scarred over the maxillary ostium. **B,** A partial middle turbinectomy with an endoscopic middle meatus antrostomy.

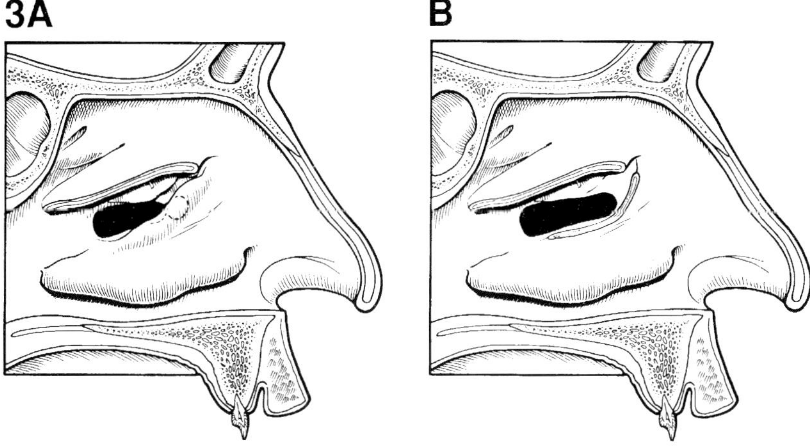

Fig. 2–3. **A,** The unicate is scarred over the maxillary ostium. **B,** The uncinate is removed and the maxillary ostium is connected to the antrostomy. **C,** Scarring or incomplete connection of the antrostomy to the maxillary ostium is present. The two openings need to be joined.

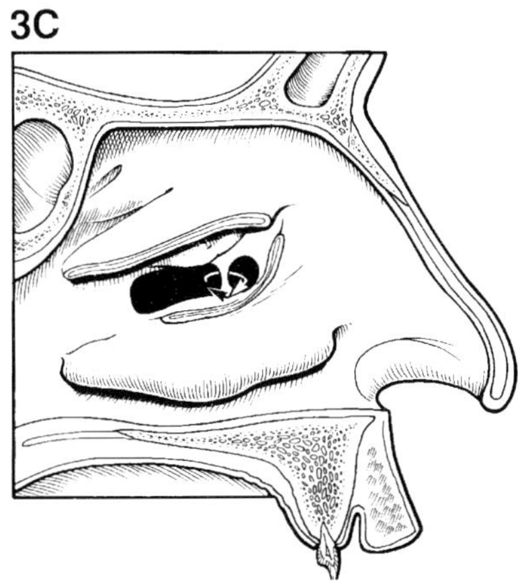

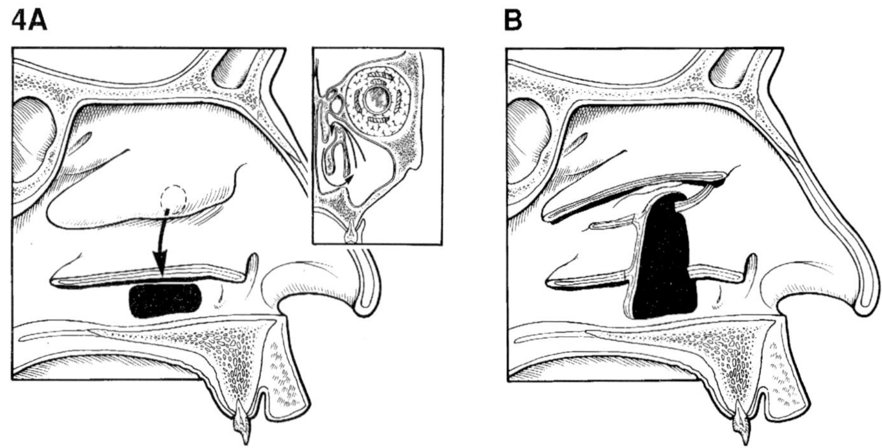

Fig. 2–4. **A,** The patient has had a previous partial inferior turbinectomy and an inferior meatus antrostomy. Many times there will be drainage from the middle meatus antrostomy into the inferior meatus antrostomy. **B,** The two antrostomies are joined and the intervening segment of inferior turbinate has been removed.

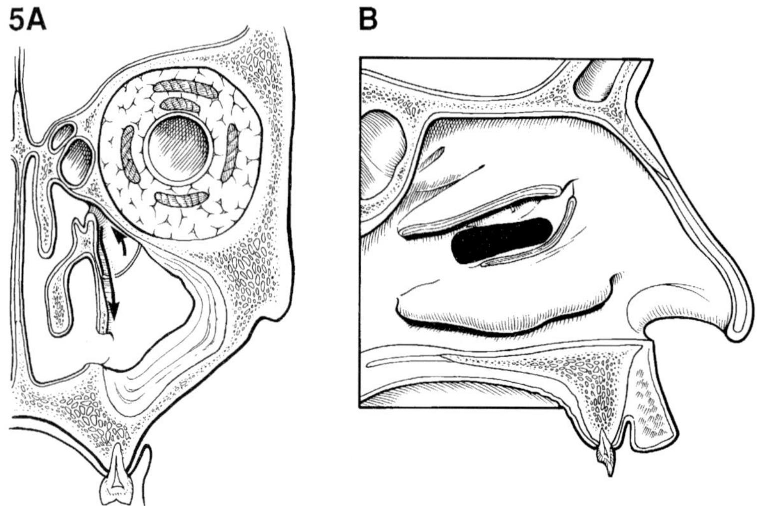

Fig. 2–5. **A,** After a Caldwell-Luc with an inferior meatus antrostomy the maxillary ostium is still obstructed. **B,** An endoscopic middle meatus antrostomy is placed.

surgery to be sure the maxillary ostium is included in the antrostomy. If there is not an antrostomy, I place a middle meatus antrostomy endoscopically (Fig. 2–2).

3. The scarring of the uncinate over the maxillary ostium is managed by endoscopic removal of the residual uncinate and connection of the ostium to the antrostomy (Fig. 2–3A, B). The same connection is made when the ostium and antrostomy exhibit circular flow (Fig. 2–3C).
4. An uncommon problem I have observed is circular flow between a middle meatus and inferior meatus antrostomy usually with a small inferior turbinate between. I correct this problem by connecting the middle and inferior meatus antrostomy with removal of the intervening wall or partial removal of the inferior turbinate. This results in a partial medial maxillectomy (Fig. 2–4).
5. After a Caldwell-Luc procedure, some patients do not improve. I believe residual

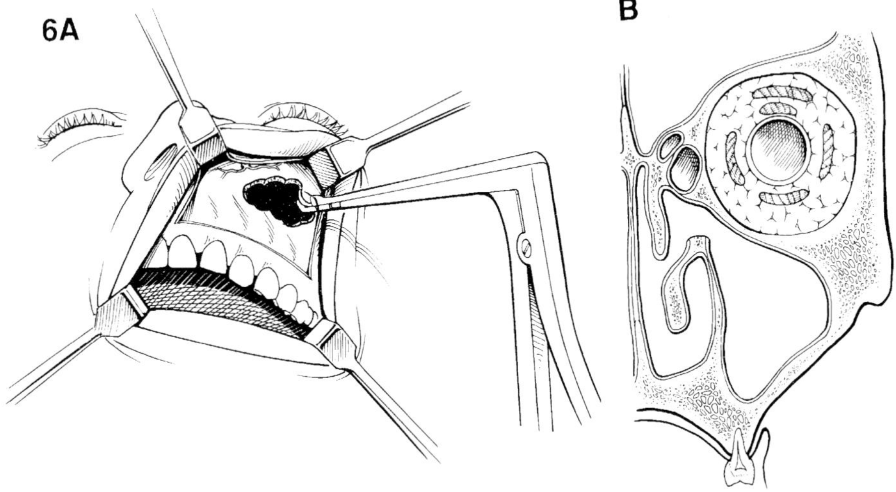

Fig. 2–6. **A,** A Caldwell-Luc with removal of the irreversibly diseased mucosa may be necessary. **B,** With a Caldwell-Luc and removal of diseased mucosa, always place an endoscopic middle meatus antrostomy.

respiratory epithelium in the area of the maxillary ostium begins to function. If the maxillary ostium is not functional, the patient will still have symptoms of maxillary sinusitis. I treat this with an endoscopic maxillary antrostomy (Fig. 2–5).

6. When all the previously described abnormalities have been eliminated and all positive bacterial cultures have been treated with an appropriate antibiotic, I will consider a Caldwell-Luc approach with removal of the maxillary mucosa. Our data would suggest that irreversibly diseased maxillary mucosa and intrinsic chemical mediators may render the maxillary sinus nonfunctional.[3] The resulting aggressive removal of maxillary sinus lining results in contraction of the maxillary lumen and ingrowth of nondiseased nasal lining with a resultant noninfected maxillary sinus. I always include an endoscopically placed middle meatus antrostomy with the Caldwell-Luc approach (Fig. 2–6).

Summary

The surgical treatment of maxillary sinusitis with an endoscopically placed middle meatus antrostomy must always include as part of the antrostomy the maxillary ostium.

REFERENCES

1. Lang J. *Clinical Anatomy of the Nose, Nasal Cavity and Paranasal Sinuses.* New York, NY: Thieme Medical Publishers, Inc. 1989.
2. Kennedy DW, Zinreich SJ, Kuhn F, et al. Endoscopic middle meatal antrostomy: Theory, technique, and patency. *Laryngoscopy* 1987:43:1–9.
3. Raghbe S, Duncavage JA. Maxillary sinusitis: Value of endoscopic middle meatus antrostomy versus Caldwell-Luc procedure. *Operative Techniques in Otolaryngology-Head and Neck Surgery* 1992:(2):129–133.

3

Endoscopic Frontal Sinus Surgery

John P. Bent, III and Frederick A. Kuhn

In the last decade, many otolaryngologists have accepted functional endoscopic sinus surgery (FESS) as the procedure of choice for the surgical treatment of chronic sinusitis. The basic philosophy of FESS is to remove only the tissue necessary to relieve obstruction, restoring natural sinus drainage, ventilation, and physiology. The expectation is that some diseased tissue will return to normal under these conditions. This surgical technique has been supported by rapid technological advances, including radiographic imaging, sinus endoscopes, video equipment, and a wide array of versatile sinus instruments. Consequently, a revolution is underway in the approach to chronic sinusitis.

These changes have had a significant impact on the management of frontal sinus disease. Surgeons can now remove tissue obstructing the frontal recess under direct vision via an intranasal approach. However, the frontal sinus is the most challenging of the four paranasal sinuses to treat endoscopically. Its superior and anterior location makes visualization difficult. The relatively narrow size of the frontal recess predisposes it to stenosis. Furthermore, the proximity of the frontal recess to the anterior ethmoid artery, orbit and anterior cranial fossa portends potentially grave complications. Yet with full knowledge of sinus anatomy and potential pitfalls, as well as a thorough preoperative evaluation, the endoscopist can safely and successfully restore normal frontal sinus physiology.

Anatomy and Physiology

The frontal sinus is simply an anterior ethmoid cell which has grown into the frontal bone.[1] This growth begins in the second trimester of fetal life and continues into adolescence. The size of the frontal sinus varies significantly, ranging from aplasia to near total aeration of the frontal bone. From one to four "frontal pits"[2] grow cephalad from the middle meatus to form the anterior ethmoid cells and pneumatize each half of the frontal bone; generally, the second frontal pit becomes the frontal sinus. Other frontal pits that do not become the frontal sinus may develop into agger nasi cells, frontal cells, supraorbital ethmoid cells, or intersinus septal cells (Fig. 3–1). These cells may become primarily infected or obstruct frontal sinus drainage.

The frontal recess is an inverted funnel shaped space which connects the frontal sinus ostium to the middle meatus. Rarely is it a duct or tube shaped structure, hence the common term "nasofrontal duct" is most often incorrect. The frontal recess is not universally defined. However, the clinical concept of a space connecting the frontal sinus with the anterior ethmoid region, as well as the vulnerability of this space to obstruction, is more important than the precise anatomic defini-

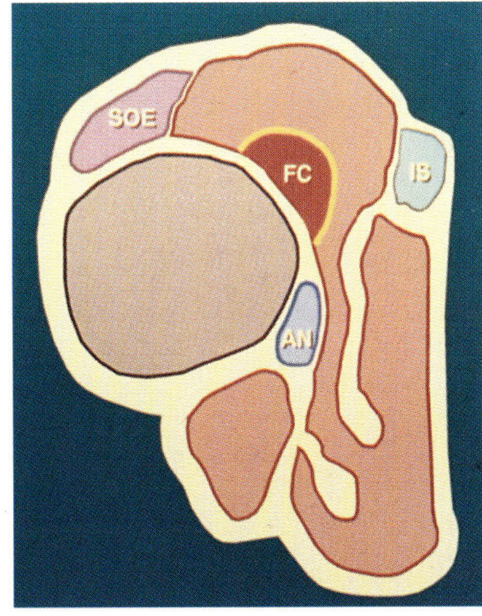

Fig. 3–1. Right paranasal sinuses at the level of the frontal recess demonstrating supraorbital ethmoid (SOE), intersinus septal (IS), agger nasi (AN), and frontal (FC) cells.

tion. It is accepted that the frontal recess usually enters the middle meatus medial to the ethmoid infundibulum, either anterior (55% of cases) or superior (30% of cases) to the superior attachment of the uncinate process on the lateral nasal wall[3]; occasionally, it drains directly into the ethmoid infundibulum (15% of cases) or posteriorly to the uncinate process.[2,3] The frontal recess boundaries are the middle turbinate medially, the orbit laterally, the agger nasi region anteriorly, and the skull base posteriorly (Figs. 3–1 to 3–3). The lateral lamella of the cribriform plate is immediately medial to the frontal recess. This extremely thin bone extends vertically from the vertical attachment of the middle turbinate to the cribriform plate and connects to the orbital plate of the frontal bone (Fig. 3–4). Some authorities consider the ethmoid bulla, rather than the skull base, the posterior landmark for the frontal recess.[4] The anterior ethmoid artery generally is the posterior boundary of the frontal recess. It may be protected by the ethmoid bulla lamella as it attaches to the skull base. However, this relationship is unpredictable, because in some cases the superior lamella of the ethmoid bulla does not insert on the anterior skull base, leaving the anterior ethmoid artery exposed in front of the ethmoid bulla.

The frontal sinus itself is bounded by the anterior and posterior tables, with the orbital roof inferiorly and an intersinus septum medially. The blood supply derives from the supraorbital and supratrochlear branches of the ophthalmic artery, while venous drainage travels into the superior ophthalmic vein en route to the cavernous sinus. Sensory innervation arises from the supraorbital and supratrochlear branches of the trigeminal nerve.

The frontal recess connects internally with the inferior and medial region of the frontal sinus. This internal frontal sinus ostium is not always the most inferior or gravitationally dependent region of the frontal sinus. However, the frontal sinus mucous membrane cilia transport the mucous blanket over the grooves and crevices of the sinus until it reaches the ostium. In 1932, Hilding demonstrated that the mucous blanket travels in a spiral towards the internal ostium in a way that effectively defies gravity.[5] Messerklinger confirmed Hilding's work 35 years later; he made the

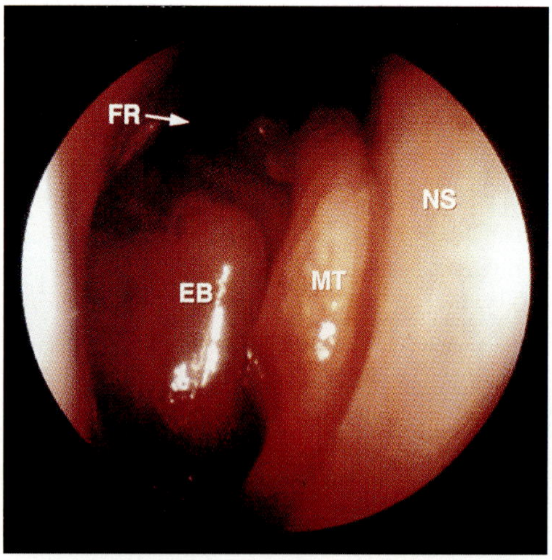

Fig. 3–2. Endoscopic view of right middle meatus with an intact ethmoid bulla (EB) posterior to the frontal recess (FR). The nasal septum (NS) and middle turbinate (MT) are seen medially.

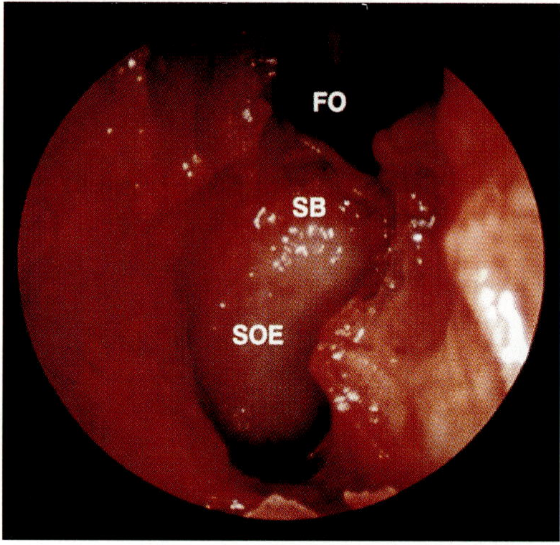

Fig. 3–3. Endoscopic view of left middle meatus with the ethmoid bulla removed to the skull base (SB), exposing a supraorbital ethmoid cell (SOE) and a widely patent frontal sinus ostium (FO).

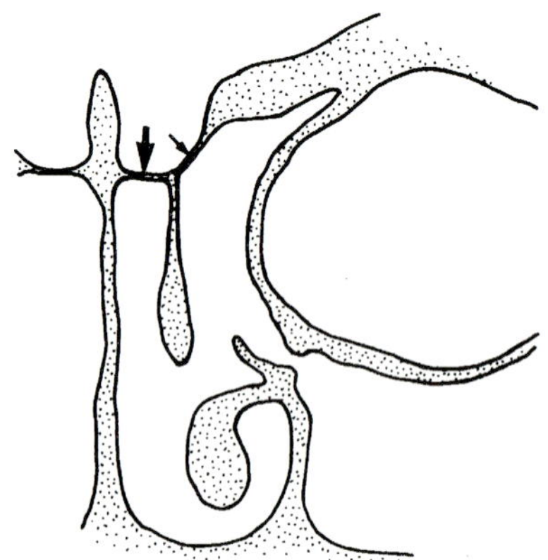

Fig. 3–4. Medial boundary of the frontal recess: cribriform plate (large arrow) separated from the lateral lamella of the cribriform plate (small arrow) by the attachment of the middle turbinate.

additional discovery that a portion of the mucous blanket actually recirculates within the frontal sinus and frontal recess while the remaining mucus enters the middle meatus.[6]

The frontal sinus has several hypothetic functions. It serves as a buffer for the brain in forehead trauma, contributes to forehead contour, reduces the weight of the skull, and adds resonance to the voice. Mucociliary clearance mechanisms help keep the sinus aerated and prevent airborn particulate contamination and fluid collection. However, the frontal sinus is rarely significant unless it becomes obstructed or infected. Typical symptoms of frontal sinusitis include headache, rhinorrhea, and fever, often accompanied by signs of nasal mucosal edema and erythema with purulence draining into the middle meatus. If neglected, acute or chronic frontal sinusitis may progress to osteomyelitis, cellulitis, or subperiostial (Pott's puffy tumor), intracranial, or intraorbital abscess.

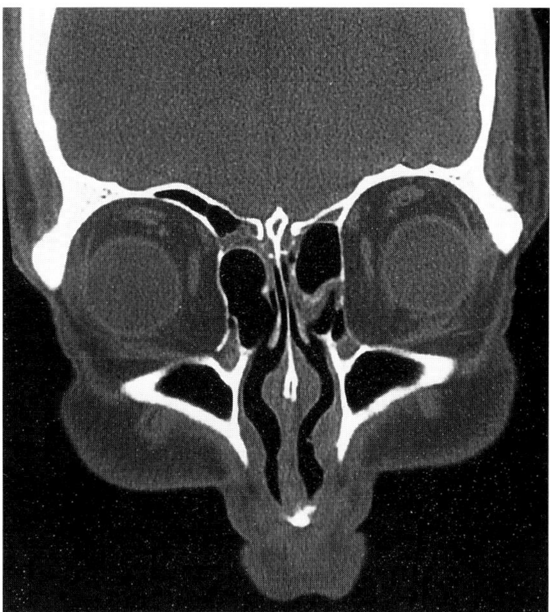

Fig. 3–5. Bilateral agger nasi obstruction of the frontal recess.

Pathophysiology

Frontal sinusitis is directly related to either impaired mucociliary clearance or anatomic obstruction. Causes of impaired mucociliary function include cystic fibrosis, immotile cilia syndrome, tobacco smoke or pollutant exposure, rhinitis medicamentosa, and allergic rhinitis. These conditions generally require medical treatment or behavior modification. FESS can be used as an adjunct to medical treatment in these instances if there exists concomitant anatomic obstruction.

Because the frontal sinus drains into the middle meatus via the anterior ethmoid system, the patency and lack of disease in this region is critical to normal frontal sinus function.[7] Air cells obstructing mucociliary clearance, soft tissue obstruction, and postsurgical scarring are the most common reasons for surgical intervention. Frontal and nasoethmoid trauma are less frequent causes of frontal recess obstruction. The obstructing frontal recess cells are of anterior ethmoid origin. These include the agger nasi cell, frontal cells, and supraorbital ethmoid cells.

The agger nasi region is an eminence on the lateral nasal wall anterior–superior to the origin of the middle turbinate. When pneumatized, this most anterior of the ethmoid cells is termed the agger nasi cell (see Fig. 3–1).[8] It has been shown to be present in up to 98.5% of individuals.[9] It may obstruct the inferior aspect of the frontal recess where it enters the middle meatus (Fig. 3–5). The supraorbital ethmoid cell aerates the orbital plate of the frontal bone, lateral and posterior to the frontal sinus. The supraorbital ethmoid cell may

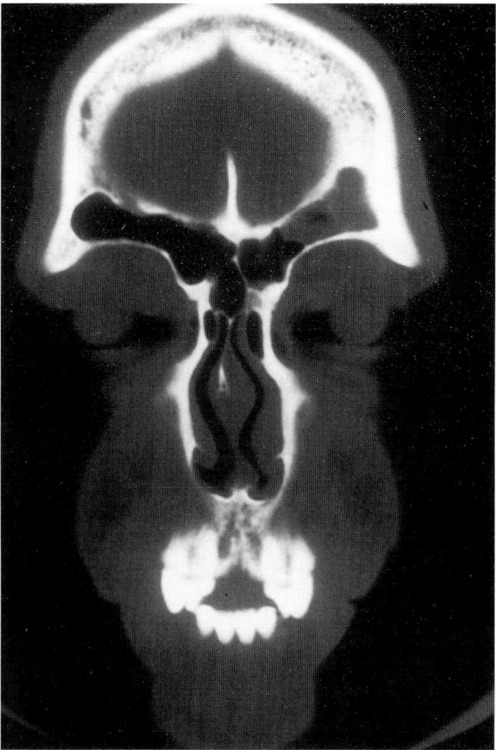

Fig. 3–6. Opacification of the left supraorbital ethmoid cell with a well aerated frontal sinus medially.

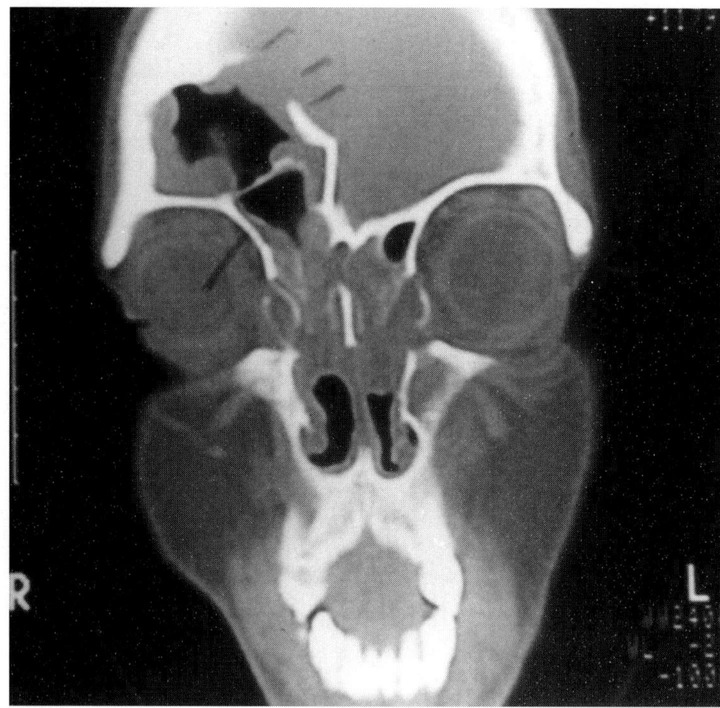

Fig. 3–7. Right frontal cell impinging upon the frontal recess causing a mucocele of the frontal sinus.

either become primarily opacified (Fig. 3–6) or obstruct the frontal sinus, leading to a secondary frontal sinus infection. A third cell which may obstruct the frontal sinus is the frontal cell, described in two different reports earlier this century,[3,10] and recently appreciated as an endoscopic obstacle to frontal recess patency.[11] It lies superior to the agger nasi cell and may impinge upon either the frontal recess (Fig. 3–7) or the frontal sinus (Fig. 3–8). Finally, large cells within the frontal sinus septum may block the internal ostium of the frontal recess (Fig. 3–9).

Chronic inflammatory tissue may also occlude the frontal recess. Many viral and bacterial infections will respond to medical therapy. On the other hand, allergic fungal sinusitis (AFS), at our current state of knowledge, always requires surgical debridement to alleviate the problem. Bone erosion or displacement, as well as recurrent disease, both common with AFS, can make this a particularly difficult disease to treat (Fig. 3–10).[12] Polyp formation is frequently associated with chronic inflammation, and may play a significant role in obstructing frontal sinus drainage. This necessitates identification of the underlying cause of polyp formation, with initiation of appropriate treatment. However, the etiology is often elusive and the response to medications incomplete, necessitating surgical removal in

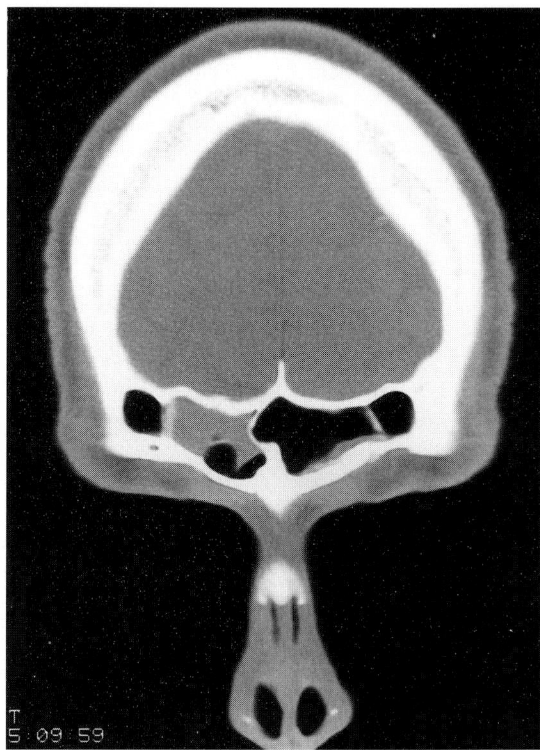

Fig. 3–8. Right frontal cell obstructing the frontal sinus superior to the frontal recess.

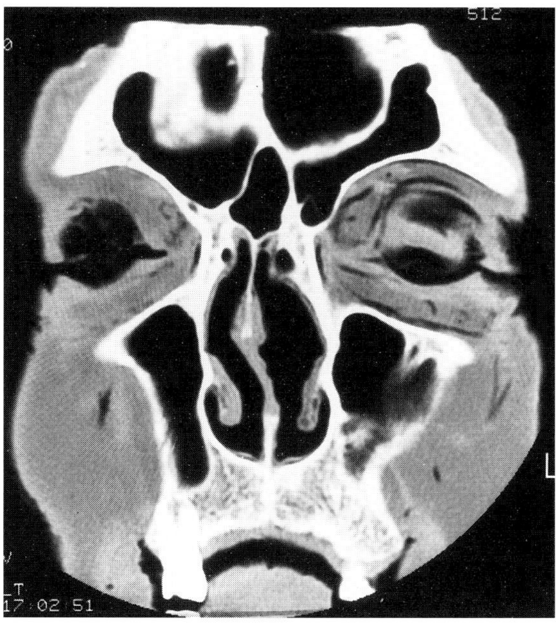

Fig. 3–9. Cadaveric example of a large intersinus septal cell.

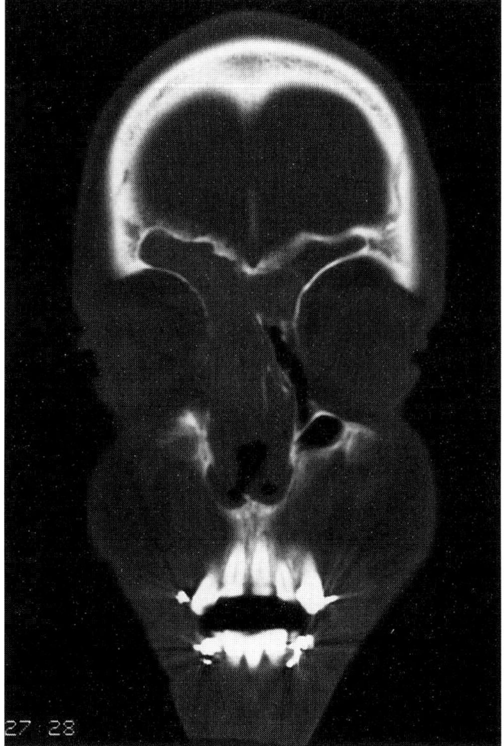

Fig. 3–10. Allergic fungal sinusitis with typical heterogeneous opacifications in both frontal recesses. Impacted fungal debris and mucin on the right side has caused deviation of the nasal septum to the left.

the majority of cases. Frequently, anatomic abnormalities contribute to the polyp formation, and this possibility should be addressed during polypectomy.

Traumatic and iatrogenic factors also contribute to frontal sinus pathology. One large series of frontal sinusitis demonstrated that 15 of 25 (60%) patients suffering frontal sinus trauma developed chronic frontal sinusitis.[13] The frontal sinus is also the most common site of residual disease following intranasal sinus surgery. This disease is usually persistent, rather than recurrent, due to incomplete removal of ethmoid cells during the initial procedure.[14] Partially removed anterior ethmoid cells, particularly the agger nasi cell, are the primary culprits.[8] In experienced hands, dissection in the frontal recess will lead to recurrence in approximately 12% of routine cases and in up to 27% in patients with diffuse polyposis.[15] Examination of the frontal recess at the end of an endoscopic ethmoidectomy is therefore essential to minimize postsurgical frontal sinus obstruction.

Surgical Treatment

Any patient presenting with chronic frontal sinusitis must undergo a thorough evaluation before being considered a surgical candidate. During the initial encounter, the otolaryngologist should try to elicit symptoms of frontal sinusitis, such as rhinorrhea, postnasal drainage, intermittent fever, or a frontal pressure headache. Existence of other medical disorders, such as allergies, asthma, congenital illnesses, or immune deficiencies, and their relation to the sinus symptoms, should be documented. The patient's history may point toward the aforementioned mucociliary clearance disorders, or previous surgery may suggest an iatrogenic frontal recess obstruction. The office endoscopic exam may identify septal deviation, polyps, purulence, concha bullosa, postoperative scarring, or the absence of landmarks. In a patient with a previous uncinectomy, direct examination of the frontal recess may be possible using the 30° or 70° telescopes. If purulence is identified, endoscopic culture may help direct antibiotic therapy.

All patients with chronic frontal sinusitis should be given a substantial trial of medical therapy. Several lengthy trials of culture-directed antibiotics used with combinations of decongestants, mucolytics, topical or oral steroids, or antihistamines may be indicated. Immunotherapy should be considered in patients with an allergic component to their sinusitis. Failure of extensive, individualized medical therapy to alleviate symptoms within 2 to 3

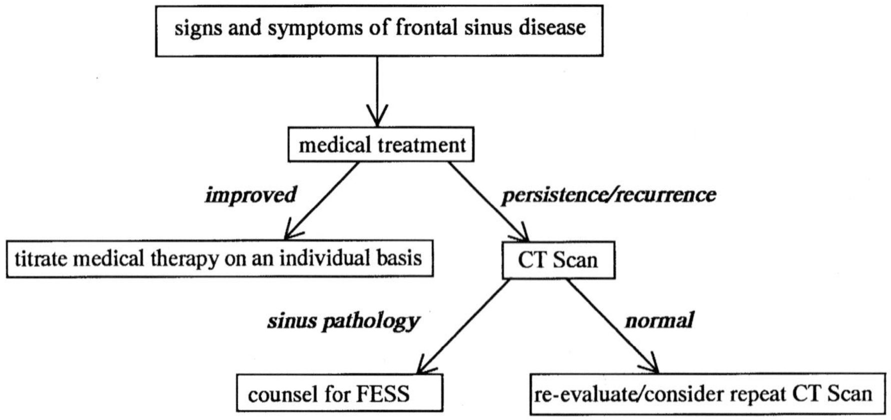

Fig. 3–11. Work-up of frontal sinus disease.

months warrants a CT scan to rule out an anatomic obstruction. If frontal recess disease is identified endoscopically or radiographically, then the patient is counselled about the potential risks and benefits of FESS (Fig. 3–11).

Nonendoscopic surgical approaches to the frontal sinus include simple trephination and drainage, external frontoethmoidectomy, frontal sinus obliteration through an osteoplastic flap, and frontal sinus cranialization. Compared with these procedures, FESS removes *only* the diseased tissue while restoring *natural* mucociliary clearance and ventilation pathways. The procedure has less morbidity than nonendoscopic sinus procedures, can be done on an outpatient basis, has a shorter convalescent period, and leaves no external scarring on facial skin. In preserving normal frontal sinus anatomy, future radiologic or endoscopic evaluation is not distorted. The disadvantages of FESS are that additional surgical expertise and diligent postoperative care are required and, in rare instances, a nonendoscopic procedure may ultimately be necessary.

Functional endoscopic frontal sinus surgery utilizes many of the same instruments used for an endoscopic ethmoidectomy, but requires new instruments to reach into the frontal recess. The frontal recess instruments developed in conjunction with Karl Storz (1989) solve this problem (Fig. 3–12). A frontal sinus ostium seeker helps palpate and identify the opening of the frontal recess. Additional necessary instruments include 45° and 90° curettes and giraffe forceps: the forceps must be available in side-to-side and front-to-back biting orientation. The curettes are extremely useful for dissecting soft tissue and bone cells out of the frontal recess to a position where they may be grasped and removed. Occasionally, the surgeon can visualize the frontal recess with the 30° endoscope, but often the 70° scope is required.

An endoscopic frontal sinusotomy begins with adequate anesthesia. In properly selected patients, local anesthesia with sedation has several advantages over general anesthesia. One retrospective analysis of intranasal ethmoidectomies in 180 patients demonstrated a 27% decrease in blood loss under local anesthesia.[16] Furthermore, an awake patient's feedback may alert the surgeon if the dissection abuts orbital periostium or dura. Injection sites for an ethmoidectomy are adequate for the frontal recess, although an effort should be made to infiltrate the most superior and anterior aspect of the middle meatus. While awaiting vasoconstriction, the nose is examined endoscopically, correlating endoscopic and CT findings. If a concha bullosa of the middle turbinate exists, it is removed by excising the lateral half of the turbinate with a sickle knife and turbinate scissors. The middle turbinate is always preserved, consistent with the philosophy of functional endoscopic sinus surgery. The first step of the procedure usually consists of identification and complete removal of the uncinate process. This should yield wide exposure of the middle meatus, enabling the surgeon to identify the ethmoid bulla posteriorly and the lamina papyracea laterally. Obstructing agger nasi cells are exenterated by fracturing the posterior wall anteriorly or laterally. Great care is taken to avoid injuring the lamina papyracea laterally and the vertical lamella of the cribriform plate medially. The weakest point of the entire anterior skull base is at the roof of the ethmoid where it is penetrated by the anterior ethmoid artery.[17] This corresponds to the lateral lamella of the cribriform plate depicted in Figure 3–4. Pediatric sinus for-

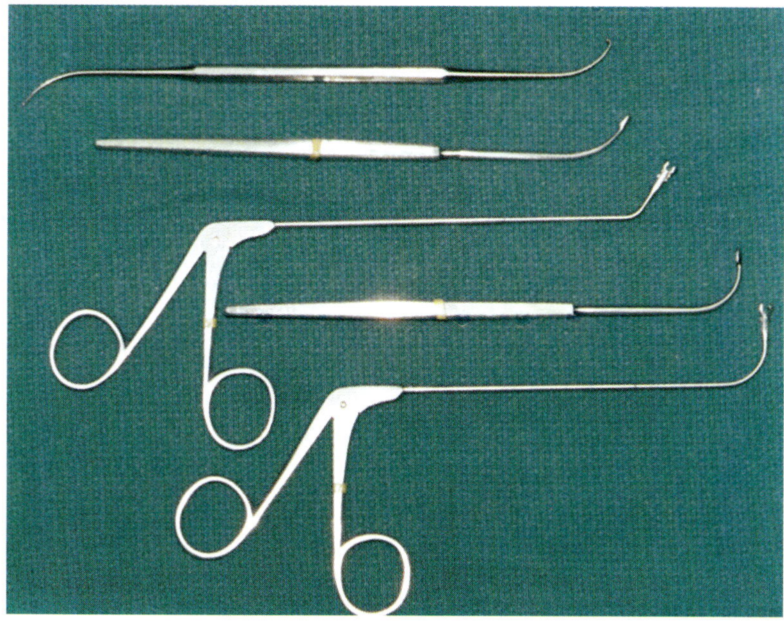

Fig. 3–12. Kuhn-Bolger frontal recess instruments (from top to bottom): frontal sinus ostium seeker (including a hooked end), 45° curette, 45° giraffe forcep, 90° curette, and 90° giraffe forcep.

ceps often facilitate gentle, atraumatic dissection. Once the uncinate and agger nasi cells have been removed, the frontal recess, perhaps with assistance of the 70° endoscope, may be identified. Any remaining obstruction should be mobilized with the instruments shown in Figure 3–12. The surgeon's movements should be from posterior to anterior, with very limited side-to-side action, thus protecting the orbit and anterior cranial fossa. If obstruction persists, the ethmoid bulla can be removed to the skull base posteriorly, which is then followed anteriorly to the frontal recess. Removal of the ethmoid bulla exposes the anterior ethmoid artery, mandating great care in this region. Once the frontal recess is identified, it can be inspected visually and carefully palpated with the frontal sinus currettes or ostium seeker to verify its patency. Aspiration of mucus or purulence may help confirm the proper location. Mucosal trauma has been shown to contribute to frontal recess synechiae that prohibit natural mucus transport,[18] so unnecessary mucus membrane trauma, removal, and instrumentation should be avoided. Intranasal endoscopic ethmoidectomy and identification of the frontal sinus ostium will result in the resolution of most cases of frontal sinusitis. [7,15,20,21] Further manipulation of the frontal recess should be done with caution, and only for a very stenotic or closed pathway.

In the unusual case where instrumentation of the frontal recess is necessary, removal of bone must come from the anterior wall. The posterior and posterior–medial walls abut dura, and the lateral wall is shared with the orbit. The posterior mucosa of the frontal recess must be preserved to serve as a framework for mucosal regeneration and to minimize the risk of stenosis. Polyps and bone fragments can be gently retracted into an accessible position using the hooked end of the frontal sinus ostium seeker. The 45° and 90° frontal sinus currettes are extremely useful for dissecting soft tissue as well as bone cells out of the frontal recess. Once the obstructing tissue is fully identified and isolated, it may be removed with the appropriately angled and oriented frontal recess giraffe forcep. Occasionally, the bone obstruction is so dense that it cannot be gently removed. In 1914, Lothrup reported drilling away the frontal sinus floor via an external frontal sinusotomy to create a wide intranasal drainage.[19] He experienced great success with this technique for chronic frontal sinusitis patients, but the procedure never attained widespread acceptance. In the last decade, Draf has introduced a frontal sinus procedure which is essentially an intranasal modification of the Lothrup technique. He describes an extensive experience enlarging the frontal recess by drilling away its anterior wall under endoscopic vision, in some cases removing the anterior floor of the frontal sinus and the anterior-superior nasal septum to create wide intranasal frontal sinus drainage.[20] We have not used these techniques, but generally employ a combined external and endoscopic intranasal approach when bone drilling is necessary.[21] Several manufacturers are attempting to develop and attain FDA approval for drills designed for intranasal use, which would certainly augment the endoscopist's armamentarium.

Bleeding with subsequent impaired visibility is the endoscopist's chief hazard and frustration. In cases of revision surgery or nasal polyposis, the KTP/532 laser may be extremely useful in maintaining hemostasis. Polyp and scar vaporization cause simultaneous photocoagulation and minimize blood loss. The recently introduced Xomed–Treace endoscrub sleeves allow rapid cleaning of the endoscope without removal from the nose. This feature can be especially valuable in the frontal recess, where exposure in a bloody field can be quite difficult. If bleeding cannot be controlled and threatens safe, accurate visibility, the procedure should be terminated and rescheduled for a later date.

Computer assisted intraoperative three-dimensional CT localization is a highly specialized technology marketed by ISG (Toronto, Canada). It has been demonstrated to be very helpful in identifying intranasal landmarks, particularly in revision cases. In our experience with multiplanar two-dimensional and three-dimensional CT reconstruction, another ISG capability (Allegro system), has been extremely valuable in preoperative planning.[22] We use 1.5 mm axial sinus CT sections to reconstruct coronal, sagittal, or three-dimensional images, often demonstrating critical sites of frontal recess obstruction (Fig. 3–13). A recent study has demonstrated that this technique poses minimal radiation hazard to the patient.[23] However, because this technology is not available in most medical centers, a more feasible option is to reconstruct the 1.5 mm axial scan data on the original CT scanner immediately after the study is performed. Another radiographic alternative is the cross-table lateral plain film. When taken intraoperatively with a probe in the frontal sinus, such a film can localize the radiopaque instrument and prevent errant dissection (Fig. 3–14).

In some cases the endoscopic approach, by itself, is insufficient. For instance, revision cases may be complicated by dense bone and soft tissue frontal recess scarring, prohibiting intranasal identification of the frontal ostium. Frontal cells or postsurgical changes within the frontal sinus itself also may be unreachable endoscopically. In these cases an endoscopic intranasal frontal sinusotomy may be combined with an endoscopic external frontal sinusotomy. This is usually achieved with a frontal sinus trephine, approximately 5 to 6 mm in diameter, through which endoscopes, curettes, and forceps can be passed to remove obstruction (Figs. 3–15, 3–16). When wider exposure is necessary, as after failed fat obliteration of the frontal sinus, an osteoplastic flap may be necessary rather than a trephine. Locating the frontal recess when there are no intranasal landmarks may be very difficult. A red rubber catheter passed from the frontal sinus into the nose may make intranasal identification easier. Dissection can then proceed more safely through the soft tissue and bone cells immediately adjacent to the catheter. Although the quality of mucosal regeneration is unclear in the de-epithelialized frontal recess and frontal sinus,[24] these combined "above and below" approaches may provide the only opportunity to restore normal sinus ventilation and drainage. Our experience with 16 combined external and endoscopic intranasal frontal sinusotomies indicates that function can be improved in 87.5% of cases.[25]

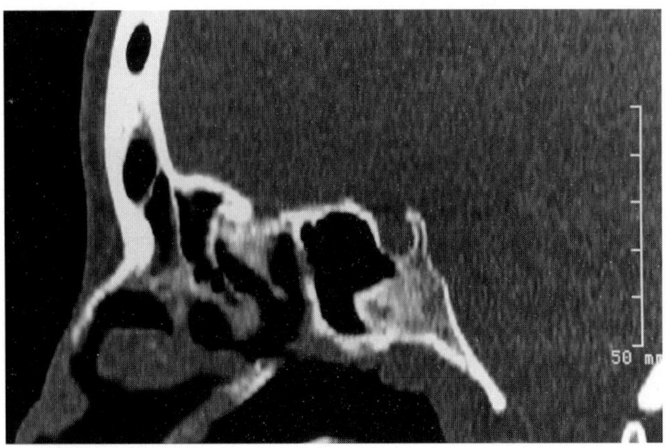

Fig. 3–13. Sagittal image of frontal sinus using ISG multiplanar two dimensional reconstruction.

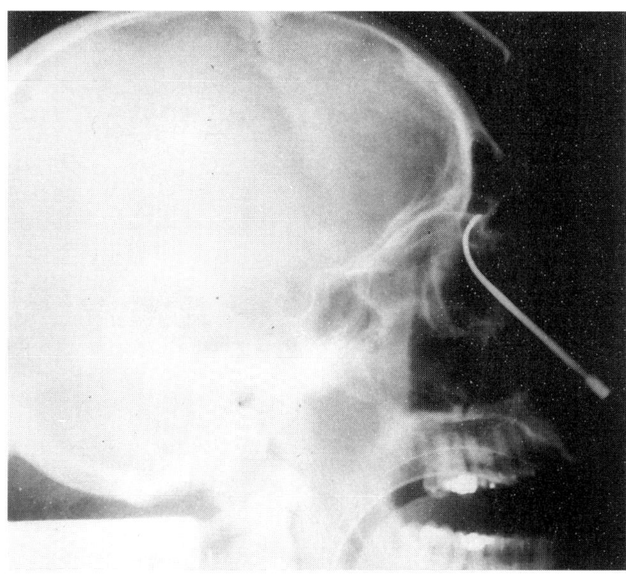

Fig. 3–14. Lateral plain film with probe in frontal sinus.

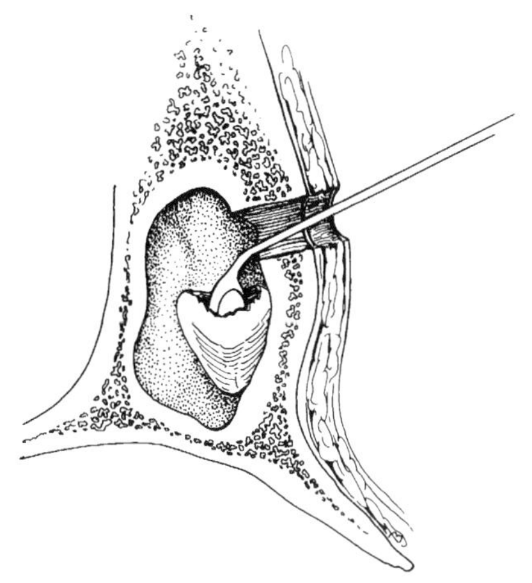

Fig. 3–15. Currette passed through frontal sinus trephine.

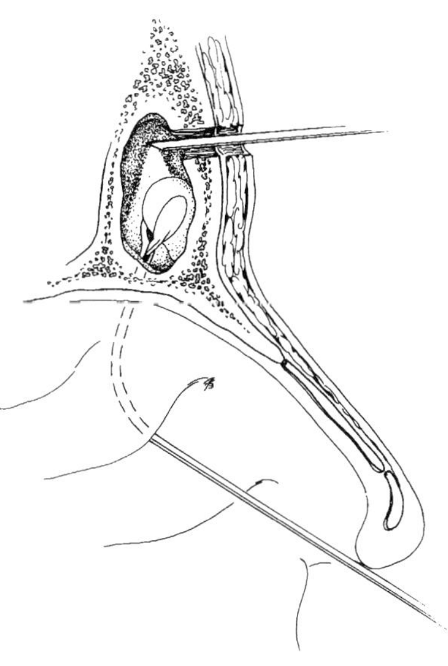

Fig. 3–16. Giraffe forcep passed through frontal recess, visualized by endoscope inserted through trephine.

If the dissected frontal recess is too narrow, stenting may prevent scarring. The frontal recess lumen diameter necessary to restore sinus function has not been determined. Wigand and Hosemann's experience with over 500 endoscopic frontal sinus procedures has led them to believe that "if a probe of 2.5 mm diameter can be inserted into the frontal sinus there is no concern about adequate ventilation and drainage."[26] Schaefer and Close reported stenting the frontal recess with a 4 mm silastic catheter when the diameter was as narrow as 4 to 6 mm; they had satisfactory results in 2 of 4 patients.[27] Animal studies have suggested that soft, rather than rigid, stents yield the best results.[28] Gelfilm rolled into a tight stent provides soft support of the surgically manipulated frontal recess, and can be removed either during the postoperative cleaning or allowed to resorb. A polyethylene tube formed into an "umbrella" shape reportedly functions well to preserve the frontal recess lumen postoperatively.[29]

Postoperative Care

Routine postoperative care includes vigorous normal saline irrigations of the nasal cavity at least 4 time per day for several weeks. Antibiotics are only used if active infection was identified intraoperatively, directed by culture results, or if marked polyposis was present. Topical steroids are recommended for nasal polyposis or allergic rhinitis. A tapering dose of oral steroids is prescribed for massive polyposis if not medically contraindicated. A maintenance antibiotic and steroid dose are continued until healing is complete with polyp resolution. There is no prospective data to substantiate or refute the routine use of antibiotics or steroids after FESS. Consequently, these agents are used sporadically, as necessary in each case. A steroid and antibiotic treatment regimen is certainly validated whenever the patient's presentation suggests possible underlying osteitis.

Physician cleaning of the nasal cavity is individualized for each patient, but is generally performed between postoperative days 2 to 4. The patient then returns weekly for endoscopic exams until all coagulum, purulence, desquamated polyps, bone flakes, and other debris have cleared. If packing has been required for hemostasis, it is generally removed within 3 days. Children too young to cooperate with endoscopic exams in clinic are reexamined approximately 2 weeks after surgery under general anesthesia.

Complications

Surgery of the frontal recess is more dangerous than maxillary and anterior ethmoid endoscopy because of the very close proximity of the laminea papyracea and anterior cranial fossa. Potential immediate complications include bleeding, CSF leak, and a floppy middle turbinate. Periorbital ecchymosis or crepitance are probably the most common early complications, but should occur less than 1% of the time. Other possible early complications include intraorbital hematoma and intranasal bleeding. Synechia between the middle turbinate and the lateral nasal wall is one of the most common late complications; this can be reduced by minimizing trauma to the lateral middle turbinate surface during insertion of the endoscopes and instruments. Encephalocoele formation due to a defect in the anterior skull base is a reported late complication. All patients are advised of the risk of recurrent or persistent sinusitis and the possible need for additional surgery.

Conclusions

The vast majority of frontal sinus disease patients can be treated endoscopically. Intimate knowledge of intranasal anatomy and the various instruments, combined with a careful preoperative evaluation, is essential for success. We recommend extensive cadaver dissection as a means of refining surgical technique. With patience, persistence, and a commitment to functional surgery, the results should be very rewarding.

REFERENCES

1. Schaeffer JP. The genesis, development and adult anatomy of the nasofrontal region in man. *Am J Anat.*1916;20:125–146.
2. Kasper KA. Nasofrontal connections: a study based on 100 consecutive dissections. *Arch Otol.*1936; 23:322–343.
3. Van Alyea OE. Frontal sinus drainage. *Ann Otol.* 1946; 55:267–278.
4. Loury MC. Endoscopic frontal recess and frontal sinus ostium dissection. *Laryngoscope.* 1993; 103:455–458.
5. Hilding A. The physiology of drainage of mucous. *Am J Physiol.* 1932;100:664–670.
6. Messerklinger W. On the drainage of the frontal sinus in man. *Acta Otolaryngol.*1967;63:176–181.
7. Stammberger H. Endoscopic endonasal surgery—concepts in treatment of recurrent rhinosinusitis. Part I. Anatomic and pathophysiologic considerations. *Otolaryngol—Head & Neck Surg.*1986;94:143–146.
8. Kuhn FA, Bolger WE, Tisdal RG. The agger nasi cell in frontal recess obstruction: an anatomic, radiologic and clinical correlation. *Oper Techni Otolaryng—Head & Neck Surgery.*1991;2:226–231.
9. Bolger WE, Butzin CA, Parsons DS. Paranasal sinus bony anatomic variations and mucosal abnormalities: CT analysis for endoscopic sinus surgery. *Laryngoscope.* 1991; 101:56–64.
10. Lillie HI, Simonton KM. Developmental extension of an anterior ethmoid cell within the frontal sinus. *Arch Otol.*1940;32:32–37.
11. Bent JP, Cuilty-Sillers C, Kuhn FA. The frontal cell as a cause of frontal sinus obstruction. *Amer J Rhinology.* 1994;8:185-191.
12. Bent JP, Kuhn FA. The diagnosis of allergic fungal sinusitis. *Otolaryngol—Head Neck Surg.* 1994; in press.
13. Hardy JM, Montgomery WW. Osteoplastic frontal sinusotomy: an analysis of 250 operations. *Ann Otol.* 1976;85:523–532.
14. Kuhn FA, Kennedy DW, Hassab MH. Persistent or recurrent sinus disease after intranasal ethmoidectomy. Presented at the VIII International Symposium on Infection and Allergy in the Nose, Baltimore, MD, June 1989.
15. Kennedy DW. Prognostic factors, outcomes, and staging in ethmoid sinus surgery. *Laryngoscope.*1992;102(12, part 2):1–18.
16. Stankowitz JA. Complications in endoscopic ethmoidectomy: an update. *Laryngoscope.*1989;99:686–690.
17. Stammberger H. *Functional Endoscopic Sinus Surgery.* Philadelphia, PA: BC Decker;1991:70–76.
18. Hilding A. Experimental surgery of the nose and sinuses. *Arch Otol.* 1933;47:321–327.
19. Lothrup HA. Frontal sinus suppuration with results of a new procedure. *JAMA.* 1915;65:153–160.
20. Draf D. Endonasal micro-endoscopic frontal sinus surgery: the Fulda concept. *Oper Tech Otolaryng—Head & Neck Surg.*1991;2:234–240.
21. Metson R. Endoscopic treatment of frontal sinusitis. *Laryngoscope.*1992;102:712–716.
22. Kuhn FA, Cuilty-Sillers C, Vickery CL, Figueroa RE. Three-dimensional imaging in the evaluation and management of the frontal sinus. Presented at the International Advanced Sinus Symposium, Philadelphia, PA, July 23, 1993.

23. Vickery CL, Kuhn FA, Davis JS. Sagittal computerized tomography reconstruction of the paranasal sinuses and cataract risk. Presented at the Annual Meeting of the American Rhinologic Society, Minneapolis, Minnesota, October 1, 1993.
24. Forsgren K, Stierna P, Kumlien J, Carlsoo B. Regeneration of maxillary sinus mucosa following surgical removal. Eperimental study in rabbits. *Ann Otol.* 1993;102:459–466.
25. Bent JP, Spears R, Kuhn FA. An alternative to frontal sinus obliteration. Presented at the Southern Section of the Triologic Society, Marco Island, FL, January 14, 1994.
26. Wigand ME, Hosemann WG. Endoscopic surgery for frontal sinusitis and its complications. *Am J Rhinol.* 1991;5:85–89.
27. Schaefer SD, Close LG. Endoscopic management of frontal sinus disease. *Laryngoscope.* 1990;100:155–160.
28. Neel BH, Whicker JH, Lake CF. Thin rubber sheeting in frontal sinus surgery: animal and clinical studies. *Laryngoscope.*1976;86:524–536.
29. Wolf G, Stammberger H. Personal communication.

4

Sphenoid Sinus Surgery

James A. Stankiewicz

The sphenoid sinus is involved in sinus disease by itself or more commonly as part of a pansinusitis. In an anatomically spacious nose, the sphenoid sinus can be approached directly medial to the middle turbinate, and sphenoidotomy is usually straightforward. Unfortunately, such a straightforward approach is often not possible. The sphenoethmoid recess can be compromised by a deviated septum, large middle turbinate, or both, making a direct approach to the sphenoid very difficult. In a revision sinus surgical case, the landmarks are often distorted, making the sphenoidotomy hazardous. This chapter discusses various aspects of sphenoid sinus surgery which are very helpful in both isolated disease and pansinusitis.

Isolated Sphenoid Sinus Disease

As mentioned above, for symptomatic sinusitis or mucocele, the sphenoid sinus can be approached directly medial to the middle turbinate or lateral to the middle turbinate through the ethmoid sinuses. The approach medial to the middle turbinate is the safest because it brings the surgeon directly onto the sphenoid ostia which in most cases of sinusitis can be easily identified. However, in markedly inflamed or reactive noses, the mucosa may be so edematous to make that approach problematic. It is, therefore, important to utilize every effort to identify the anterior sphenoid wall and ostia prior to opening the skull base. In small children, with their variable anatomy, the sphenoid sinus is even more difficult to find than in the adult.

If, however, a direct medial approach is possible, the steps taken to open the sphenoid are usually straightforward. Unless the sphenoid ostia is directly visualized, penetration into the sphenoid sinus should always be preceded by measurement of distance to confirm the sphenoid anterior wall. This is important in mucocele or polyp surgery where landmarks are distorted. A measuring instrument, which can be a beaded probe (7, 9, 11 cm marks), a marked suction, etc., is placed on the anterior sphenoid wall (Fig. 4–1). This distance should measure 7 cm (varying about 0.5 cm longer in the very tall patient and 0.5 cm shorter in the very small adult patient). In the child, the measurement is taken just superior to the choana, which will provide a good estimate of the anterior sphenoid wall.

For all approaches to the sphenoid, the finding of the ostia is the safest way to enter the sphenoid sinus. Once the measurement is taken, a search for the ostia is begun medially and adjacent to the septum at the lower level of the superior turbinate (medial to the middle turbinate). When the ostia is cannulated, it is safe to enter the sphenoid. A Frazier suction is used to enter the sphenoid to fracture the anterior sphenoid wall adjacent to the ostia. In most cases, the anterior wall ostia is eggshell thin and fractures readily. Rarely, in extensive disease, the anterior wall is thickened and may present a problem. Provided the ostia is identified and measurements are accurate, even a thick wall can be fractured with a Frazier suction. A straight forceps can then be placed into the sphenoidotomy, opened in the sinus, and pulled back anteriorly. This will effectively push the anterior wall nasally, allowing for safe removal of the anterior wall. A sphenoid punch, either alone or as part of a universal set, is a great help in making a large sphenoidotomy (Fig. 4–2). The sphenoid can be opened medially and inferiorly without concern. The lateral extent is to the lateral wall of the sphenoid, not ethmoid. Superiorally, care is taken when removing the superior overhang of the anterior wall, which is aided by utilizing a curved suction, spoon curette, or punch to fracture the bone outward. A biting forceps may not only remove the overhang but also open the skull base above the opening, creating a cerebrospinal fistula.

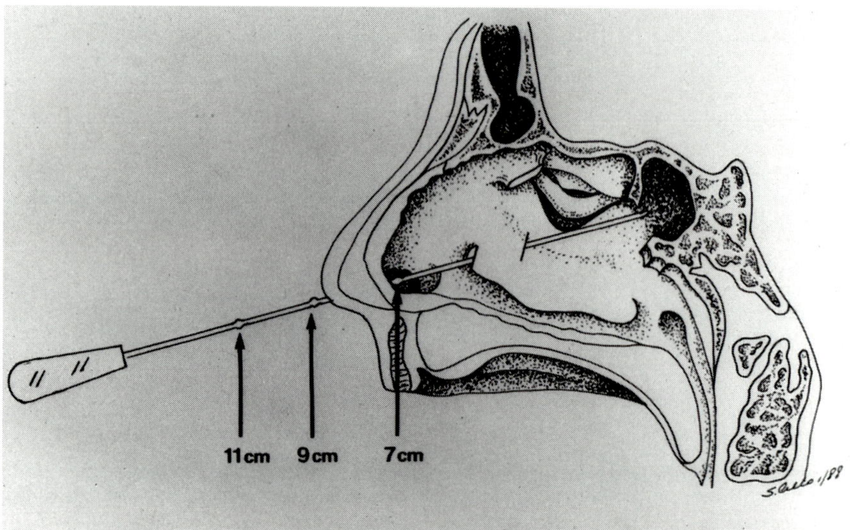

Fig. 4–1. Measuring probe to accurately assess distance to sphenoid sinus. From Stankiewicz JA: The endoscopic approach to the sphenoid sinus, *Laryngoscope* 99(2):218–221, 1989. By permission.

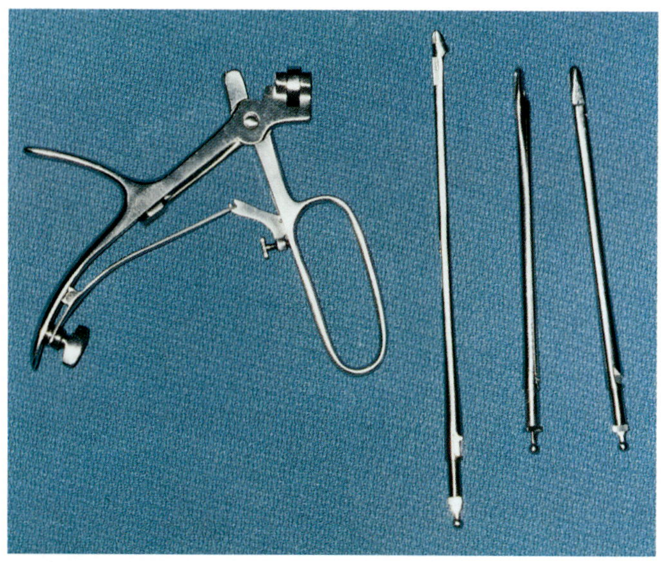

Fig. 4–2. Sphenoid punch instrument used in creating wide sphenoidotomy.

In the case of chronic disease in which the anatomy, including the ostia, is indistinct, reference to the CT scan is important. The sphenoid is often very small on one side and may, in essence, be an extension of the posterior ethmoid, measuring 7.5 to 8 cm. It is important to recognize this. If uncertainty is still present, a fluoroscopic or intraoperative lateral skull x-ray can be obtained to locate exactly the skull base (Fig. 4–3). Computer assisted endoscopic measurement is also helpful, if available. Surgery should never proceed unless the anatomy is known to the surgeon. Once inside the sphenoid, a mucocele can be marsupialized, a cyst opened, and polypoid disease removed. Of concern is the fact that 20% of sphenoid sinuses have a dehiscent carotid artery.[1] It is better to leave tissue/polypoid disease on the posterior wall or roof of the sphenoid than to risk carotid rupture and a major catastrophe. Fungal disease, such as the fungal ball, should be removed totally if possible. Remember, however, the fungal ball or the mucocele may expand the sinus, greatly thinning out the skull base and making entrance into the carotid, optic nerve, or skull base a possibility (Fig. 4–4). Experience with cerebrospinal fluid (CSF) fistula repair in the sphenoid is discussed in Chapter 10.

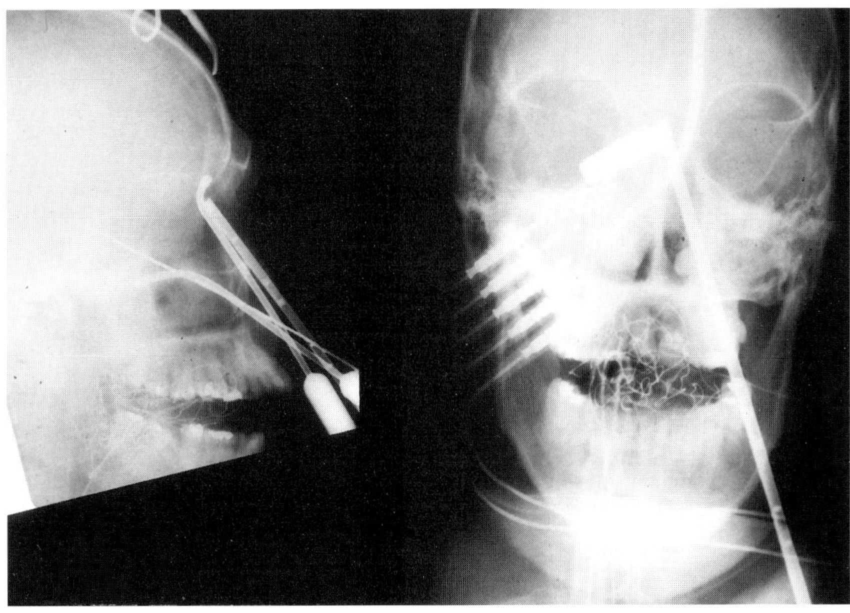

Fig. 4–3. Intraoperative lateral skull x-ray with probe on sphenoid and skull base.

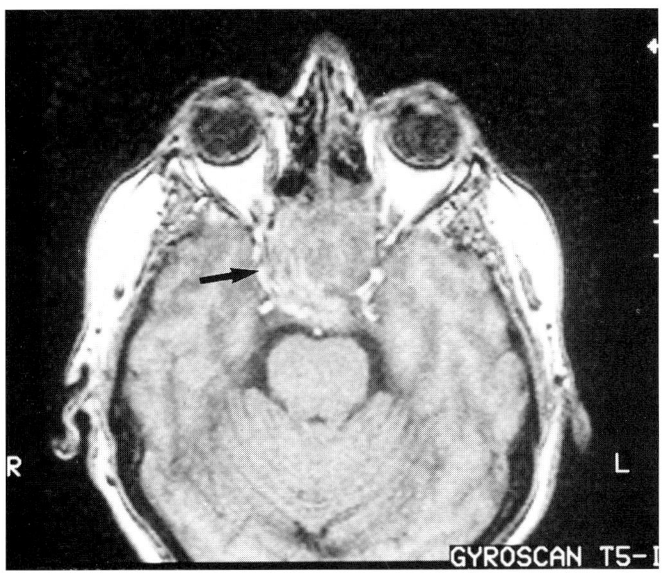

Fig. 4–4. Greatly expanded sphenoid sinus due to fungal ball and mucocele. (MRI scan)

Recently, several cases of clival lesions have been approached endoscopically through the posterior sphenoid sinus wall (Fig. 4–5). Unfortunately, for clival lesions and other problems, such as repair of CSF fistula, surgery is almost impossible to perform with the middle turbinate in place. Therefore, middle turbinate incisions are made with an endoscopic punch or scissors anterior superiorally and posterioinferiorally, and the lower body of the middle turbinate is removed (Fig. 4–6). This immediately places the surgeon at the level of the posterior ethmoid sinus and skull base.[2] Since most patients with isolated disease have normal sinuses, the opening of the posterior ethmoid is quick and unproblematic. The sphenoid sinus ostia is identified and probed as described earlier. A wide sphenoidotomy is performed as described and the sphenoid disease handled as necessary taking into consideration concerns for the carotid artery, optic nerve, and skull base as discussed.[3] The limitation of clival lesions and posterior wall sphenoid sinus surgery is the

A

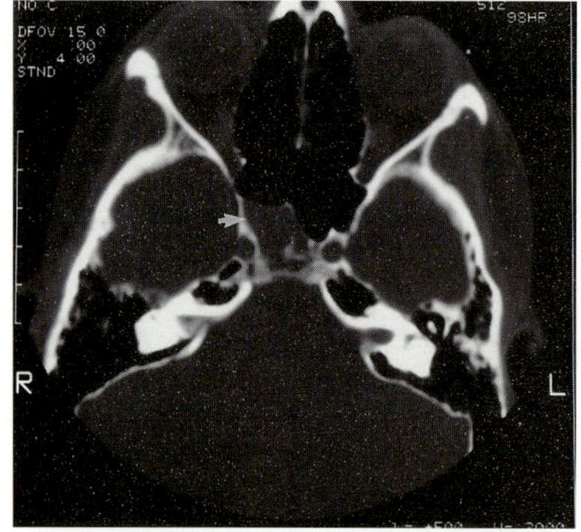

B

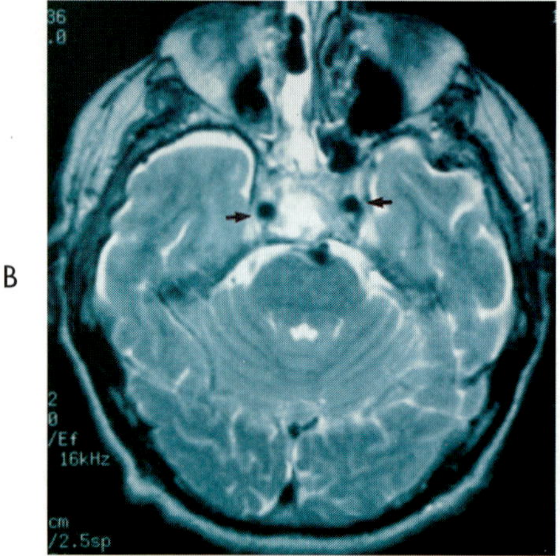

C

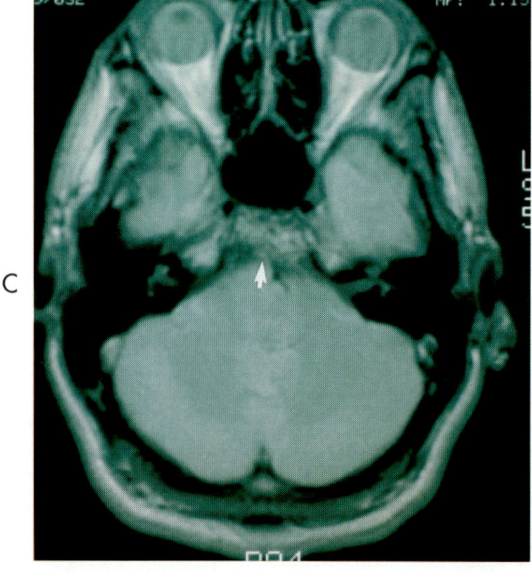

Fig. 4–5. Clival lesions including: **A,** Cyst (CT scan); **B,** pituitary tumor (MRI scan); **C,** fibrous dysplasia (MRI scan).

anatomy and available instrumentation. Forceps, knives, probes, and drills have to reach to 9 cm or more. Endoscopic sinus instrumentation is limited in this regard, and neurosurgical pituitary or laryngeal microinstruments may be helpful. Lesions in the clivus often will thin out or erode the posterior wall, allowing exposure without using a drill. Biopsy or cyst drainage can be accomplished taking care to stay inferomedially to avoid the dura high and the carotid laterally. If marked bleeding is experienced upon entering the sphenoid sinus or upon tumor biopsy, packing is placed. Certain tumors such as metastatic renal cell carcinoma are very vascular and can give the impression of carotid-like bleeding. Usually this bleeding will occur upon first entrance into the sphenoid ostia with a suction and can be readily packed off. It is suggested that the H & P and laboratory data be scanned closely with the isolated sphenoid/clival lesions preoperatively to rule out evidence of metastatic tumor. In the situation with renal cell carcinoma above, review of the lab data showed hematuria. A renal ultrasound was obtained and was positive for a left kidney lesion positive for renal cell carcinoma. MRI and angiography may be necessary to more accurately identify the vascularity and nature of the clival lesion.

Sphenoid Sinus and Pansinusitis

Surgery on the sphenoid sinus in the patient with pansinusitis, especially with extensive polyposis, is approached in a somewhat different manner than for isolated sinus disease (Fig. 4–7).[4] In many of these patients, surgical landmarks are not present. This is especially true in the revision patient, and presents a true challenge.

In pansinusitis without polyposis the sphenoid sinus can be approached in different ways. One commonly recommended way is to open directly into the sphenoid through the posterior ethmoids without finding the sphenoid ostia. After entering the posterior ethmoids through the basal lamella, the anterior wall of the sphenoid and skull base are encountered. Measurement should indicate that this is 7 cm in distance. Staying at a level no higher than the lower portion of the middle turbinate, the sphenoid anterior wall is pressed inward with a forceps or suction tip. The anterior wall is usually very thin and fractures easily. Hard bone means either chronic disease or skull base/brain, and further advancement needs to be reassessed by means of measurement techniques or radiologic techniques, as noted previously.

My preference is to find the sphenoid ostia to ensure the correct sphenoid location. Once the

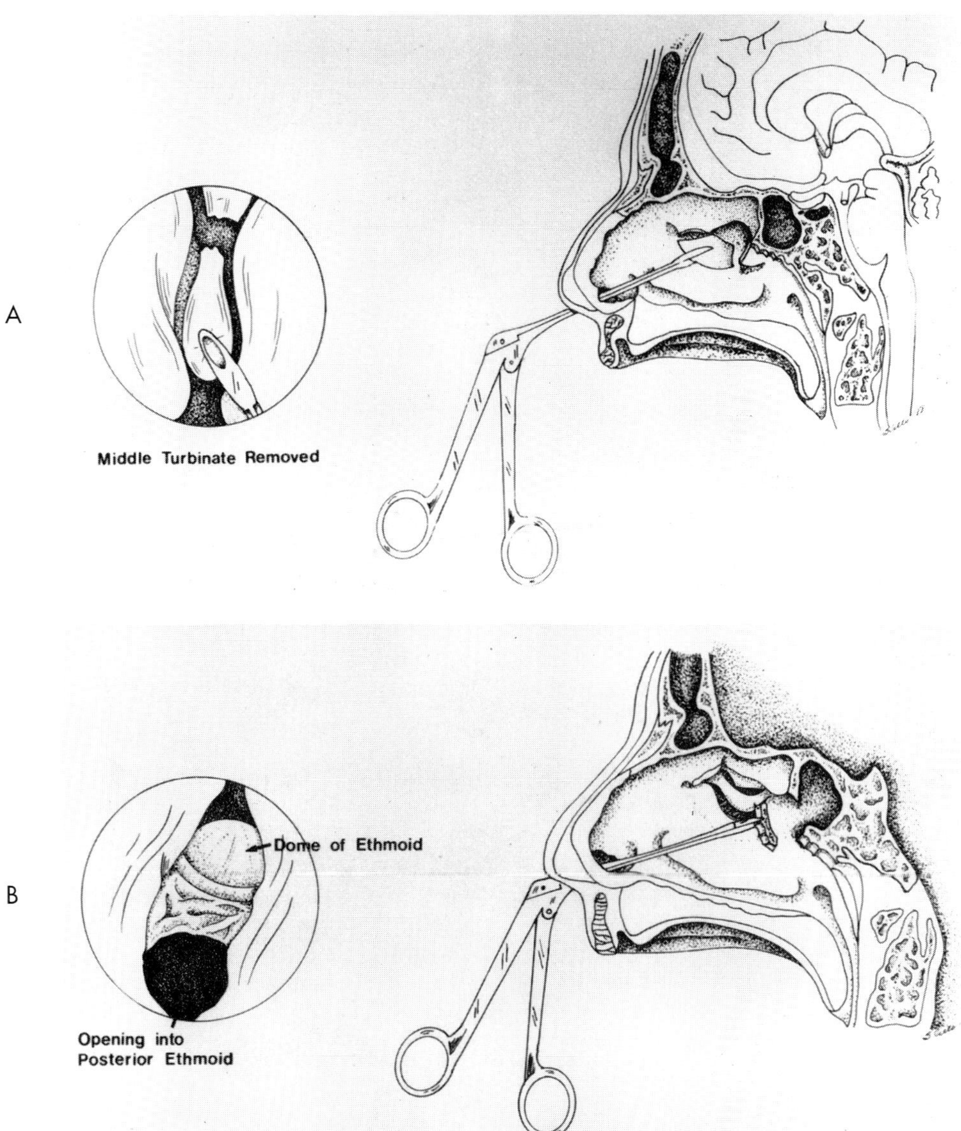

Fig. 4–6. **A,** Incisions in middle turbinate. **B,** Middle turbinate removal with view to the posterior ethmoid and skull base. From Stankiewicz JA: The endoscopic approach to the sphenoid sinus. *Laryngoscope* 99(2):218–221, 1989. By permission.

basal lamella is breached and the posterior ethmoid cells are cleaned of debris and disease, the membranous posterior part of the middle turbinate through which the posterior ethmoid drains is identified. The lower part of the membrane is removed moving posteriorly. After this is done, the superior turbinate comes into view, and the sphenoid ostia can be probed and identified. Once this is done, the sphenoid can be opened widely using the same techniques as noted in the isolated sinus. The suction, straight forceps, and sphenoid punch are used. The lower part of the superior turbinate is pushed medially or removed and a wide antrostomy is created. An alternative way of entering the sphenoid is described by Parsons. The anterior wall is identified and "hugged" as a probe or elevator is moved medially. A "ridge" is encountered which is the lateral part of the sphenoid ostia.[5] The ostia is entered and the superior turbinate is pushed medially. A wide sphenoidotomy can then be created. Again, disease in the sphenoid is removed carefully avoiding the posterior and superior walls as much as possible.

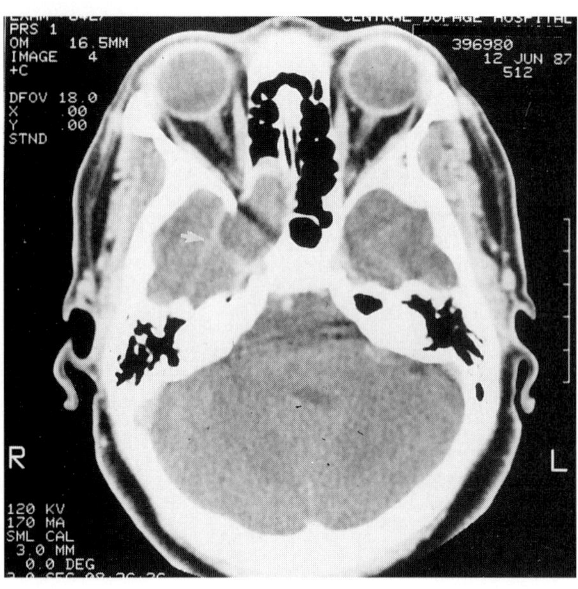

Fig. 4–7. Sinusitis with sphenoid sinus and mucocele (CT scan). From Stankiewicz JA: Sphenoid sinus mucocele. *Arch Otolaryngol Head Neck Surg* 115:735–740, 1989. By permission.

Revision surgery is the most difficult approach to the sphenoid sinus because in most cases landmarks are compromised. In this scenario the finding of the sphenoid serves two purposes: 1) removal of disease, and 2) as a landmark for surgery in the posterior superior ethmoids and skull base.[6] This is especially important in the patient with extensive recurrent polyps. A true marsupialization of the sphenoethmoid sinuses cannot be done without opening widely the sphenoid sinus. The maxillary antrostomy and sphenoidotomy are the keys to this surgery. Typically, I clean out all inferior polypoid disease first and then perform anterior ethmoidectomy. The maxillary antrostomy is created which identifies the lamina papyracea. The bulla ethmoidalis and basal lamella are entered and inferior disease is cleaned from the posterior ethmoids. All superior disease is left until the sphenoid is identified. When the sphenoid ostia is located via probing and measurement, a wide sphenoidotomy is created. Disease is removed and the superior disease is attacked. The skull base is identified with the sphenoidotomy. Using a small curved suction as a cell finder, the posterior superior ethmoid disease is dissected out laterally. Disease removal is from posterior to anterior. The agger nasi cells and the frontal recess are the last cells to be opened. This helps with removal of disease and prevents troublesome bleeding.

Patients with previous surgeries including sphenoidotomy may present with severe pain requiring revision sphenoidotomy. The key is always finding the sphenoid opening or ostia utilizing probing, measurement, or radiologic techniques. It is very rare that the sphenoid sinus cannot be entered if all the above are considered.

Clinical Correlation

In over 750 sphenoidotomy procedures, 3 CSF fistulas have occurred, none with meningitis or brain injuries. These 3, and 10 other CSF fistulae related to neurosurgical procedures, have been controlled endoscopically. No carotid artery or optic nerve injuries occurred. Only one sphenoid surgery had to be stopped because of marked bleeding and this involved a tumor with a clival metastatic renal cell carcinoma. No patient has had bleeding as a result of partial middle turbinate removal to approach an isolated sphenoid sinusitis or mass.

Operating Room Considerations

When surgery on the sphenoid sinus is contemplated, instrument preparation is important. A sickle cell knife or spoon curette can be used to push sphenoid fragments out of the sinus into the nose. A curved small suction can be used to break down the anterior wall and push it nasally. The curved suction is also helpful in freeing up and removing fungal disease or a fungus ball. Beaded probes or measured suctions marked at 7, 9, and 11 cm are absolutely necessary (see Fig. 4–2). Sphenoid punches or universal sets are extremely helpful. Unfortunately, these instruments are not available in endoscopic sinus sets, and may thus require scavenging from rhinology/sinus and neurosurgery trays. Smaller, precise punches, elevators, and forceps are required for intrasphenoid and clival surgery. The neurosurgery hypophysectomy tray is helpful. All patients should have a throat pack or a nasopharyngeal foley in place in case of massive bleeding from the carotid. Large Merocel sponges or nasal packing also should be in the operating room in case a massive carotid hemorrhage occurs. If the nose can be packed and bleeding controlled, the patient should survive.

The Carotid Drill (Sofferman)

Entrance into the carotid artery during sphenoid surgery may kill a patient. However, if quick action is taken to stop the hemorrhage, the patient may survive. In the outpatient setting, steps delineated in Table 4–1 should be followed.[7] In the inpatient setting, the approach outlined in Figure 4–8 is recommended. A close working relationship with neurosurgery and neuroradiology is the key to success in this terrible complication.

Conclusion

Surgery of the sphenoid sinus in advanced sinusitis/polyposis and isolated sphenoid/clival disease can be quite challenging. The surgeon has to be aware of all of the endoscopic techniques available and know how to locate the sphenoid when landmarks are not present. This chapter has outlined exactly how to approach the sphenoid in all circumstances.

Table 5–1 Outpatient carotid drill

1. Pack nose and throat
2. Call neurosurgery immediately
3. Expose carotid artery in the neck
4. Temporarily occlude carotid with vascular clamp or tape
5. Ligate carotid if neurosurgery approves
6. Get patient to inpatient hospital immediately
7. If distance is too great, neurosurgery to perform a "trapping procedure." The carotid is clipped below the anterior communicating artery to isolate this segment from blood flow.

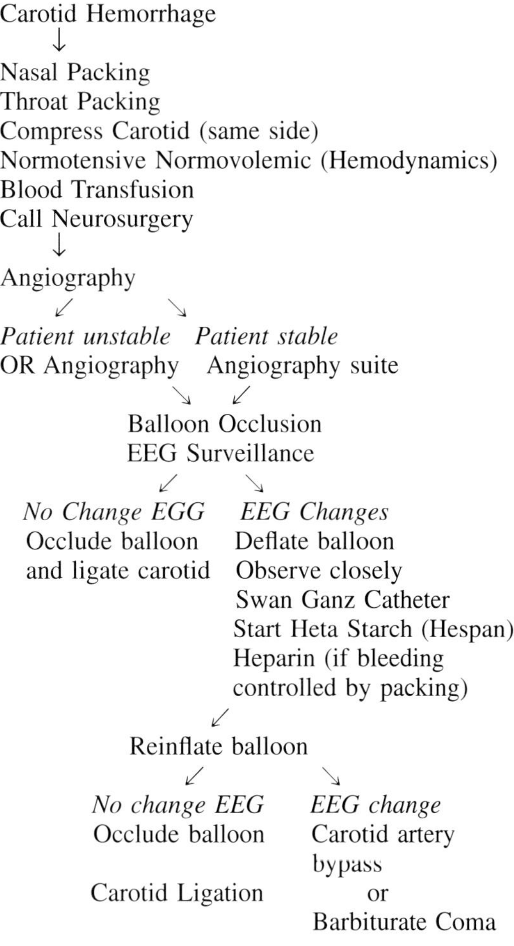

Fig. 4–8. Decision tree for treatment of arterial hemorrhage in an inpatient setting.

REFERENCES

1. Kennedy DW, Zinreich SJ, Hassab MH. The internal carotid artery as it relates to endonasal sphenoethmoidectomy. *Am J Rhinol.* 1990; 4:7–12.
2. Stankiewicz JA. The endoscopic approach to the sphenoid sinus. *Laryngoscope.* 1989; 99:218–221.
3. Stankiewicz JA. Sphenoid sinus mucocele. *Arch Otolaryngol Head Neck Surg.* 1989; 115:735–740.
4. Kennedy DW, Josephson JS, Zinreich SJ. Endoscopic sinus surgery for mucoceles. *Laryngoscope.* 1989; 99:885–895.
5. Parsons D, Bolger W, Boyd E. The 'Ridge'—A safer entry to the sphenoid sinus during functional endoscopic sinus surgery in children. *Oper Techn Otolaryngol Head Neck Surg.* 1994; 5:43–44.
6. Wigand ME. Transnasal ethmoidectomy under endoscopic control. *Rhinology (Eur).* 1981; 19:7–15.
7. Sofferman R. Optic nerve decompression and sphenoid sinus hemorrhage. Presented at Sisson International Head Neck Conference. Vail, CO, Feb 1991.

5

The Care of Children with Sinusitis

David S. Parsons and David W. Chambers

The evaluation and treatment of sinusitis in children has changed dramatically over the past decade because of the development, refinement, and widespread availability of computed tomography (CT) scanning and rigid nasal endoscopes. Until recently, pediatricians and otolaryngologists were taught that sinusitis in the pediatric population was uncommon. Now with the increased availability and use of CT imagery, the diagnosis of sinusitis is being made with greater frequency. Consequently, otolaryngologists are seeing a growing number of children with recurrent or chronic sinusitis.

Because young pediatric patients' midfacial structures are dynamically developing, their anatomy is not the same as that of adults. Consequently, their evaluation and treatment are different. The surgeon should verify that the child's disease is not responding to optimal and prolonged medical therapy prior to consideration of surgical intervention. Endoscopic techniques have made surgery safer and more effective for the treatment of children with recalcitrant recurrent or chronic sinus disease.

History

A thorough history is the single most important aspect of the evaluation of pediatric sinusitis. The most important and sometimes the most difficult portion of the history is distinguishing symptoms of sinus disease from those of nasal disease. The average toddler will have six to eight upper respiratory infections (URIs) per year.[1] Symptoms of URI, particularly rhinitis, may last up to 2 to 3 weeks. Therefore, many normal toddlers may have rhinorrhea for more than 4 months each year.

To help the physician distinguish nasal symptoms from sinusitis, studies have been done to determine the most common symptoms of sinusitis. One study reported that rhinorrhea, cough, and fetid breath were the most consistent symptoms of *acute* sinusitis.[2] This report also found fever to be an inconsistent finding, while headaches and facial pain appeared to be prominent symptoms only in older children. A second study of *chronic* sinusitis consistently demonstrated seven cardinal symptoms in children (Table 5-1).[3] Any infant or child with a majority of these symptoms should be considered for treatment of sinusitis. Other symptoms that appear less frequently but may be helpful in making the diagnosis include: sore throat, hoarseness, fever, facial puffiness or edema, facial tenderness, epistaxis, recurrent otitis media, asthma exacerbations, and nausea or vomiting of mucus.[4]

Chronic nasal obstruction is the most consistent complaint of children with chronic sinusitis.[3] *Purulent nasal discharge* is often treated with antibiotics, with frequent resolution of the symptom or thinning of the nasal discharge. Children occasionally will have recurrence of these symptoms after the course of antibiotics has been completed. This nasal discharge is closely related to nasal edema and nasal obstruction. Because of the small size of the child's nose, a small amount of nasal edema can create marked nasal congestion. Consequently, unlike adults who tend to complain more of postnasal drainage, nasal obstruction and purulent nasal discharge are the predominant complaints in children with sinusitis.

Postnasal drainage and *cough* are also major complaints of children with sinusitis. Many young children are not aware of drainage down the back of their throats, as it is always there; that is, it is "normal" to them. However, if the physician directly asks the parent or child if drainage is present in the back of the throat, the response is often affirmative. Cough is frequently related to postnasal drainage, especially in children who do not have any chest congestion. The cough is usually worse at night or in the early morning. The

Table 5-1 The seven cardinal symptoms of chronic sinusitis in children with the frequency in which they were identified when a careful history was obtained.[3]

Symptoms	% of Cases
1. Chronic nasal obstruction	100%
2. Prolonged purulent nasal discharge	90%
3. Postnasal drainage	63%
4. Chronic cough	71%
5. Malodorous breath	67%
6. Headaches	90%
7. Behavioral changes	63%

drainage and cough often improve with antibiotic therapy, but return after discontinuation of medications in chronic disease.

Malodorous or *fetid breath* is only rarely offered as a complaint by parents. However, when specifically asked, the parents often recall that the children have markedly foul breath poorly responsive to proper oral hygiene. Unlike the cough and nasal discharge, fetid breath may continue even during antibiotic treatment.

There has been debate about *headaches* as a symptom of sinusitis. Some have suggested that headaches in small children with sinusitis are uncommon. Parsons and Phillips identified small toddlers who often complained of the associated symptoms of head pain with exacerbations of sinusitis. The parents had to be asked the appropriate questions to identify these symptoms.[3] The head pain was manifested by a variety of different actions including: head holding, rubbing of cheeks, head banging, hair pulling, putting face into the lap of a parent or onto a cool surface. This symptom was commonly identified with appropriate questioning.

As is the case with malodorous breath, complaints of *behavior changes* in children are rarely offered by the parents as a symptom of sinusitis. If questioned appropriately, parents will regularly describe behavioral or personality changes which coincide with the onset of other symptoms of sinusitis. These behavior changes may be subtle but, to the parent, will seem out of character. Manifestations that coincide with sinus infections include: fussiness, whining, irritability, lethargy, impatience, crankiness, and hostility.[4]

The importance of the history cannot be overemphasized. Asking appropriate questions of children and parents is critical when trying to distinguish sinusitis in a child from other etiologies of nasal rhinitis. Adequate time spent with the patient and family obtaining a thorough history is imperative for the diagnosis of sinusitis.

Physical Examination

The most common physical findings in children with sinusitis are purulent nasal discharge, malodorous breath, and pharyngeal findings consistent with chronic cough and postnasal drainage. These findings are not pathognomonic of sinusitis. In fact, no finding will consistently make the diagnosis, except when complications exist such as subperiosteal edema or abscess. Despite the unrewarding findings on the physical examination, a complete head and neck examination should always be performed to rule out any other possible etiology for the patient's symptoms.

Findings with anterior rhinoscopy are usually not overly productive. Information, however, can be gained about the degree of nasal congestion, deviated nasal septum, turbinate hypertrophy or erythema, the presence of purulence, or nasal polyps. Other methods of evaluating the paranasal sinuses have proven ineffective in children. These methods include percussion of the face to illicit tenderness or transillumination of the sinuses.[5] Even the use of telescopes in the cooperative patient is of limited value. It is important, however, to perform a thorough examination to eliminate other etiologies of sinus or nasal disease such as allergy, deviated septum, foreign body, tumor, or congenital atrophic rhinitis.

Predisposing Factors of Pediatric Sinusitis

The diagnosis of sinusitis in children can be strongly suspected from the history obtained during the work-up. Many diseases or abnormalities can lead to or mimic sinusitis (see Table 5-2). These factors must be addressed in the history, physical exam, and laboratory work-up of the patient. Any disorder that leads to the obstruction of sinus ostia has the potential to cause sinusitis. Obstruction may be due to bony structural abnormalities or mucosal edema. Whatever the underlying cause of sinusitis, these predisposing factors must be identified and maximally treated prior to consideration of surgical intervention.

Allergies and URIs are the most common causes of chronic nasal symptoms in children. It is reported that 58% to 81% of all patients treated for chronic sinusitis had a positive allergy work-up.[3,6] Any child suspected of having sinus disease severe

Table 5-2 Predisposing or associated factors

1. Allergies
2. Recurrent upper respiratory tract infection
3. Asthma
4. Adenoidal hypertrophy
5. Bony abnormality of sinuses
6. Immunodeficiency (including AIDS)
7. Deviated nasal septum
8. Cystic fibrosis
9. Posttraumatic deformities
10. Nasal foreign body
11. Primary ciliary dyskinesia
12. Choanal atresia or stenosis
13. Nasal mass

enough to warrant surgery should have an allergy assessment. Allergies to milk proteins are the most common allergies seen in small children. Therefore, any toddler being evaluated for surgery should be considered for a milk-free diet trial. Recent reports have also implicated secondhand smoke as a major contributor to otitis media, allergies, and sinusitis in children. We now recommend that the house and car of the child be smoke free. This means that parents either stop smoking or at least refrain from smoking in the house and car. We have seen numerous examples of this small intervention reversing the child's sinus disease and obviating the need for expensive medical care or surgical intervention.

Recurrent URIs can also contribute to chronic sinus infections. As mentioned previously, the average toddler may have nasal rhinitis for up to one-third of the year. Because of the immature nature of the immune system in toddlers, they may have a more difficult time clearing their upper respiratory tracts. This problem is magnified if the child attends a large day care center where there is greater exposure to a great variety of viruses. The child no sooner fights off one infection than he or she is exposed to yet another virus. Sometimes removal of a child from a large day care setting will reduce the exposure and allow the child to clear the recurrent or chronic infections. In today's society, in which day care has become a necessity for many families, smaller day care settings are recommended.

The possibility of asthma associated with sinus disease should be investigated. Asthma is not an etiology of sinus disease but sinusitis has clearly been associated with worsening of bronchospasm. Approximately two-thirds of sinus surgical patients also had asthma.[3] Surgical intervention has a remarkably positive effect on pulmonary symptoms in the vast majority of patients.[7]

Adenoidal hypertrophy as a cause of sinus disease has been debated for years. Anecdotal information has been handed down for decades, but no scientific study has documented a correlation between adenoidal hypertrophy and sinusitis. Further, it is difficult to explain how a posterior nasal pharyngeal obstruction can produce obstruction of the ostiomeatal complex. However, enlarged adenoids may in fact produce nasal obstruction with stasis of nasal secretions and cause nasal symptoms mimicking sinusitis. Adenoidectomy usually relieves the obstruction and thereby alleviates the symptoms in patients with simple adenoidal hypertrophy. There is, however, another population of patients who have adenoidal hypertrophy secondary to chronic adenoiditis related to chronic sinusitis. It appears that a simple adenoidectomy will not relieve these patients' symptoms, and they will require definitive treatment of their sinusitis prior to resolution of their symptoms.[3] One must always consider adenoidal hypertrophy as either a cause of nasal symptoms or a potential complication of sinusitis.

Another factor which contributes to chronic sinusitis is immunodeficiency. Hypogammaglobulinemia may be present in toddlers and is of questionable significance. However, IgG subclass deficiency may manifest as chronic sinusitis. The work-up for immunodeficiencies includes total immunoglobulins and IgG subclasses, but the rate of clear findings of immunodeficiency remains low.

Acquired immunodeficiency syndrome (AIDS) can manifest in children as unremitting otitis media or sinusitis. While taking a patient history, parents should be questioned on possible exposure to AIDS. If any finding in the history or physical exam suggests possible exposure, HIV studies should be conducted.

Cystic fibrosis (CF) must also be considered in the differential diagnosis of children with chronic sinusitis. Patients with CF tend to have a history of chronic lower respiratory infections as well as sinonasal disease. Otitis media is not common in CF. Children suspected of having CF should undergo a sweat chloride determination or DNA study to diagnose the disorder.

Primary ciliary dyskinesia (PCD), like CF, is a hereditary disease which also must be considered as an underlying etiology of sinus disease. Although less common than CF, PCD presents an equally complex problem. These children tend to have recurrent pneumonias, chronic sinonasal disease, and unremitting problems with otitis media. Patients who have histories consistent with PCD should undergo a nasal or corina biopsy to evaluate the mucosa for deficiency of dynein in the cilia.

Further, physicians must consider various structural abnormalities in the differential for sinusitis. These include nasal foreign body, choanal atresia or stenosis, nasal mass, posttraumatic nasal deformity, or dental anomalies. All these conditions are rare but can be diagnosed with a thorough nasal exam including nasal endoscopy.

A thorough history and physical examination will help determine the possible involvement of these contributing factors. Consistently ask those questions which are appropriate for assessing which factors are important for each patient. A thorough head and neck exam is essential with anterior rhinoscopy and, where possible, nasal endoscopy.

Treatment

Every attempt should be made to cure sinusitis in these patients with medical management. Children are still growing and anatomically different from adults. Their anatomy is fragile, and the potential for surgical complications is significantly elevated. To avoid the risks associated with surgery, the otolaryngologist must assure that the pediatric patient has received all available medical therapy for an appropriate duration, prior to consideration of surgery.

Initial medical treatment includes appropriate antibiotic therapy. The pathogenic organisms in acute and subacute sinusitis in children have been identified as *S. pneumoniae, H. influenzae,* and *M. catarrhalis.*[8,9] Generally, any antibiotic which is effective for acute otitis media should provide adequate coverage. As is true with adults, a simple 10-day course of antibiotics may not be an adequate dose to cure sinusitis in children, particularly in cases with a high number of recurrences. The pathogenic organisms in chronic sinusitis are not yet well documented. In addition to the organisms involved in acute sinusitis, *S. aureus* and alpha hemolytic strep have also been identified as consistent pathogens in chronic sinusitis.[10,11] Most authorities agree upon broad spectrum antibiotic therapy covering both *S. aureus* and anaerobes. In addition, therapy should be continued for at least 3 to 4 weeks in recalcitrant cases. The role of anaerobic organisms in pediatric chronic sinusitis is unclear.

In addition to antibiotic therapy, nasal irrigation has proven to be of great value in treating chronic sinusitis. Saline irrigations are very useful in school-age children, but may be difficult or even impossible to administer in toddlers. The use of buffered hypertonic saline has been even more effective than normal saline irrigations.[12] The hypertonic solution draws fluid from the mucosa, thereby shrinking the membrane and opening up the sinus ostia to promote drainage. If buffered hypertonic saline or normal saline irrigations are not tolerated, the same solutions from a mist spray bottle should be encouraged.

The use of nasal steroids in children is inadequately studied. Many experts feel nasal steroids clearly are effective. While a short course of oral steroids has been found to transiently reduce symptoms, its use is generally limited to those children with polypoid changes.

Radiology

The coronal CT scan has now become the standard radiographic evaluation of sinuses in children. Routine sinus radiographs are difficult to read, and significant sinus disease can be misinterpreted.

The timing of the CT scan in children is critical. The optimal time is at the conclusion of maximal medical therapy, but only when a positive outcome is not observed. This usually means the sinus CT scans should be obtained after a minimum 3- to 4-week course of appropriate antibiotics with simultaneous use of buffered hypertonic saline irrigations and nasal steroids. This will provide the surgeon with a picture of the patient's sinuses at a point of maximal medical "wellness." If the patient has been effectively treated, this is theoretically as good as the sinuses will get.

Children who have significantly improved sinus symptoms with antibiotic therapy should be managed medically without surgery. If patients improve while on therapy but redevelop a sinus infection off therapy, a long-term trial of antibiotic prophylaxis should be considered. When the child returns with a poor response to maximal prolonged medical therapy and has a CT scan obtained at maximal wellness which shows disease, surgical intervention may be considered.

Preoperative Preparation

Only after maximal medical therapy has been tried and failed should surgical intervention be considered. The physician must meet with the parents and thoroughly discuss the realistic benefits and potential complications of the procedure. Parents need to understand that surgery will not prevent the child from getting sick again. With or without surgery, the child will still be exposed to and may contract the same number of URIs. The child may even have periodic episodes of sinusitis. However, the child's symptoms should be less severe and respond better to medical therapy after surgery.

Prior to performing functional endoscopic sinus (FES) surgery on children, the surgeon must have an understanding of the anatomy of their paranasal sinuses. It is imperative to remember that the anatomy is small and exceedingly fragile. Small children should never be the first patients on whom surgeons learn to do FES. Surgeons should first learn proper surgical techniques with extensive cadaveric laboratory experience and refine their skills on adults or adolescents. The operative field in children is extremely small and delicate, and precise surgery is essential. Consequently, pediatric FES should be performed only by specially trained endoscopic surgeons.

The preoperative work-up must include a thorough hemostatic evaluation. This should include CBC, with platelets, and an Ivy bleeding time. A complete history directed at possible bleeding disorders and recent use of aspirin, ibuprofen, or NSAIDs is essential. The number one cause of complications with FES surgery is poor visualization due to bleeding. With the small operative fields in children, even a small amount of blood can obscure the surgeon's visualization. Of pediatric surgical cases, 10% will be cancelled due to laboratory abnormalities; 50% of these patients have transient inhibitors due to medical therapy (aspirin, antibiotics, etc.) or mild viral illnesses.[13]

A short course of oral steroids may also be given preoperatively for children with visible polyps. Prednisone (1 to 2 mg/kg/day) given 10 to 14 days prior to surgery will reduce the size of large polyps and thus improve visualization and decrease blood loss. This will mean improved surgical results and safety for the child.

Operative Technique

The goal of FES surgery in children is to remove any bony or mucosal abnormality which is obstructing the ostiomeatal complex (OMC) and natural ostia outflow tracts. FES should create a patent communication to the diseased paranasal sinuses and restore ventilation and drainage, allowing recovery of the sinuses. Care is taken to preserve the normal mucociliary action and drainage. A conservative approach is emphasized in which the extent of surgery is dictated by the extent of disease.

Prior to entering the operating room, the child receives an intranasal spray with a decongestant. Oxymetazoline is preferred over other intranasal decongestants (i.e., phenylephrine) because it has fewer systemic side effects and has been shown to be a more effective vasoconstrictor.[14] Pediatric FES surgery is almost always performed under general anesthesia. A pharyngeal pack is placed to limit the amount of blood which is ingested by the child and to prevent bubbling of bloody secretions onto the telescope.

A transoral sphenopalatine block through the greater palatine foramin is then performed using 1% lidocaine with 1:100,000 epinephrine. The total of all injections for the FES should never exceed 7 mg/kg of lidocaine with epinephrine. This solution is then injected intranasally at the attachment of the middle turbinate. Cottonoids soaked with oxymetazoline are then placed in the middle meatus. All these steps help to optimize hemostasis and minimize blood loss.

The patient is prepped and draped with eyes remaining untaped. This allows for monitoring of the globes for movement to prevent an orbital complication. The patient's CT scan should be on the view box opposite the surgeon for reference during the procedure.

Again, the surgeon should make every attempt to keep the procedure as functional as possible. The turbinates should not be removed in children. The surgeon must always remember that the lacrimal duct is just lateral to the anterior uncinate and the sac is lateral to the agger nasi cell. Use of a sickle knife can easily injure the lacrimal drainage system and cause postoperative epiphora. The use of a sickle knife is strongly discouraged in children.

Prior to initiating any surgical steps, the CT scan should be reexamined for evidence of concha bullae. These are usually bivalved when present in the small, pediatric nose. Removing only the lateral portion of the concha bulla substantially improves visibility.

The next critical step is to identify the uncinate. A curved ball-tip seeker is placed within the hiatus semilunaris.[15] The uncinate is then gently displaced anterior and medially. Adhesions between the uncinate and lateral wall are often identified in patients with diseased OMCs. A pediatric back-biter is placed in the middle meatus through the hiatus semilunaris with the blade advanced into the infundibulum. Multiple bites are taken from the inferior uncinate, removing it entirely to its anterior insertion. This creates a "window" to optimally view the natural ostium of the maxillary sinus with a 30 or 70 degree telescope (Fig. 5–1). The action of the back-biter blade is lateral to medial, thus reducing potential for injury to the lacrimal duct or sac.

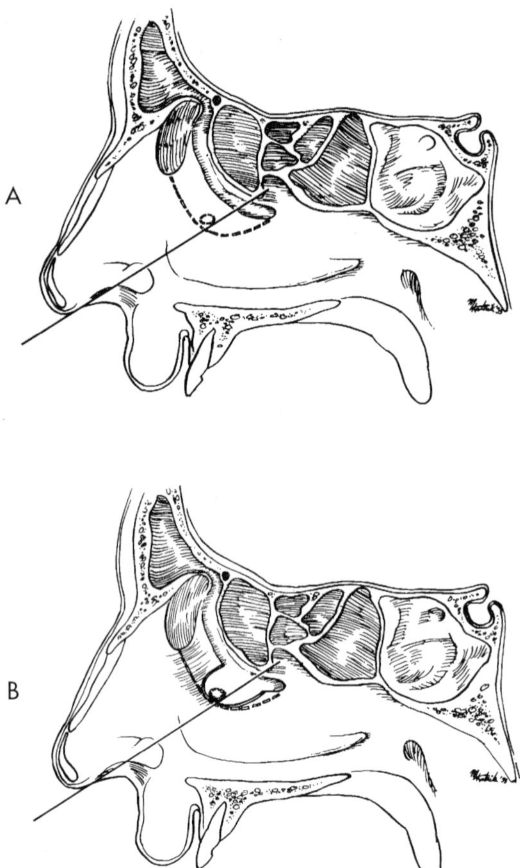

Fig. 5–1. **A,** The natural ostium to the maxillary sinus (dotted oval) is consistantly found 1 to 2 mm posterior to the anterior extent of the uncinate process as it inserts into the lateral nasal wall. The solid line represents the telescopic alignment when looking at the inferior aspect of the bulla ethmoidalis. The natural ostium is generally superior to this line. **B,** A back-biter is used to remove the lower half of the uncinate. When the entire anterior extent is resected, a 30 or 70 degree telescope will identify the natural ostium. The authors would like to thank Mark Katnik for his assistance with medical illustrations.

The maxillary ostium is identified and checked for patency. Often the ostium is adequate and the obstruction is due to a lateralized uncinate with adhesions to the lateral wall obstructing the infundibulum. These ostia are not enlarged. However, if the ostium is small or obstructed, it is enlarged only by removing the posterior fontanelle *in continuity* with the natural ostium. Failure to include the natural ostium in the created middle meatus antrostomy is the number one cause of failure of FES in patients of any age.

The natural ostium is consistently found in the anterior-superior portion of the fontanelle, usually within 1 to 2 mm of the anterior insertion of the uncinate. It is critical that all the lower uncinate be removed, to its anterior limit. This cannot be done effectively with a sickle knife. It is this lower anterior portion of the uncinate that covers the natural ostium and is frequently found during revision surgeries for failed FES surgery.

When attempting to identify the natural ostium of the maxillary sinus, accessory ostia also may be visualized. Confusion may then exist regarding the location of the *natural* ostium. The surgeon should remember three simple guidelines. First, accessory ostia are in the same plane as the lateral nasal wall. The natural ostium is in an oblique plane. The anterior lip of the natural ostium is more lateral than the posterior lip. Second, accessory ostia tend to be perfectly circular, while the natural ostium is more oval. Third, the natural ostium is anterior-superiorly located in the fontanelle. Any ostia found in the inferior or posterior portion of the fontanelle are most certainly accessory ostia.

The removal of the uncinate, along with soft tissues in creation of a maxillary antrostomy and ethmoidectomy, has recently been facilitated by the use of a powered rotory microdebrider (the "Hummer" in Chapter 20).[16] This instrument has been adapted from temperomandibular joint surgery. It provides a precise removal of soft tissue and bone with less bleeding and improved visualization. It has proven extremely useful in the removal of nasal polyps and is the instrument of choice for pediatric FES.[17]

The ethmoid sinuses are approached by removing the inferiomedial wall of the bulla ethmoidalis. Dissection should continue posteriorly to include the natural ostium of the bulla and laterally to identify the lamina papyracea which represents the lateral margin of the dissection. If the mucosa encountered in the bulla is normal, no further dissection is necessary. This constitutes a "Mini-FES."[15] If the mucosa of the bulla is diseased, the procedure may be extended for more complete removal of the anterior and posterior ethmoids. However, in children, opening the ostiomeatal complex (OMC) with a Mini-FES often may allow resolution of disease in the frontal, posterior ethmoid or sphenoid sinuses so that more extensive surgery is not required.

Once the dissection is completed, a rolled stent is placed in the middle meatus to prevent lateral movement of the middle turbinate and obstructive adhesions. Gelfilm is the preferred material. If proper hemostatic techniques are employed, nasal packing is not required.

Nasal surgeries concurrent with FES are discouraged. Middle turbinectomies are also discouraged because the long-term complications are unknown. With proper surgical techniques and patience, FES can be performed without sacrifice of the turbinates. Septoplasties should be performed at an earlier stage. When performed simultaneously, bleeding is increased and postoperative middle meatal and septal scarring is increased. This condition will not be identified in children who will not cooperate with nasal endoscopy in the office. As the scar matures, its contraction will deviate the septum, producing marked obstruction.

Adenoidectomy may be indicated in a patient with sinus disease and should be performed *prior* to the FES. Because of the close relationship of symptoms with adenoiditis and sinusitis, an adenoidectomy may relieve the patient's need for sinus surgery. However if the sinus symptoms persist after adenoidectomy, an FES procedure may be necessary.

Postoperative Care

Gelfilm remains in place for approximately 2 weeks. Because children do not tolerate nasal endoscopy in the office, it is usually necessary to return to the operating room 2 weeks after surgery to remove the stent and perform any cleansing and removal of adhesions.

Postoperatively, patients are placed on a 3 to 4 week course of antibiotics. Patients begin with buffered hypertonic saline nasal irrigations 1 day after surgery and continue these, twice daily, as long as necessary to help clean the sinonasal passages. Nasal steroids are used until symptoms resolve.

Patients are then followed-up in the office and evaluated clinically, not radiographically. Routine repeat sinus CT scans or plane x-rays are rarely indicated. If a patient clinically shows signs of repeated recurrence of disease, a CT scan may be required, but is again obtained at a point of maximal wellness.

After surgery, families need to be reminded that the healing process takes several months. They also need to know that sinus disease may recur and that the child may require revision surgery. In children, it is far better to offer conservative surgical therapy with a subsequent revision procedure than to offer aggressive surgery with complications.

Conclusion

The incidence of chronic sinusitis in the pediatric population is greater than previously thought. The diagnosis and treatment of sinus disease have dramatically changed with the advances in CT scans and nasal endoscopes. However, the main emphasis in treatment of sinus disease in children continues to be medical. In those select cases where medical therapy is ineffective, functional endoscopic procedures have proven effective.

REFERENCES

1. Dingle JH, et al. *Illness in the Home: A Study of 25,000 Illnesses in a Group of Cleveland Families.* Cleveland, OH: Press of Western Reserve University; 1964.
2. Wald ER, et al. Acute maxillary sinusitis in children. *N Engl J Med.* 1981; 304:749–754.
3. Parsons DS, Phillips SE. Functional endoscopic surgery in children: a retrospective analysis of results. *Laryngoscope.* 1993; 103:899–903.
4. Parsons DS, Pransky SM. Functional endoscopic sinus surgery in infants and young children. Instructional Courses of the AAO-HNS, Vol 5, Chap 18, 159–164, 1992.
5. Otten F, Grote JJ. The diagnostic value of transillumination for maxillary sinusitis in children. *Int J Pediatr Otorhinolaryngol.* 1989; 18:9–11.
6. Gross CW, et al. Functional endoscopic sinus disease in the pediatric age group. *Laryngoscope.* 1989; 99:272–275.
7. Nishioka GJ, et al. Functional endoscopic sinus surgery in patients with chronic sinusitis and asthma. *Otolaryngol Head Neck Surg.* In press.
8. Wald ER, et al. Treatment of acute sinusitis in childhood: a comparative study of amoxicillin and ceclor. *J Pediatr.* 1984; 104:297–302.
9. Wald ER, et al. Subacute sinusitis in children. *J Pediatr.* 1989; 115:28–32.
10. Brook WE. Bacteriologic features of chronic sinusitis in children. *JAMA.* 1981; 246:967–969.
11. Muntz HR, Lusk RP. Bacteriology of the ethmoid bullae in children with chronic sinusitis. *Arch Otolaryngol Head Neck Surg.* 1991; 117:179–181.
12. Parsons DS, Wilder BE, Davis WE. Buffered hypertonic saline nasal irrigation. Submitted.
13. Bolger WE, Parsons DS, Potempa L. Preoperative hemostatic assessment of the adenotonsillectomy patient. *Otolaryngol Head Neck Surg.* 103:396–405.
14. Riegle EV, et al. Comparison of vasoconstrictors for functional endoscopic sinus surgery in children. *Laryngoscope.* 1992; 102:820–823.
15. Parsons DS, Setliff R, Chambers D. Special consideration in pediatric functional endoscopic sinus surgery. *Op Tech Otolaryngol Head Neck Surg.* In press.
16. Setliff RC, Parsons DS. "The hummer"—new instrumentation for FES surgery. *Am J Rhino.* In press.
17. Parsons DS, Setliff RC "The hummer"—innovative instrumentation for sinonasal surgery in children. Publication submitted.

6

Revision Endoscopic Sinus Surgery in the Pediatric Patient

Rodney Lusk

Indications for Primary Ethmoidectomy

The indications for performing pediatric endoscopic sinus surgery are controversial. Several authors[1–7] have reported series that show the procedure is safe and well tolerated. The success rate in pilot studies has also been encouraging.[1,7–9] As a matter of principle, surgical intervention should be offered only after the surgeon and parents (or guardians) are satisfied that maximum medical management has failed. Hard guidelines are not available at this time, therefore the indications for endoscopic sinus surgery remain individualized.

At a minimum, the patient should have failed several prolonged courses (4 to 6 weeks) of broad spectrum oral antibiotics. We currently use amoxicillin/clavulanate (Augmentin®—SmithKline Beecham Pharmaceuticals, Philadelphia, PA), cefuroxime (Ceftin®—Allen & Hanburys, Research Triangle Park, NC), cefprozil (Cefzil™—Bristol Laboratories, Princeton, NJ), cefpodoxime (Vantin®), loracarbef (Lorabid™—Eli Lilly and Company, Indianapolis, IN) and erythromycin plus sulfisoxazole (Pediazole®); all of which are associated with potential risks and side effects such as gastrointestinal distress and diarrhea. Adjuvant therapy with topical nasal steroid sprays is also usually recommended, but compliance in younger patients can be a problem. There are no good prospective studies that demonstrate the efficacy of topical nasal steroid sprays in chronic sinusitis. As a general rule, we do not use oral steroids except in patients with polyps or cystic fibrosis. Systemic steroids are used only for one or two weeks preoperatively and may be used for a variable period postoperatively.

Since surgery is a last resort, the patient should be symptomatic for several months prior to becoming a surgical candidate. We would consider the patient to be symptomatic if symptoms are suppressed with oral antibiotics but return within days of cessation of antibiotic therapy. Sinusitis should be documented with a coronal CT scan with the patient on full-dose broad-spectrum antibiotics for 4 weeks. Evidence of disease on the CT scan does not automatically mean that the patient is a surgical candidate. Currently, 36% of our patients have evidence of sinus disease, and we are continuing to manage them medically.

In pediatric patients who have not had ethmoid surgery, we have found that most sinusitis is located in the ethmoid sinuses and anterior portion of the maxillary sinuses. As indicated by the data in Figure 6–1A, there is no significant difference between the amount of disease in the anterior and posterior ethmoid cells. In the maxillary sinus, however, there is greater disease in the anterior portion, as shown in Figure 6–1B ($P = 0.004$). Figure 6–2 shows almost equal distribution of patients with any disease located in the ethmoid and maxillary sinuses. The surgery performed continues to be tailored to the amount of disease documented by CT scan and observed at the time of surgery. It is our recommendation that all disease be removed, but as conservatively as possible.

The parents should have realistic expectations of what the surgical procedure can accomplish. Unless appropriately counseled, they may feel surgery has failed if the child develops any purulent rhinorrhea postoperatively. It should be emphasized that the child will continue to have intermittent purulent rhinorrhea associated with viral upper respiratory tract infections. It is our belief that patients who have systemic disease, such as cystic fibrosis, allergies, or immune deficiencies, are not as effectively treated with endo-

Ethmoid Sinus Posterior

Anterior	0	1	2	3	Total
0	123	9	4	5	141
1	16	12	5	0	33
2	3	8	11	2	24
3	0	4	5	19	28
Total	142	33	25	26	226

p=0.048

A

Maxillary Sinus Back

Front	0	1	2	3	Total
0	122	14	1	0	137
1	5	9	3	4	21
2	1	0	4	2	7
3	6	10	20	27	63
Total	134	33	28	33	228

p=0.004

B

Fig. 6–1. Comparison of amount of disease in the anterior and posterior ethmoid cells and anterior and posterior portion of maxillary sinuses. The numbers 0 to 3 represent the amount of disease noted on CT scans; 0 = No disease, 1 = <50% disease, 2 = >50% disease, 3 = Complete opacification. Stippled area = no difference between the two areas compared. Squares above and to the right of the stippled line represent patients who have more disease in the posterior cells; squares to the left and below the stippled area represent patients with less disease in the posterior cells. When the two are compared with a *t*-test and when the patients with no disease are omitted, there is no significant difference ($P = 0.048$) for the ethmoid sinus disease (**A**), but there is significantly ($P = 0.004$) more disease in the anterior portion of the maxillary sinus (**B**).

Summary Table		
	Total	*Percent*
Total with disease in max. sinus	53	46.90%
Total with clear max. sinus	60	53.10%
Total maxillary observations	113	100%
Total with disease in ethmoid sinus	48	42.48%
Total with clear ethmoid sinus	65	57.52%
Total ethmoid observations	113	100%

Fig. 6–2. Summary table of the amount of disease in the maxillary and ethmoid sinuses.

scopic ethmoidectomy, and the parents should be made aware of this.

Incidence of Revision Endoscopic Sinus Surgery

Of 1264 patients we evaluated for chronic sinusitis over the past 5 years, 420 (33.23%) have undergone endoscopic sinus surgery. The incidence of nonendoscopic surgical procedures performed on these patients with revision ethmoidectomy is outlined in Table 6-1. The overall incidence of revision ethmoid surgery is 11%, which correlates well with other reported series. Lazar has reported 8% and 7.6% in children.[7,10] He noted that in adults the revision rate was higher, 10.2%.[10] Shaefer has reported a 4% revision rate in adults.[11] Kennedy[12] has reported that 49% of his patients have had previous ethmoid surgery, but this may be a reflec-

Table 6-1 Nonendoscopic sinus procedures

10	Adenoidectomies
8	Tonsillectomies & adenoidectomies
8	Nasal antral windows
3	Caldwell-Luc procedures

Nonendoscopic sinus procedures that failed to control symptoms of sinusitis.

tion of the nature of his highly referred practice and not a true indication of the percentage of patients requiring revision surgery.

Work-up for Failed Endoscopic Sinus Surgery

Assessment of the allergic status of the patient should be performed prior to the initial surgical procedure. If the interval between the initial and the revision surgery assessment has been significant or if the patient's allergic symptoms have changed, it may be appropriate to reassess the allergies. It is our experience that children who fail endoscopic sinus surgery have a much higher incidence of allergies—68% as opposed to 23%[1] of the children initially evaluated. Lazar[10] found a higher incidence of allergic patients in revision surgery as well.

As part of management during the postoperative period, most patients will remain on full-dose broad-spectrum antibiotics until the cavity is healed. Patients who undergo symptom-free intervals for weeks without antibiotics probably have recurrent acute rather than chronic sinusitis. We feel recurrent acute sinusitis is most effectively treated with antibiotic therapy, whereas chronic sinusitis is best treated with revision surgery. As with the primary procedure, the definition of surgical or medical failure must be individualized, and patients should have had persistent symptoms for a minimum of several months.

Patients deemed medical management failures after endoscopic surgery should undergo another coronal CT scan after 3 to 4 weeks of full-dose antibiotics. The second CT scan is performed to assess the extent and site of disease and to look for any sites of surgical defects, such as penetration of the lamina papyracea or the roof of the ethmoid, that would increase the chance of a surgical complication. This can be extremely important because significant alteration in the anatomy creates greater risk of surgical complication (Fig. 6–3). One should also look for evidence of obstruction of the maxillary sinus ostium or presence of residual uncinate process (Fig. 6–4).

Review of the CT scan with the parents provides an opportunity to review the anatomy of the sinuses and the extent of the disease, and to discuss the potential surgical complications. It is more likely that the patient will have an operative complication during revision surgery than during the primary procedure. Parents should understand that major complications are possible, including, 1) penetration of the lamina papyracea and trauma to the medial rectus muscle, 2) optic nerve trauma,

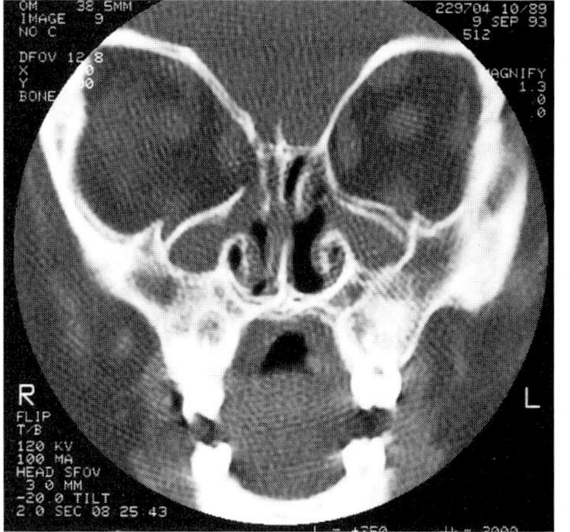

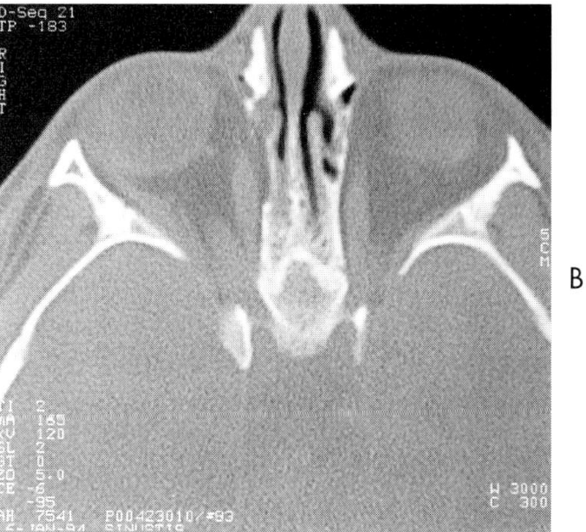

Fig. 6–3. This is the preoperative revision CT scan of a patient operated on at another institution. Note the large amount of lamina papyracea missing on the coronal **(A)** and axial **(B)** views.

3) penetration of the roof of the ethmoid with resultant CSF leak and possible meningitis, 4) trauma to the lacrimal duct, and 5) anesthetic complications. It should be well documented that these complications were discussed with the patient's guardians.

The patient should have already been assessed for evidence of systemic diseases predisposing towards sinusitis. If the patient has recurrent sinusitis, otitis media, and recurrent bronchitis or pneumonia, one must be suspicious of a systemic disease. Subtle immune deficiencies should be investigated if this triad is noted or if revision ethmoid surgery is necessary. It is our experience that patients requiring revision ethmoidectomy are more likely to have immune deficiencies. We have found the incidence of immunodeficiency in revision sinus surgery to be 20%. We currently reserve the assessment of IgG subclasses for failed eth-

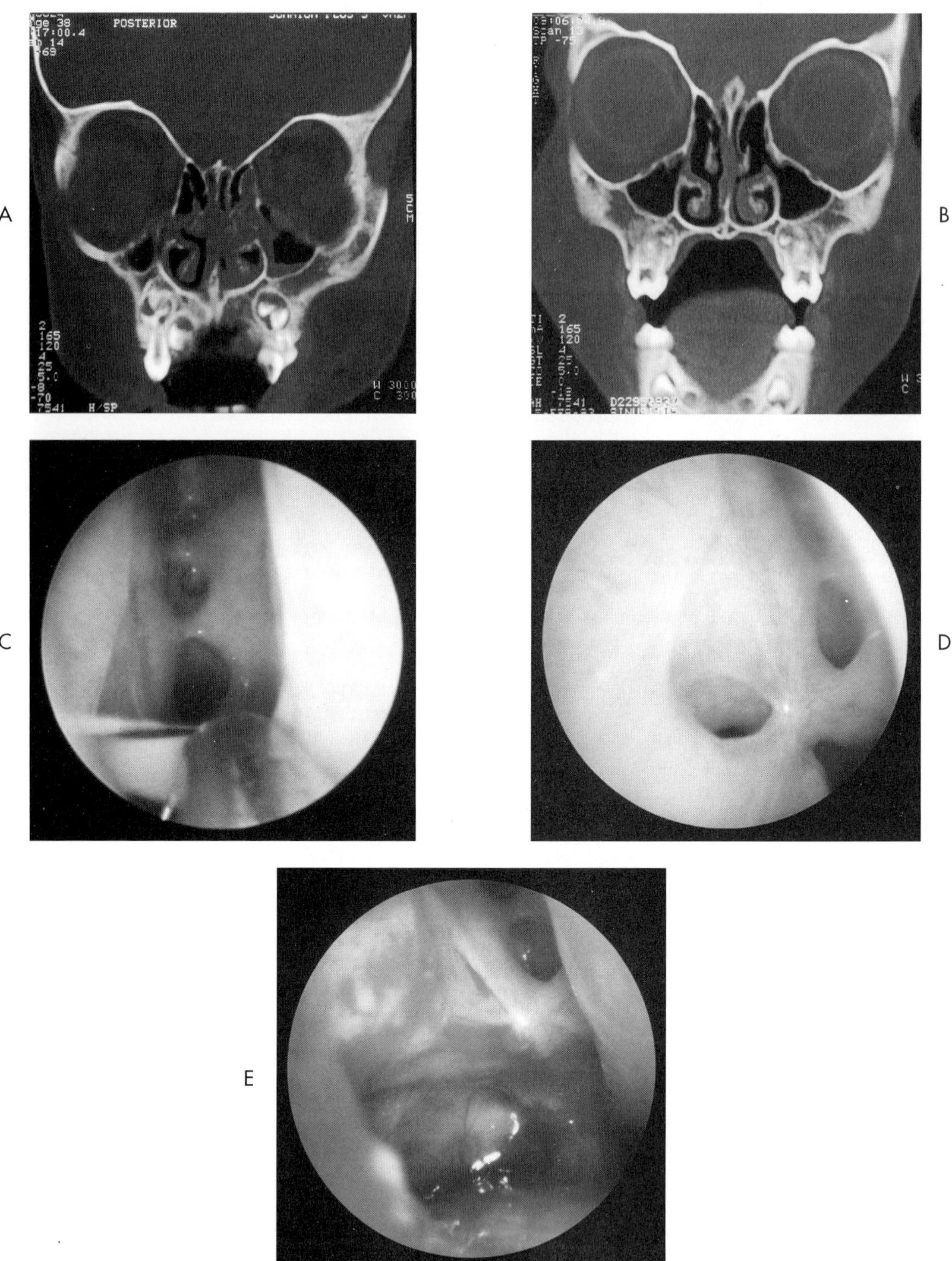

Fig. 6–4. **A,** Preoperative CT scan of a patient with anterior ethmoid disease. **B**, Postoperative CT scan of same patient showing residual uncinate process and scarring on the right side. **C**, Secretions suctioned from the obstructed ostia. **D**, Ostium after clearing as viewed with a 30-degree telescope. **E**, Ostiums after enlarging.

moidectomy because the overall incidence of abnormality is approximately 10%. The only treatment for subclass deficiency is to continue antibiotics and institute gamma globulin therapy, which is expensive and not yet of proven efficacy. Blood screens such as IgM, IgG, IgA, IgE, and a CBC with differential should be repeated. Pneumococcal and tetanus titers should be obtained. It is important for the parents to know about immune deficiencies so they will have realistic expectations regarding surgery. One should also consider performing ciliary biopsies in the most resistant cases. On rare occasions, esophageal gastric reflux can be associated with severe scarring (Fig. 6–5).

Systemic diseases should be maximally managed to minimize their effect on the sinuses and subsequent surgery. Examples are the use of systemic steroids and vitamin K supplementation in patients with polyps and cystic fibrosis. It is also important to warn parents about the use of aspirin and ibuprofen which will inhibit platelet function and increase intraoperative bleeding. It is easiest to tell the parents that they should only use Tylenol® (McNeil Consumer Products Company, Fort Washington, PA), and then no errors will be made preoperatively. If maximum medical management fails to control the disease, then the patient should be considered for revision ethmoidectomy.

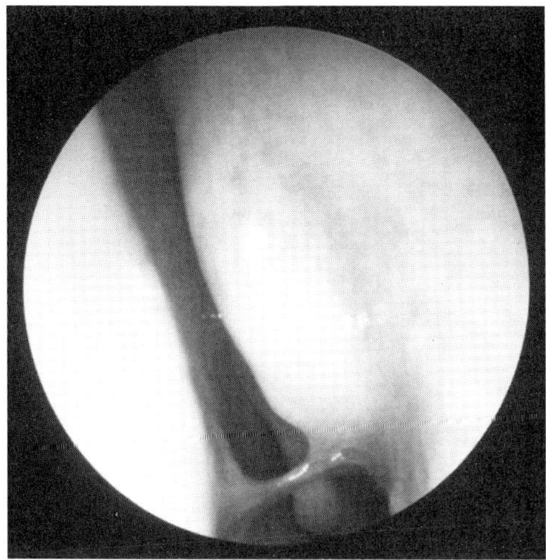

Fig. 6–5. Scarring of the middle meatus.

Surgical Procedure

Vasoconstriction of the nose is important intraoperatively. Reigle and colleagues[13] found that oxymetazoline hydrochloride (0.05%) was a better vasoconstricting agent than phenylephrine hydrochloride (0.25%) or cocaine (4%). We therefore use oxymetazoline on neuropledgets to vasoconstrict the nose prior to revision surgery, the uncinate process and perhaps some of the middle turbinate may have already been removed. In addition, there may be scar tissue throughout the middle meatus, which will make injection of local vasoconstricting agents difficult to perform (see Fig. 6–5). For approximately 2 years, we have been injecting 0.5 cc of 1% lidocaine with 1:100,000 epinephrine transorally in the sphenopalatine foramen without problems, and it is our subjective impression that this block reduces the amount of bleeding during the ethmoidectomy (Fig. 6–6).

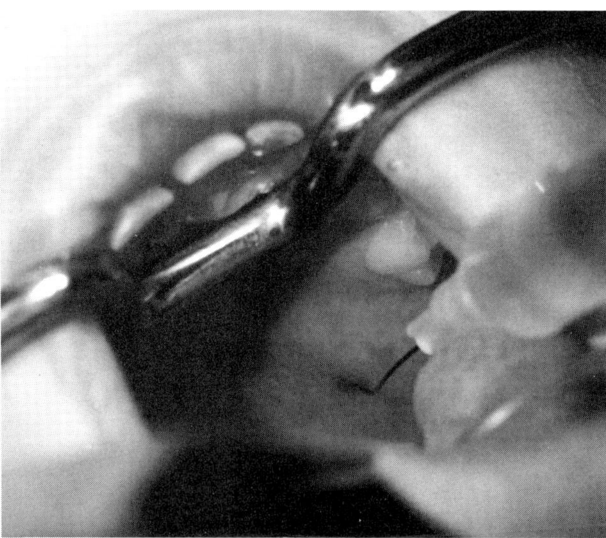

Fig. 6–6. Transoral sphenopalatine injection.

Endoscopic ethmoidectomies should be performed with minimal trauma to the lateral wall of the nose and the lateral surface of the middle turbinate. For this reason we are more inclined to use a 2.7-mm telescope whenever necessary to minimize trauma to the middle turbinate. We initially thought the use of a 2.7-mm telescope was a significant disadvantage, but with experience we no longer feel this is the case. The 2.7-mm telescope allows good visualization and causes significantly less trauma to the middle turbinate in small children. It is our feeling that exposure of the middle meatus is best accomplished by ensuring that all the uncinate process is removed laterally and not by resecting the middle turbinate. For this reason, we rarely do partial middle turbinectomies even in the smallest children.

If there is significant scarring in the middle meatus, it will have to be removed first to allow exposure of the middle meatus (see Fig. 6–5). Often it is easiest to sharply transect the scar tissue, which is most frequently located anteriorly between the lateral wall and the anterior lateral surface of the middle turbinate. If polyps are present in the middle meatus, they should be removed as a first step, under direct visualization, with small bites. A new instrument that has been particularly useful in resecting polyps is the Stryker SE4 Micro Debrider (San Jose, CA) (see chapters 5 and 20). This instrument allows polyps to be transected and suctioned away with minimal bleeding and trauma to the surrounding tissue. It is also useful with thickened mucosa, although removal of ethmoid septa is not as precise as we would like. In addition, it is not particularly useful in removing dense scar tissue or reactive bone. This instrument definitely has a place in our surgical armamentarium, and we have found it most useful with polypoid disease or, in our population, in children with cystic fibrosis.

The next most useful maneuver is to identify the maxillary sinus ostium, which in our experience is the most likely site of failure. Scarring was noted in 25% of the right maxillary ostia and 21% of the left ostia of patients who required revision surgery. Frequently there was a patent accessory ostium, but the natural ostium was scarred closed (Fig. 6–7). Some residual uncinate process was noted on both sides in 9% of patients. The most frequent problem noted was edema or recurrent polyposis at the maxillary ostia, 32% on the right and 22% on the left. The ostium, if not obviously patent, can be visualized with a 30 degree telescope and palpated with a seeker (Fig. 6–8). Once the ostium is identified, a 45 degree forceps and back biter can be used to open it. During the initial procedure, we try not to traumatize or remove the mucosal lining around the superior and anterior portion of the maxillary sinus natural ostium. We have found the straight biting Acufex® punch to be very helpful in opening the posterior fontanelle. During revision surgery, however, we are more aggressive anteriorly in an effort to ensure that the ostium is opened. Parsons[14] has noted that the ostium is usually oval in shape and not in a plane parallel to the medial wall of the maxillary sinus. If it is round and parallel to the maxillary sinus, it is most likely an accessory ostium. The natural ostium is invariably located farther anterior than suspected. It has been our experience that the orbit is most likely to be entered in the region of the junction between the roof of the ethmoid and the

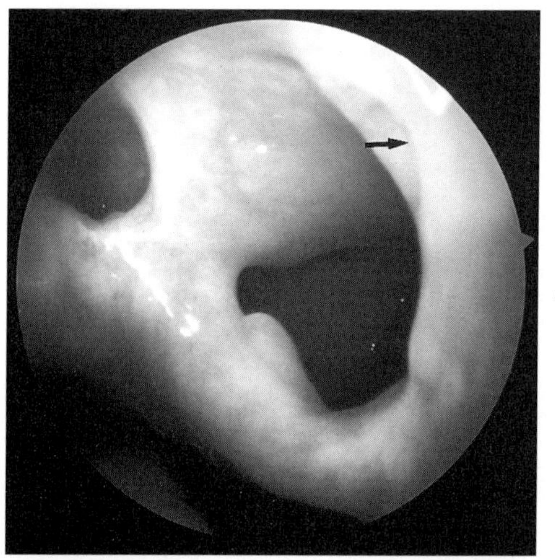

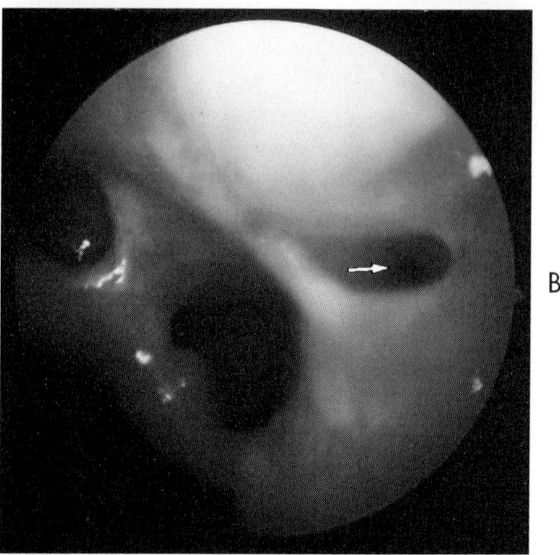

Fig. 6–7. **A,** Secretions over the natural ostium of the maxillary sinus (arrow). Note the large posterior accessory ostium. **B**, Secretions removed and the natural ostium (arrow) is readily apparent. Reprinted with permission from Lusk, Rodney. *Pediatric Sinusitis,* Raven Press, 1992.

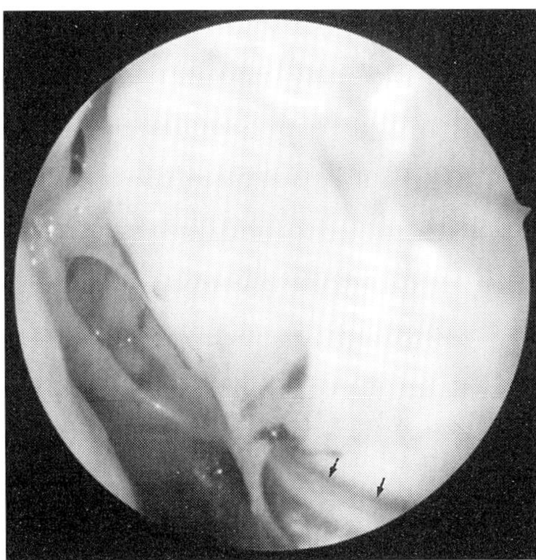

Fig. 6–8. Maxillary ostium, sinus ostium not patent but palpated with a seeker (arrows).

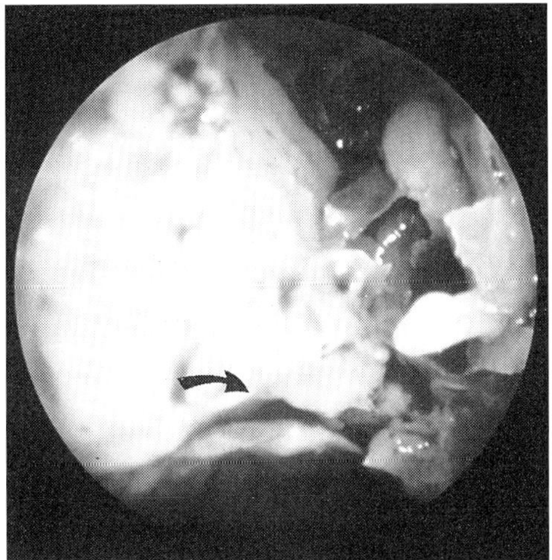

Fig. 6–9. View of left lamina papyracea with the arrow pointed at the junction of the lamina papyracea and roof of the maxillary sinus in a pediatric cadaver specimen. Reprinted with permission from Lusk, Rodney *Pediatric Sinusitis*. Raven Press, 1992.

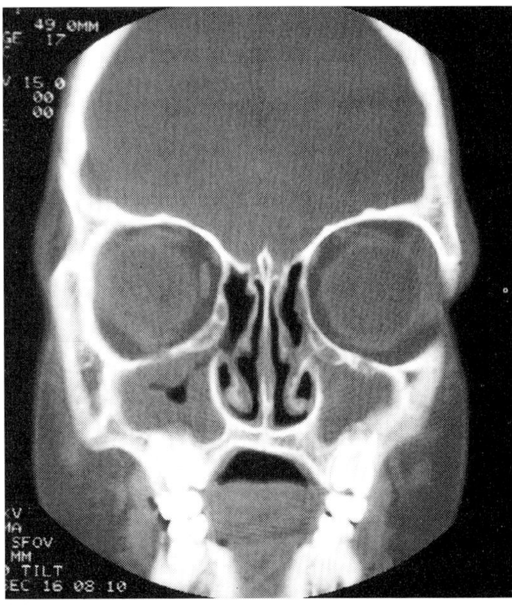

Fig. 6–10. Infraorbital cells which had not been adequately opened at the time of surgery.

lamina papyracea (Fig. 6–9) and is more likely to occur on the left than the right. Failure to appropriately open infraorbital cells (Haller cells) can result in a narrowed obstructed maxillary ostium (Fig. 6–10). During the revision surgery, care must be taken to open the entire inferior portion of the infraorbital cell. The lamina papyracea, once identified, is followed inferiorly into the infraorbital cell, and the inferior margin is removed. Once the maxillary sinus ostium is identified, it may be opened posteriorly. The roof of the maxillary sinus or the floor of the orbit can then be identified by its smooth surface and the contour followed onto the lamina papyracea. This is the first major landmark to identify. The lamina papyracea can then be followed posteriorly into the larger posterior ethmoid cells where the roof of the ethmoid is easiest to identify.

If the lamina papyracea cannot be identified, it is best to proceed to the posterior ethmoid complex to identify the roof of the ethmoid cavity. This is similar to the Wigand technique that Lazar and associates[10] proposed using when no landmarks are available. We do not remove the posterior portion of the middle meatus or the superior turbinate. Once the roof of the ethmoid is identified, careful dissection can be used along the roof towards the anterior ethmoid and frontal recess. During this dissection, small bites should be taken because scar tissue attached to the roof or the lamina papyracea can result in fracturing and removal of the bone. This increases the chance of trauma to the orbital contents, brain, and meninges. Currently we do not have the necessary instrumentation to cut precisely mucosa or scar tissue. Once this is developed, revision ethmoidectomy will be much easier to perform.

The cavity should be opened to the extent of the lamina papyracea and the roof of the ethmoid sinus. Care should be taken not to do extensive dissection into the frontal recess, even with revision ethmoid surgery, unless it is diseased. If the mucosa is normal, leave it in place and do not perform extensive surgery in this area. If there is extensive scarring or diseased tissue in the frontal recess, then the area should be carefully opened, but the surgeon must realize that the risk of persistent disease and frontal sinus growth inhibition is significant. Parsons and Muntz have indicated that they have become much more conservative in their dissection of the frontal recess.[14,15] At times this area cannot be opened endoscopically, and an external approach will be necessary (Fig. 6–11).

In children, entry to the sphenoid almost always has to be through the posterior ethmoid cells. One must be particularly mindful of the relationship between the posterior ethmoid cells and the optic nerve. Dissection in this region must take place medially and not laterally to protect the optic nerve. This includes any dissection done in the sphenoid where the optic nerve can be exposed, even in children (Fig. 6–12).

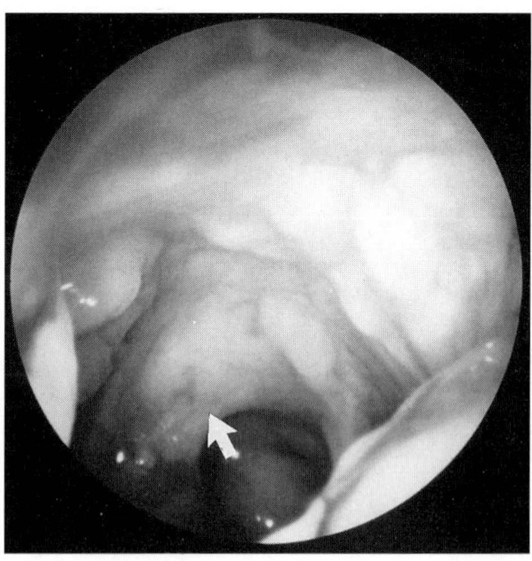

Fig. 6–12. Optic nerve (arrow) exposed in the lateral wall of an 8-year-old patient.

In general, normal mucosa should be left intact whenever possible. Our current instrumentation does not allow us to cut precisely through mucosa and not strip normal mucosa from the underlying bone. With advances in instrumentation this will be possible, and the cavities will likely heal faster and with less trauma. The Stryker SE4 Micro Debrider is useful in removing edematous tissue and polyps. It is our impression that scarring is more likely to occur with extensive dissection and stripping of mucosa in the ethmoid cavity.

Postoperative Care

We continue to use a Gelfilm stent in the ethmoid cavity postoperatively. We currently are removing the stent in 2 weeks and removing excessive granulation tissue from the regions of the frontal recess and maxillary antrostomy. We make no effort to remove all granulation tissue because this is part of the natural healing process. Once the excessive granulation tissue is removed—how much to remove is a matter of judgment on the part of the surgeon—half a Gelfilm stent is placed in the ethmoid cavity. This three-layer-thick stent will dissolve in approximately 2 weeks. Some surgeons do not place a stent in the ethmoid cavity but do remove granulation tissue at 2 weeks.[7] Others neither place a stent in the ethmoid cavity nor remove granulation tissue, with apparently equally good results. Wolf indicates that this is his practice, and his revision rate is 10%—not significantly different than our 11%.[16] The most appropriate method of stenting the cavity is yet to be defined in prospective protocols.

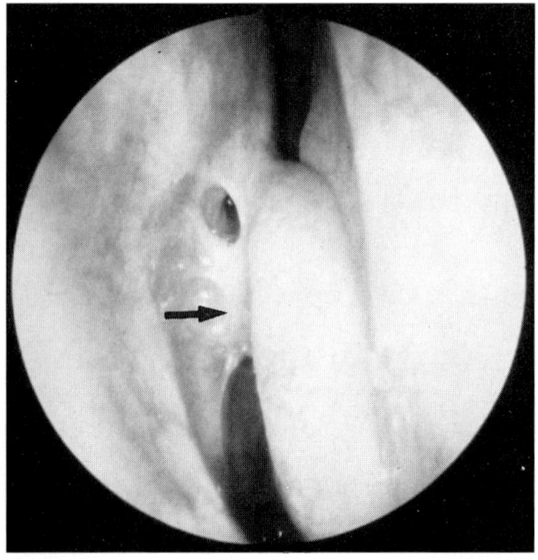

Fig. 6–11. Patient with scarring (arrow) of the right frontal recess that eventually required external frontal ethmoidectomy and subsequent obliteration.

Postoperatively, we continue the patient on full-dose broad-spectrum antibiotics and topical nasal steroid sprays. The patient is examined in the office 2 or 3 weeks after stent removal. The half Gelfilm stents will have dissolved by then, and the cavity can be examined with anterior rhinoscopy. If there is crusting in the cavity, then we maintain the patient on prophylactic doses of antibiotics and reevaluate in another 2 to 3 weeks. Once the cavity is well healed and free of crusting, we discontinue the antibiotics altogether and continue the topical nasal steroid sprays. We follow our patients at regular intervals to ensure accurate assessment of their symptoms.

Results

There is little information assessing the effectiveness of revision surgery in children. Lazar and associates[10] reported an overall success rate of 78% in their adult and pediatric revision ethmoidectomy patients. The 16 children in the study were not assessed as a separate group.

We assessed 45 children who had revision ethmoidectomies performed at our institution. In that group, 10 patients had failed adenoidectomy, 8 had failed tonsillectomy and adenoidectomy, 8 had failed nasal antral windows, and 3 had Caldwell-Luc procedures at other hospitals (see Table 1). For 22 patients, enough prospective symptom data were collected to assess their symptoms. Rhinitis, nasal obstruction, irritability, day cough, and night cough were all statistically ($P < .002$) less frequent after the revision surgery. The only symptom that was not improved was headaches ($P = 0.27$). When the parents were asked to rate their children's symptoms on a scale of 1 (worst ever) to 10 (normal) preoperatively versus postoperatively, 14 were rated improved, 2 unchanged, and 7 worse. This gave a P value of 0.02, which showed statistical improvement in the overall assessment postoperatively. By our assessment, 60% of our 45 revision patients were significantly improved or resolved after their revision surgery.

REFERENCES

1. Lusk RP, Muntz HR. Endoscopic sinus surgery in children with chronic sinusitis—A pilot study. *Laryngoscope.* 1990;100:654–658.
2. Lusk RP, Lazar RH, Muntz HR. The diagnosis and treatment of recurrent and chronic sinusitis in children. *Pediatric Clin No Amer.* 1989;36:1411–1421.
3. Lusk RP. Surgical management of sinusitis. In: Lusk RP, ed. *Pediatric Sinusitis.* New York, NY: Raven Press; 1992:77–127.
4. Lusk RP. Endoscopic approach to sinus disease. *J Aller Clin Immunol.* 1992;90:496–505.
5. Gross CW, Gurucharri MJ, Lazar RH, Long TE. Functional endonasal sinus surgery (FESS) in the pediatric age group. *Laryngoscope.* 1989;99:272–275.
6. Gross CW, Lazar RH, Gurucharri MJ. Pediatric functional endonasal sinus surgery. *Otolaryngol Clin No Amer.* 1989;22:733–738.
7. Lazar RH, Younis RT, Gross CW. Pediatric functional endonasal sinus surgery: review of 210 cases. *Head Neck.* 1992;14:92–98.
8. Parsons DS, Phillips SE. Functional endoscopic surgery in children: A retrospective analysis of results. *Laryngoscope.* 1993;103:899–903.
9. Gross CW, Gurucharri MJ, Lazar RH, Long TE. Functional endonasal sinus surgery (FESS) in the pediatric age group. *Laryngoscope.* 1989;99:272–275.
10. Lazar RH, Younis RT, Long TE, Gross CW. Revision functional endonasal sinus surgery. *Ear Nose Throat J.* 1992;71:131–133.
11. Schaefer SD, Manning S, Close LG. Endoscopic paranasal sinus surgery: indications and considerations. *Laryngoscope.* 1989;99:1–5.
12. Kennedy DW. Prognostic factors, outcomes and staging in ethmoid sinus surgery. *Laryngoscope.* 1992;102:1–18.
13. Riegle EV, Gunter JB, Lusk RP, et al. Comparison of vasoconstrictors for functional endoscopic sinus surgery in children. *Laryngoscope.* 1992;102:820–823.
14. Parsons DS. Personal Communication.
15. Muntz HR. Personal Communication.
16. Wolf G. Personal Communication.

7

Mucoceles of the Paranasal Sinuses: Endoscopic Diagnosis and Treatment

Jordan S. Josephson and Alfredo Herrara V.

Rollet was the first to introduce the term mucocele into the medical literature in 1896. However, the clinical features of frontal sinus mucoceles dates back to Langenbecks' description in 1818. The histologic features of a mucocele were not described until 1901 when they were first described by Onodi.[1,2] Despite these reports, the etiology of mucocele formation was still poorly understood.

Over the years, many radical and conservative procedures have been described.[3-10] The postoperative visualization of these slowly growing lesions is a problem. Even with the highly advanced imaging techniques of computerized tomography (CT) and magnetic resonance imaging (MRI), it is difficult to image and evaluate the sinuses for recurrence/persistence of a mucocele after an obliterative procedure.

Preservation of the mucocele mucosa with marsupialization of the mucocele has been advocated for over 70 years by many authors.[11-14] The majority of mucoceles have been shown to be accessible endoscopically. With the advent of angled endoscopes, it has been shown that clear visualization as well as complete intranasal marsupialization is possible. Functional endoscopic sinus surgery affords the potential for dramatically reducing the morbidity involved in treating mucoceles because it provides a minimally invasive approach under local anesthesia. However, the early reports emphasize that the technique requires a great deal of endoscopic expertise on the part of the surgeon. For many reasons, in the hands of the experienced surgeon, this approach appears to be a superior alternative to the more traditional approaches.

Endoscopy allows for more accurate diagnosis. In the operating room, a less invasive technique is employed with decreased morbidity. Postoperatively, endoscopic examination reveals that the mucosal lining has active mucociliary clearance. In addition, postoperative endoscopy provides the surgeon with a tool for direct visualization of the cavity for close follow-up. Early detection of recurrence can be visualized, should it occur.

In this chapter, we will briefly discuss the different radical and conservative procedures available to treat this disease. Furthermore, we will discuss the endoscopic sinus surgical approach for treating mucoceles of the paranasal sinuses.

Clinical Presentation

Mucoceles occur with approximately the same frequency in men and women. They occur most often in the frontal sinus followed in decreasing order by the ethmoid, maxillary, and sphenoid sinuses. The clinical presentation of a mucocele varies. It depends on the anatomic area involved. We will discuss each of these separately.

When the frontal sinus is involved, the mucocele usually presents with frontal headache and frequently with proptosis. Displacement of the globe in a downward and outward direction may result in diplopia. Should the mucocele erode the anterior table of the frontal sinus, Pott's puffy tumor may occur. There may be some change in the contour of the anterior frontal sinus wall, as well.

With mucoceles of the sphenoid sinus or the ethmoid sinus, the symptoms are usually more subtle. Headaches with occipital, vertex, or deep nasal pain may accompany various ophthalmologic complaints, such as diplopia, visual field disturbance, and globe displacement. Cranial nerves II–VI and the pituitary gland may be involved, causing symptoms related to these structures. These, however, are rare.

Mucoceles of the maxillary sinus may present with cheek pain, maxillary nerve hypesthesia, a feeling of fullness in the cheek, and/or dental pain. Rarely will there be a swelling of the involved cheek.

Occasionally, patients who have a mucocele present with signs and symptoms consistent with chronic sinus disease. These patients may suffer from a myriad of signs and symptoms including: low grade fevers, slightly elevated white blood cell count (WBC) and erythrocyte sedimentation rate (ESR), cervical lymphadenopathy, purulent discharge, nasal polyposis, mucosal edema, retracted tympanic membranes, middle ear disease, hearing loss, proptosis, conjunctivitis, dacryocystitis, facial pressure or pain, headaches, yellow or green mucus, postnasal drip, rhinorrhea, chronic sore throat or cough, hoarseness, fatigue, malaise, parosmia, halitosis, epistaxis, cough and/or worsening of asthma or bronchitis.

Diagnosis

The diagnosis of a paranasal sinus mucocele is based on the history and the physical examination. Confirmation of this diagnosis is accomplished with various diagnostic studies.

Although plain films may demonstrate opacification, bone erosion, or expansion caused by the mucocele, CT is necessary to accurately determine the regional anatomy and extent of the lesion.[15] This study needs to be performed in the coronal and axial planes to visualize the bony margins around the mucocele accurately. Intravenous contrast is rarely indicated. The CT study is best performed with the patient in the prone position and with the gantry angled perpendicular to the soft palate. Scanning is performed with 4–mm slices at 3–mm intervals. It is important that the images be photographed with magnification of the paranasal sinuses. Optimal windowing for the fine structures of the ethmoid sinus provides the surgeon with the best reading. Typically, this occurs with a window width of approximately 2,000 and a center in the negative range. Axial cuts are valuable for evaluating the posterior table of the frontal sinus for erosion and the sphenoid anatomy. If intracranial extension is suspected, contrast is indicated. However, bear in mind that MRI is a more sensitive study than CT for the identification of an early intracranial process.

MRI is also of significant benefit when the identity of a possible mucocele is in doubt or for differentiating tumors from mucoceles. The unfortunate drawback with MRI is that this study does not depict the bony anatomy. It is therefore valuable to obtain a CT scan, as it is extremely important for the surgeon to evaluate the bony contour for patients undergoing sinus surgery. Three-dimensional reconstructions of CT images may be of additional aid to the surgeon in some unusual lesions.

Traditional Procedures

Many radical and conservative surgical procedures have been described for treating paranasal sinus mucoceles.[3-10] There are proponents of each, despite the associated drawbacks. Difficulties with these techniques include problems with postoperative radiologic imaging, the risks of general anesthesia, significant blood loss, external scars, and various cosmetic deformities.

The objective of the more radical procedures is complete removal of the mucosa within the sinus and subsequent collapse or obliteration. The Riedel procedure collapses the soft tissues of the forehead into the frontal sinus.[3] A substantial deformity of the forehead results. This deformity can be repaired, but requires a secondary cosmetic reconstructive procedure. The osteoplastic sinusotomy with fat obliteration avoids the problem of frontal deformity; however, it is difficult for these sinuses to be visualized radiographically after surgery. The persistence of significant complaints can therefore be difficult to evaluate. Frontal sinus osteoplastic obliteration may also be associated with significant intraoperative blood loss. These procedures require general anesthesia, and the patient is therefore subjected to all of its associated risks. The more radical procedures generally involve greater surgical morbidity.[4-6]

More conservative procedures for treating mucoceles have been described. For instance, the Lynch procedure combines an external ethmoidectomy and removal of the floor of the frontal sinus, with placement of a silastic tube stent.[7] This stent is intended to form a conduit for drainage from the frontal sinus into the nose. Failure due to stenosis and lack of remucosalization of the nasofrontal recess has been recognized for a long time. Therefore, many flaps have been described to reconstruct this conduit to avoid these problems.[8-9] Many authors have stated that the lining of the mucocele should not be removed, as it forms an ideal lining for the cavity. As early as 1921, Howarth stated: "By making a very large opening into the nose and by removing the floor of the mucocele, one practically makes the mucocele part of the roof of the nose."[10] Other authors have since agreed with this, in theory and in practice.[11-14] Wolfowitz and Solomon reported marsupialization of the mucocele with an intranasal operation.[11] Follow-up of these patients was not included in this report. Nevertheless, the concept of maintaining the mucocele lining has been recognized for at least 70 years.

The Functional Endoscopic Sinus Surgical Approach

INDICATIONS

The surgeon must carefully select mucocele cases that can be treated appropriately with the endoscopic technique. Although it appears that most mucoceles may be approached endoscopically, traditional surgery is still indicated for treating some patients. Certainly the surgeon, with a surgical armamentarium of both endoscopic and traditional approaches, can successfully treat patients with this problem.

Appropriate case selection requires the surgeon to take into account the history, endoscopic examination, and the CT scan results. Some cases may need further evaluation with an MRI.

Certainly, a patient who has a mucocele that is easily accessible endoscopically and without bony erosion is the best candidate. Patients who have not undergone previous surgery generally make better candidates. Bony erosions, including orbital erosion and erosion of the posterior table of the frontal sinus, do not preclude an endoscopic approach. However, an associated severe intracranial complication is a contraindication. Any change in the patient's vision or an intraorbital complication may be a relative contraindication. The surgeon should also be aware that endoscopic exposure is more limited than that of an external approach. Thus, it may not be possible to detect an extradural collection at the time of surgery. Lateral frontal sinus mucoceles may also be difficult to reach endoscopically. However, when the frontal recess is wide, it may even be possible to remove the intersinus septum and resolve these lesions endoscopically. If any of these entities are suspected, postoperative imaging should be utilized.

Additionally, frontal sinus mucoceles limited inferiorly by a closed frontal recess or by a scarred or previously reopened frontal recess/os would appear to have a significantly increased risk of restenosis than a condition in which the mucocele extends inferiorly to the level of the frontal recess. Endoscopic treatment of this type of disease requires considerable experience on the part of the surgeon. In skilled hands, it may be possible to reopen the internal os, extending the opening anteriorly with a curette. The endoscopic use of a drill has been successful in some cases.

In those patients who have diplopia as a result of globe displacement, the diplopia usually resolves within 24 hours of mucocele decompression. In those patients who have bony erosion (posterior table of the frontal sinus or of the skull base in the ethmoidal or sphenoidal area with/without dural adherence to the lining of the mucocele), wide marsupialization is best, as dural exposure and/or removal is associated with a higher morbidity rate. In these cases, preservation of the mucocele lining may actually protect the dura.

When treated endoscopically, all of these cases require a significant commitment on the part of both the patient and the surgeon. Uncertainty regarding patient compliance or lack of appropriate office equipment for postoperative cleaning of the frontal recess favors a definitive traditional approach.[16]

THE ENDOSCOPIC TECHNIQUE

The surgical procedure is performed in the operating room under local anesthesia with intravenous sedation, when possible.[17-19] With local anesthesia, blood loss is minimized. Since both the orbital contents and the skull base in the area of the anterior and posterior ethmoidal nerves are sensitive to pain, important additional feedback during the surgery is maintained. In children and adults who are not able to tolerate local anesthesia, general anesthesia is administered.

Topical cocaine solution (200–300 mg) is applied to the nasal mucosa using cotton applicator sticks under direct visualization with a 0° 4.0-mm endoscope. The lateral nasal wall and the middle and inferior turbinates are then injected with 1% lidocaine with 1:100,000 or 1:200,000 epinephrine using a 3-cc syringe and a tonsil needle. Occasionally, if diffuse polyposis is also present and precludes visualization, intraoral injection of the sphenopalatine nerve may be performed.

The precise surgery performed depends on the mucocele site and extent of any associated sinus disease. The technique for treating frontal, ethmoid, and sphenoid sinus mucoceles will be discussed separately.

Surgery for frontal sinus mucoceles

An infundibulotomy incision is performed under the direct visualization of a 0° 4.0-mm endoscope. The uncinate process is then removed with a Blakesly forceps, taking care not to tear the mucosa of the lateral wall. The ethmoidal bulla is then infractured and removed with a straight biting

Blakesly forceps. The anterior ethmoidal area is cleaned back to the ground lamella. The medial orbital wall and the skull base (with the anterior ethmoidal neurovascular bundle) are identified. The anterior skull base can be differentiated by its shape, its slightly different color, and by recognizing the canal of the anterior ethmoidal vessels.

After these landmarks are identified, a 30° 4.0-mm endoscope is used to perform a retrograde dissection along the skull base into the frontal recess. The anterior ethmoidal neurovascular bundle is the chief landmark. The artery usually lies in a bony canal in the roof of the sinus (skull base) inferior to the dome. Occasionally, the artery may pass in a canal below the skull base or in between the frontal recess and a supraorbital ethmoid cell. Care is taken during this part of the dissection to keep the tip of the forceps pointing laterally to avoid the thin medial portion of the ethmoid roof adjacent to where the anterior ethmoidal artery exits from its intracranial course. If there is bleeding in this area, an upbiting suction forceps may be used for this dissection.

The inferior aspect of the mucocele typically will be visualized bulging into the frontal recess. This is located anterior to the dome of the ethmoid. It is not infrequent that the mucocele will be covered with bone. When approaching the mucocele, there may be a marked clear fluid. This may actually give the appearance of a CSF leak. However, it is just the mucus which has been pooling around the confines of the mucocele. After carefully identifying the relevant landmarks, including the skull base and the anterior ethmoidal artery, the mucocele is opened at its protruding base. A sickle knife is first utilized to open the mucocele by cutting the opening into four quadrants (Fig. 7–1). The four quadrants are then removed with an upbiting Blakesly forceps so that the flaps join the surrounding mucosa. The mucus or mucopus is then aspirated and sent for aerobic and anaerobic culture. All residual bony septate are removed while the skull base is visualized. When the angle or distance precludes dissection with direct visualization and the upbiting forceps, a 70° 4.0-mm endoscope with giraffe forceps may need to be employed.

The ostium/frontal recess is generally displaced medially. It is important to ensure that the mucociliary clearance is reestablished. Should there be a bony partition between a supraorbital ethmoid cell and the frontal recess, then these bony fragments must be removed carefully. To prevent restenosis, the mucosa of the frontal recess/sinus/os is to be preserved. The flaps of the opened mucocele should be appropriately placed so that reepithelialization occurs between the marsupialized edges and the mucosa of the frontal recess and the ostiomeatal complex.

Surgery for ethmoidal sinus mucoceles

Mucoceles of the ethmoid can arise from any of the ethmoid cells or from the concha bullosa. Depending on the location of the mucocele, a surgical procedure will be employed to marsupialize or remove the mucocele. Because of their location, access to these mucoceles is easier than to those of the frontal and/or sphenoid sinus.

Should the mucocele arise in the concha bullosa, a sickle knife is used to make an incision into the anterior portion of the middle turbinate. This is done under the direct visualization of a 0° 4.0-mm endoscope. A scissor is used to make a superior and inferior incision. The lateral aspect of the middle turbinate is removed, which widely marsupializes the mucocele by removing the lateral wall of the mucocele.

Mucoceles arising from an ethmoidal cell are approached by first making an infundibulotomy incision. If the mucocele is in the anterior ethmoidal area, an anterior ethmoidectomy is performed back to the ground lamella. Most of these mucoceles can be totally removed. The medial orbital wall is skeletonized.

Should the mucocele arise from a posterior ethmoidal cell, the dissection is carried through the ground lamella. The posterior ethmoidal cells are cleaned, removing the mucocele. The dissection needs to be carried back to the most posterior cell, which can be recognized by its pyramidal shape. This cell (Onodi cell) very often pneumatizes posteriorly, laterally, and superiorly to the sphenoid sinus. It is closely related to the optic nerve. The medial orbital wall and the skull base (with the posterior ethmoidal neurovascular bundle being identified) need to be skeletonized. Osteitic bone is usually evident around the confines of the mucocele. This bone should be removed.

Surgery for sphenoidal sinus mucoceles

These mucoceles may or may not be associated with ethmoidal sinus disease. Should ethmoid disease be present, an ethmoid procedure needs to be performed prior to the marsupialization of the sphenoid sinus mucocele. The sphenoid can then be approached through the most posterior ethmoidal cell or can be approached medial to the middle turbinate. The sphenoid is most commonly identified inferiorly and medially to the most posterior aspect of the ethmoid. Almost uniformly the sphenoid ostium is found more medially and inferiorly than anticipated.

The vital structures surrounding the sphenoid sinus necessitate review of the CT scan anatomy

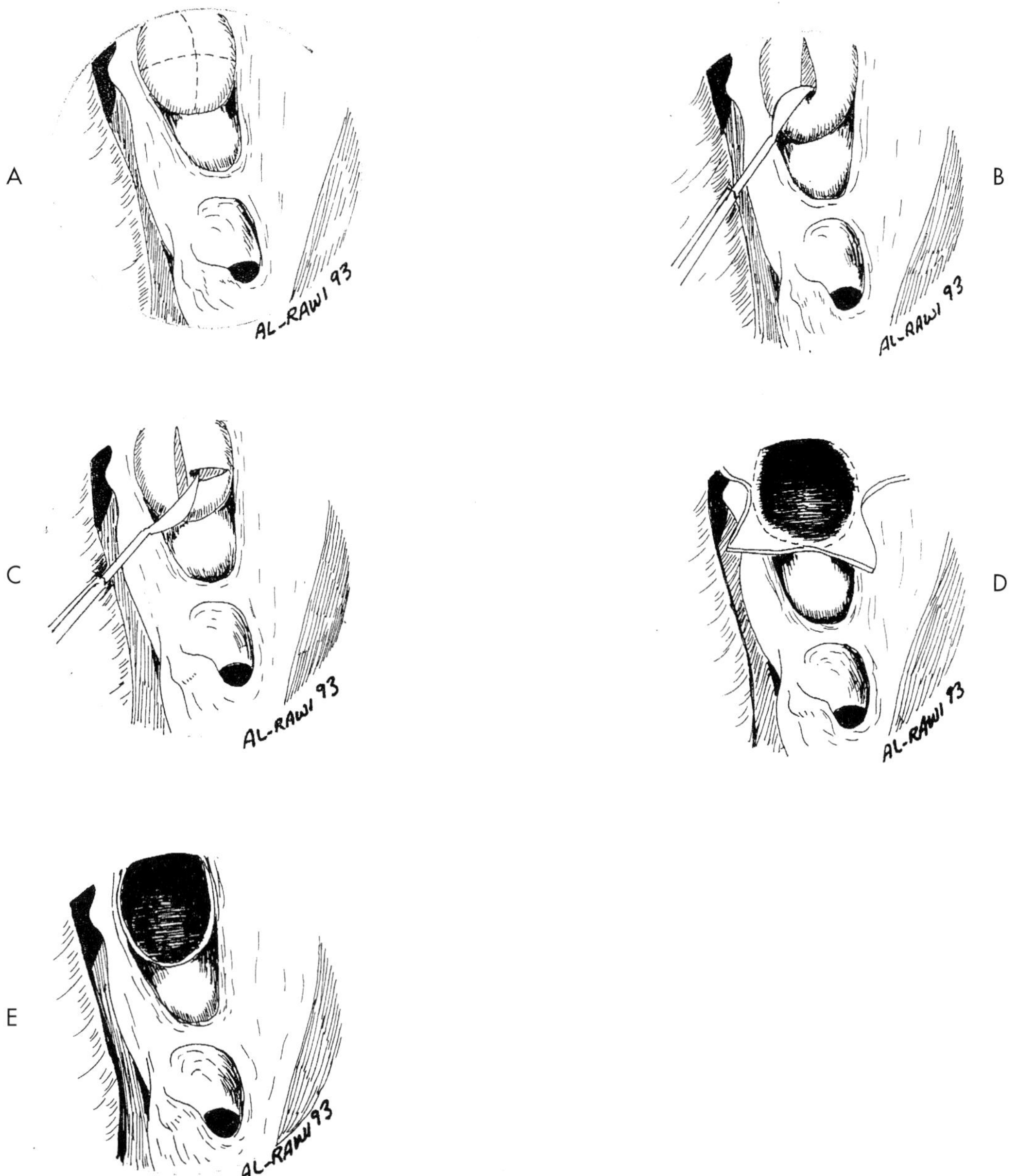

Fig. 7–1. **A,** The mucoceles extending into the frontal recess. **B,** The sickle knife makes the incision into the mucocele lining. **C,** Completion of the incision of the mucoceles performed. **D,** The flaps are marsupialized. **E,** The corners of the flap are removed allowing complete marsupialization (illustrations by Al-Rawi, M.D.)

before performing the surgical procedure. The relationship between the sphenoid sinus, the carotid arteries, and the optic nerves needs to be established. The carotid canal has been reported to be dehiscent in 23% of cadaver specimens. Protrusion of the carotid with or without a bony canal can also be present. The intersinus septa should be located, and, occasionally, the sphenoid sinus may be poorly pneumatized. This needs to be clearly identified. Although a coronal CT scan is appropriate, axial views through the sphenoid sinus can be invaluable in showing the relationship among these structures.

When the ethmoids are not involved, the sphenoid sinus may be entered directly. This is best done medial to the superior turbinate in the area of the sphenoid ostium. In addition to injecting the lateral nasal wall as previously described, it is important for the surgeon to inject the septum and the sphenoid rostrum in patients with sphenoid involvement. The sphenoid natural ostium is identified 30° from the floor of the nose. If it is difficult to visualize, then the middle turbinate may need to be displaced laterally in some cases. If the anatomy is not clearly defined, so that the area of the ostium can be identified, another approach (transseptal or transethmoid) may be required.

A small punch, a trocar, or various forceps may be employed to enter the sphenoid. The safest point of entrance is inferior and medial to the area of the natural ostium. The opening may then be widened with a sphenoid punch. A drill can be utilized if the bone is thick and difficult to penetrate with other instruments. The opening into the sphenoid, as with the other sinuses, must include the area of the natural ostium, otherwise recirculation of mucus can occur. Additionally, the chances of restenosis with recurrence of symptoms is greater should the surgically created opening not connect with the natural ostium.

Surgery for maxillary sinus mucoceles

A mucocele of the maxillary sinus can be approached endoscopically by first performing an infundibulotomy. An anterior ethmoidectomy may be required depending on the associated disease and anatomy. At times, an ethmoidectomy may not be required, or a simple limited ethmoidectomy may be all that is required for exposure. Once the ethmoid work is completed and infundibulotomy is performed, 30° and 70° 4.0-mm endoscopes are utilized with various forceps to open the maxillary middle meatal antrostomy. It is extremely important to ensure that the mucocele lining has been entered and that flaps are placed so as to marsupialize the mucocele. Backbiting forceps are employed to perform the dissection anteriorly. Care must be taken not to traumatize the nasolacrimal duct which is encased in hard bone. Upbiting forceps and a curved curette aid in the dissection posteriorly and allow the inferior flap to be placed appropriately. Occasionally, variously angled giraffe forceps are needed when the mucocele wall retracts laterally from the opening of the bony middle meatal antrostomy. A 120° 4.0-mm endoscope is utilized to visualize the anterior portion of the maxillary sinus.

It is very important for the natural ostium of the maxillary sinus to be incorporated into the middle meatal antrostomy to prevent recirculation of mucus and/or reclosure of the maxillary sinus. Wide marsupialization of the mucocele is important to prevent recurrence.

Mucoceles with more diffuse disease

Associated sinus disease needs to be treated both medically and surgically, as indicated. The procedure chosen by the surgeon needs to be customized according to the location and extent of the disease. For extensive panpolyposis, aggressive medical therapy needs to be initiated. A complete endoscopic sphenoethmoidectomy with polyp removal may be required. In this instance, long-term postoperative care in the office needs to be performed to obtain optimal results. Most likely long-term postoperative medical management will be necessary. For further information on this topic, we refer you to Josephson.[20]

POSTOPERATIVE CARE

To obtain the best possible result and to decrease the chances of scarring and mucocele reformation, postoperative care is extremely important. The patient should be seen soon after surgery and then approximately once a week for about 4 weeks. The visits can become biweekly and then monthly as needed until the patient heals completely. During these visits, the endoscopic procedure should include removal of scar bands, polyps, bone, and infectious debris. The surgeon needs to ensure continuously that the mucocele remains patent.

During each visit, the patient's nasal cavity is sprayed with 0.25% phenylephrine, and 4% lidocaine. Pontocaine, cocaine, and other similar agents may be utilized as needed. A 30° 4.0-mm endoscope is utilized with a combination of forceps (including upbiting and straight Blakesly forceps, giraffe forceps, backbiting forceps, etc.). Clots are suctioned from the various sinus cavities. Recurrent polyps, cellular debris, and crusts are removed. Osteitic bone is cleaned. Scar bands are lysed and removed. The goal of endoscopic sinus surgery is to return the mucociliary clearance patterns of flow and to alleviate the obstruction blocking this flow. Should obstructive scar bands be allowed to form, then the blockage reoccurs. Thus, the extreme importance of these meticulous postoperative procedures.

Case Studies

Case 1

A 47-year-old man treated with multiple sinus surgeries at another institution was referred to our service. The patient complained of severe headaches with frontal swelling and tenderness despite intravenous antibiotics and previous sinus surgery. The CT scan revealed a lateral frontal sinus mucocele (Fig. 7–2).

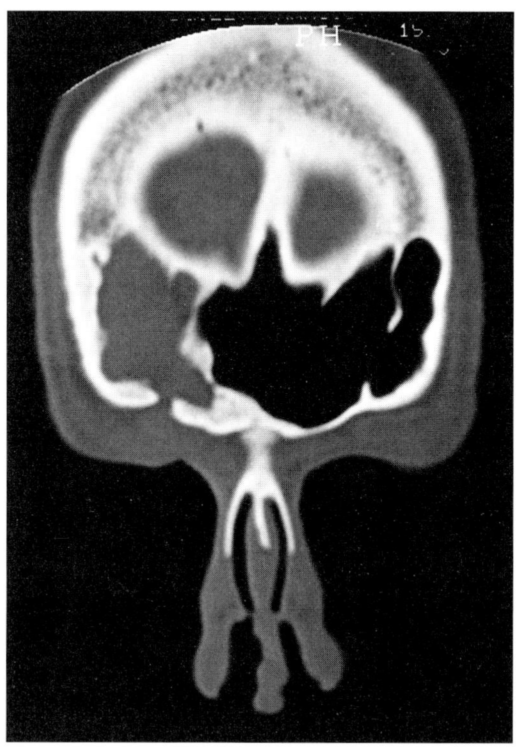

Fig. 7–2. The preoperative CT scan reveals a lateral frontal sinus mucocele.

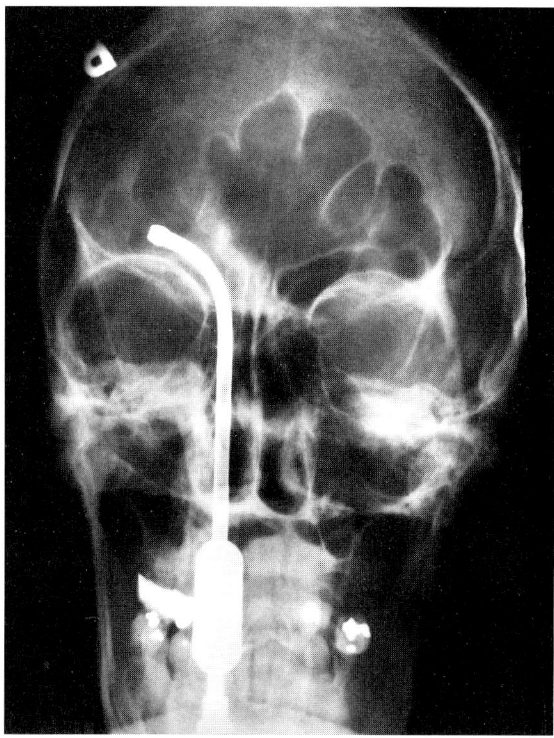

Fig. 7–3. An intraoperative plain film of the sinuses reveals a curved suction in the frontal sinus after marsupializing and decompressing the mucocele.

The patient subsequently underwent an endoscopic sinus surgery with marsupialization of the mucocele. A plain film of the sinuses revealed the curved suction to be in the mucocele itself, proving its decompression (Fig. 7–3).

Four months have now passed since surgery and the patient is free of headaches. Endoscopic examination and cannulation of the sinus in the office revealed that the mucocele had been successfully decompressed and marsupialized.

Case 2

A 61-year-old man presented with progressively worsening double vision, displacement of his left eye, left forehead numbness, and headaches over a 6-week period. A previous history of chronic sinusitis with intermittent frontal headaches and nasal discharge was elicited.

Physical examination showed a left-sided proptosis with evidence of a left supraorbital mass displacing the globe (Fig. 7–4). Endoscopic examination showed a septal deviation narrowing the right nasal passage. The middle meatus on this side was unremarkable. Endoscopic examination of the left side showed fullness in the area of the frontal recess. The left frontal sinus mass was confirmed by CT (Fig. 7–5).

A left endoscopic ethmoidectomy and intranasal frontal sinusotomy with decompression of the mucocele and a middle meatal antrostomy was performed. Ophthalmologic examination on the day following surgery showed resolution of the diplopia, and the proptosis was improved (Fig. 7–4). The patient was placed on postoperative broad spectrum antibiotics and underwent routine postoperative endoscopic cleanings.

Endoscopic follow-up with a 30° 4.0-mm endoscope demonstrated that the frontal recess and sinus were well epithelialized and patent (Fig. 7–6). To date, the frontal sinus has remained patent without evidence of renewed stenosis, and the patient is asymptomatic.

Discussion

The functional endoscopic sinus surgery approach affords the potential for improved diagnostic accuracy and for dramatically reducing the operative morbidity of surgery for paranasal sinus mucoceles by offering a minimally invasive approach under local anesthesia.

Improved diagnostic accuracy is possible as a result of improved visualization using angled telescopes, which can be used in the office, and advanced CT imaging.

The concept of marsupializing a mucocele, rather than completely removing it and obliterating the cavity, is not a new one and has been advo-

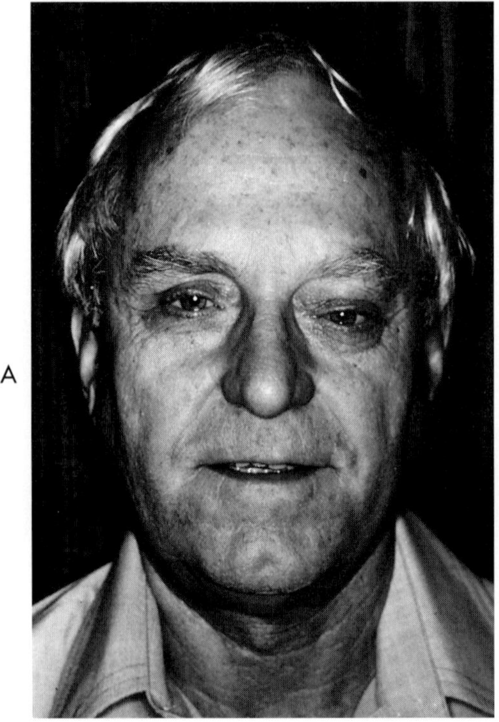

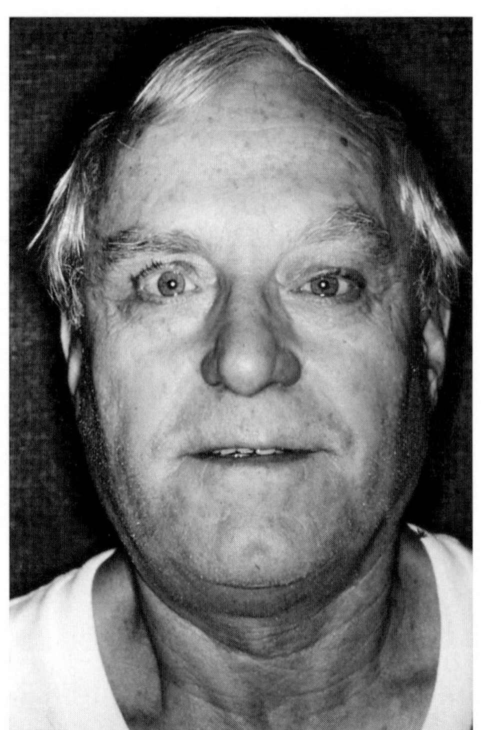

Fig. 7–4. **A,** Preoperatively, there is inferolateral displacement of the left eye and bulging of the left upper lid. **B,** On the first postoperative day, the eye has returned to a more normal position and the lid swelling has resolved. Eye motion has returned to normal. (From Kennedy DW, Josephson JS, Zinreich SJ, et al: Endoscopic sinus surgery for mucoceles: A visible alternative. The Laryngoscope. 1989, pp 885-895.)

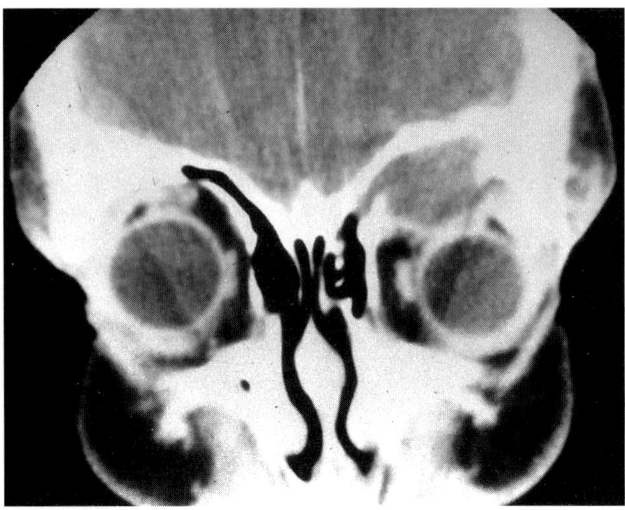

Fig. 7–5. Coronal CT showing a left frontal sinus mass (triangle) and inferolateral displacement of the left globe. (From Kennedy DW, Josephson JS, Zinreich SJ, et al: Endoscopic sinus surgery for mucoceles: A visible alternative. The Laryngoscope. 1989, pp 885-895.)

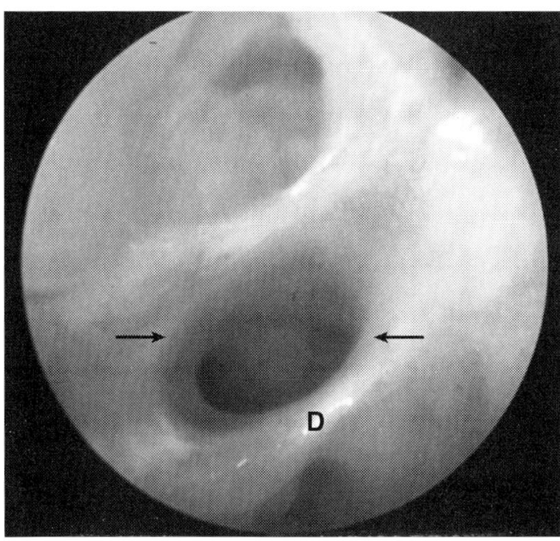

Fig. 7–6. Postoperative endoscopic view (70° telescope) shows normal appearing mucosa and a widely patent frontal sinus internal os (arrows). D, dome of ethmoid. (From Kennedy DW, Josephson JS, Zinreich SJ, et al: Endoscopic sinus surgery for mucoceles: A visible alternative. The Laryngoscope. 1989, pp 885-895.)

cated for many years. With the advent of nasal endoscopes marsupialization can now be performed with decreased morbidity. Further, endoscopy during surgery supports the concept that the mucosal lining of the mucocele has active mucociliary transport. Postoperative endoscopy further reveals that the lining of the mucocele takes on the appearance of normal mucosa.

Both the patient and the physician must be committed to long-term postoperative follow-up. Significant cleaning may be necessary to prevent recurrence of the mucocele. In addition, endoscopic follow-up in the office enables the surgeon to visualize directly the sinus cavity. As a result, diagnosis of early recurrence of these slow-growing lesions can be detected. Unlike sinus obliteration, the ability to image the sinus by CT is also preserved.

Endoscopic surgery for mucoceles may be difficult and can require considerable skill on the part of the surgeon. This approach may not be for every surgeon, even some who perform routine endoscopic procedures. However, it appears to offer the patient an approach with a dramatically reduced morbidity. The surgery can be performed under local anesthesia, with minimal blood loss, while avoiding external incisions. Packing is rarely required, and the patient can usually be discharged within less than 24 hours.

REFERENCES

1. Canalis RF. Frontal mucoceles. In: English GM, ed. *Otolaryngology, Vol 2.* Philadelphia, PA: Harper & Row; 1982:1–11.
2. Evans C. Aetiology and treatment of front-ethmoidal mucocele. *J Laryngol Otol.* 1981; 95:361–375.
3. Riedel R. *The Paranasal Sinuses: Surgery and Technique.* 2d ed., FN Ritter. St Louis, MO: CV Mosby; 1978:136–145.
4. MacBeth RE. The osteoplastic operation for chronic infection of the frontal sinus. *J Laryngol Otol.* 1954; 68:465–477.
5. Bergara AR, Itoiz AO. Present state of the surgical treatment of chronic frontal sinus. *Arch Otolaryngol.* 1955; 61:616–628.
6. Hardy JM, Montgomery WM. Osteoplastic frontal sinusitis: An analysis of 250 operations. *Ann Otol.* 1976; 85:523–532.
6. Lynch RC. The technique of a radical frontal sinus operation which has given me the best results. *Laryngoscope.* 1921; 31:1–5.
8. Sewall EC. Frontal-ethmosphenoidectomy: Further experience with this operation performed under local anesthesia. *Arch Otolaryngol.* 1928; 8:144–150.
9. Boyden GL. Surgical treatment of chronic sinusitis. *Ann Otol Rhinol Laryngol.* 1952; 61:558–566.
10. Howarth WG. Mucocele and pyocele of the nasal accessory sinuses. *Lancet.* 1921; 2:744–746.
11. Wolfowitz BL, Solomon A. Mucoceles of the frontal and ethmoid sinuses. *J Laryngol Otol.* 1972; 86:79–82.
12. Goodyear HM. Mucocele in frontal and ethmoidal sinuses. Simplified surgical treatment. *Ann Otol Rhinol Laryngol.* 1944; 53:242–245.
13. Kennedy DW, Josephson JS, Zinreich SJ, et al. Endoscopic sinus surgery for mucoceles: A viable alternative. *Laryngoscope.* 1989; 99:885–895.
14. Josephson JS, Kennedy DW. Surgery of Paranasal Sinus Mucoceles. *Oper Tech Otolaryngol Head Neck Surg Vol.1, No.2.* 1990; 133–141.
15. Zinreich SJ, Kennedy DW, Rosenbaum AE, et al. Paranasal sinuses: CT imaging requirements for endoscopic surgery. *Radiology.* 1987; 163:769–775.
16. Josephson JS, Linden BE. The importance of postoperative care in the adult and pediatric patient with functional endoscopic sinus surgery. *Oper Tech Otolaryngol Head Neck Surg Vol.1, No.2.* 1990; 112–116.
17. Kennedy DW. Functional endoscopic sinus surgery technique. *Arch Otolaryngol.* 1985; 111:643–649.
18. Josephson JS. Insights in Otolaryngology: Functional endoscopic sinus surgery. In: Goebel JA. *Insights in Otolarynogology* 1991; 6(2):1–8.
19. Kennedy DW, Zinreich SJ, Shaalan H, et al. Endoscopic middle meatal antrostomy: Theory, technique, and patency. *Laryngoscope.* 1987; 43 (Suppl):1–9.
20. Josephson JS. The role of endoscopic sinus surgery for the treatment of nasal polyposis. *Otolaryngol Clin North Am.* 1989; 22:831–840.

8

Extensive Nasal Polyposis

James A. Stankiewicz

There is no more difficult sinus surgery to perform than that for patients with extensive nasal polyposis. This is especially true in revision patients. It is important that the surgeon develops an approach to these patients that can be applied repeatedly. This chapter will describe the author's approach to these challenging patients, an approach that has been successful in over 300 patients with extensive nasal polyposis.

Preoperative Considerations

MEDICAL HISTORY

The most important questions deal with the primary disease and associated problems, for example, "Is this the first surgery or one of several?" Primary surgery in the patient with extensive polyposis is usually a straightforward surgery because all of the anatomic landmarks are present, and the polyps are almost gelatinous (not fibrous), making removal very easy. Longstanding primary polyposis and revision polyps are more fibrous and vascular and, thus, much more problematic.

Does the patient have asthma and/or aspirin sensitivity? This group of patients is the most difficult to control. In almost every classification of sinus disease, these patients are classified in the lowest class because of disease recurrence.[1,2] For best control, special consideration for preoperative and postoperative nasal and oral steroids is necessary in these patients.

Is the patient on long-term steroidal or anti-inflammatory agents? These patients have greater problems with bleeding and will tend to ooze throughout surgical treatment. It is important to consider autologous transfusion in this instance; particularly in recurrent nasal polyposis, although, in reality, the transfusion technique is rarely used. All anti-inflammatory medication except steroids should be stopped prior to surgery and in the special case of aspirin at least 10 days before. On the other hand, patients who receive a Medrol® dose pak of cortisone a few days prior to surgery do not have an increased problem with bleeding. The patient should be asked about any other medication that affects bleeding and discontinue its use prior to surgery.

Medications, past and present, including antibiotics and steroids (oral, intramuscular, nasal) should be listed in the chart so it is evident that the patient has failed appropriate medical therapy.

PHYSICAL EXAM

An attempt to quantitate the extent of obstruction by the polyps should be made. Anterior rhinoscopy and nasal endoscopy is appropriate. If infection is present, antibiotics should be given prior to surgery to reduce inflammation and, thus, bleeding during surgery. Septal deviation is often difficult to assess in the case of massive polyposis. In reality, it is uncommon to find a septal deviation because of the nasal expansion due to the polyps. Other nasal landmarks, such as middle turbinates, are not often seen or have been removed in previous surgery. A closed eye examination for evidence of bony erosion on the nasal bones, lamina papyracea, and superior orbital rim and roof is performed. The eye is pushed laterally or inferiorally if erosion is present from intraorbital polyps. Frank proptosis may be noted (Fig. 8–1).

A CT scan is the most appropriate study to determine the extent of nasal and sinus disease. It can also reflect nasal septal deviation in massive polyposis. Coronal and axial views are recommended to best evaluate advanced polyposis, especially if previous surgery has been performed. This study gives the best information regarding the skull base, sphenoid sinus, and orbits (Fig. 8–2). If there is any evidence of bony erosion on exam or CT scan, an MRI may give additional information about the extent of disease into the orbit or skull base/brain. MRI can also provide informa-

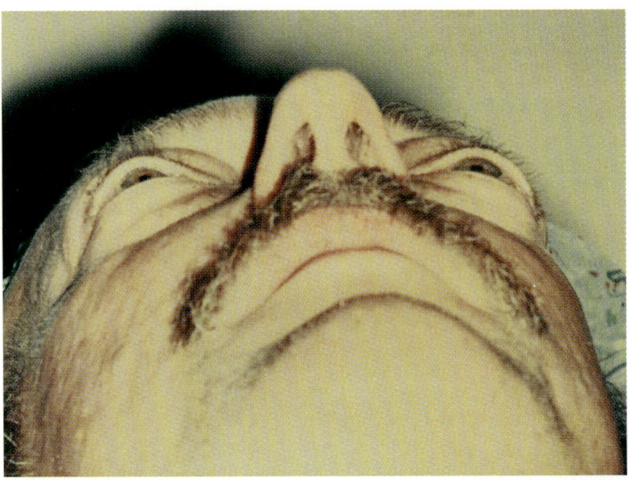

Fig. 8–1. Patient with extensive polyposis with orbital invasion causing bilateral proptosis.

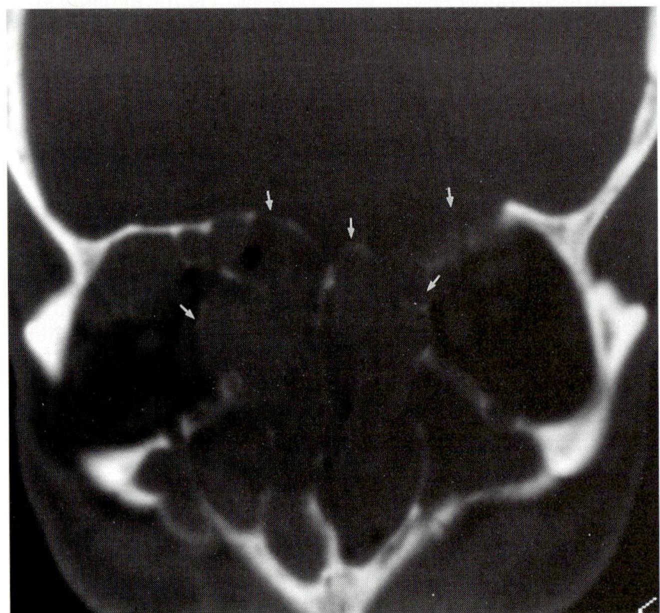

Fig. 8–2. CT scan of patient in Figure 8-1 showing extensive bony erosion.

tion about air fluid levels and fungal disease, which is helpful in treatment planning (Fig. 8–3).

Surgical Considerations

Although endoscopic sinus surgery can be used to marsupialize extensive nasal polyposis and sinus disease, this extensive surgery should be attempted only by experienced surgeons, especially in revision cases. Consideration for combination procedures—including frontal sinus osteoplastic flaps, trephination, Caldwell Luc, and, occasionally, external ethmoid surgery—is important depending on individual case circumstances. Patients with frontal sinus erosion require an external procedure, usually an osteoplastic flap (Fig. 8–4). Patients with orbital erosion should have an external ethmoidectomy as a backup procedure if endoscopic sinus surgery cannot be performed safely.

Patients with extensive disease have an increased risk of complications, especially in revision surgeries.[3,4] Patients should be made aware that the disease process may have sufficiently thinned or eroded bone at the skull base or orbit to make surgical entrance into these areas a real

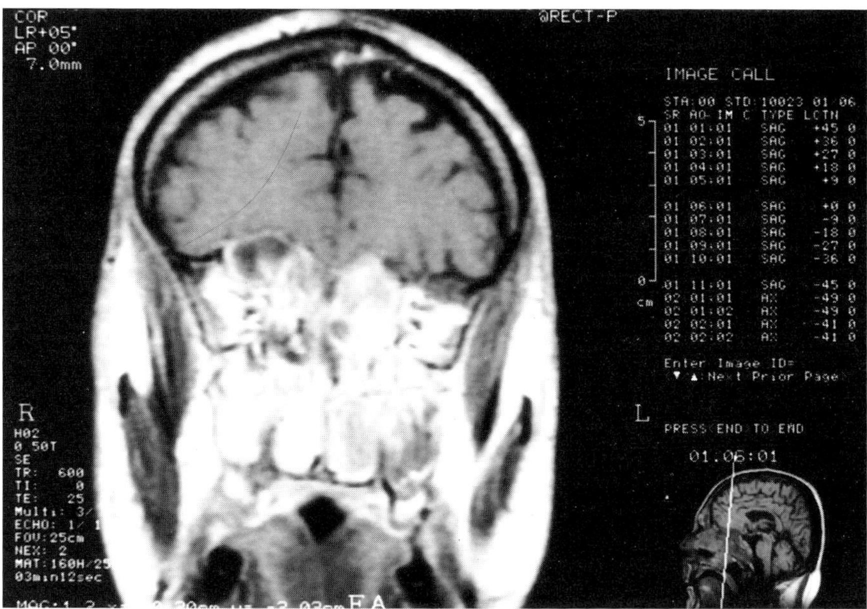

Fig. 8–3. MRI scan of patient in Figure 8-1 showing no evidence of dural or brain involvement, discriminating infection/polyposis from tumor.

possibility. CSF leak, (rarely) meningitis, and/or brain injury, blindness, double vision, and orbital hematoma are potential hazards. These risks are minimal, however, with an experienced surgeon who has planned carefully.

The choice of anesthesia is important. It is very difficult to perform surgery in patients with extensive or massive polyposis under a local standby anesthesia. Perhaps for first-time patients this may be considered, but in most cases a general anesthesia is preferred. Discussion with the anesthesiologist preoperatively is important. It is very difficult to control the asthmatic patient under local standby anesthesia and, again, general anesthesia is preferred. Hypotensive anesthesia, keeping systolic blood pressure below 100, is very helpful. Great care is taken surgically with general anesthesia because patient pain threshold feedbacks are gone, making it easier to inadvertently enter into the orbit or skull base. Increased diligence and care are necessary.

Bleeding can often be controlled from the beginning of surgery using accurate injection of local anesthesia. The posterior septal artery and the sphenopalatine branch to the middle turbinate are the two most troublesome vessels and can usually be controlled by either oral greater palatine foramen injections or intranasal turbinate injections, paying particular attention to the lower part of the basal lamella where these vessels occur.[5] Once appropriate attention is given to obtaining good vasoconstriction, surgery is begun. Longstanding or revision surgery for extensive disease will cause oozing. While suction forceps are helpful, other measures are needed to control bleeding. The use of intranasal suction cautery is helpful in controlling brisk arterial bleeding from the sphenopalatine, posterior septal, and anterior and posterior ethmoid arteries. Topical Avitene® or pledgets are beneficial. Topical ephedrine or epinephrine sprays are also helpful in controlling oozing. A 1/10,000 solution of epinephrine (9 cc saline to 1 cc epinephrine 1/1,000) in a spray bottle is used as needed. No changes in blood pressure have been noted while using this spray. Bleeding is not usually a problem with a first time surgery. If bleeding is troublesome, it usually means a larger vessel has been traumatized or the skull base may have been breached. Oozing may often occur in revision cases despite all efforts, and on occasion the nose has to be packed. In this case, either the opposite side is then operated on or surgery is cancelled and finished another day. No endoscopic surgeon should attempt meaningful surgery in a blood-filled nose, especially in extensive disease cases. When I have not completed a case because of bleeding, I have noted two things postoperatively. One is that often I have removed enough disease that repeat surgery is not necessary. Second, the repeat surgery is not as bloody as the initial surgery because of better preparation.

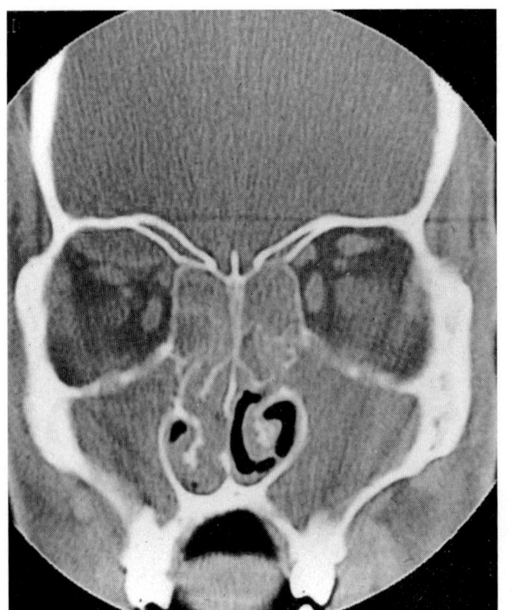

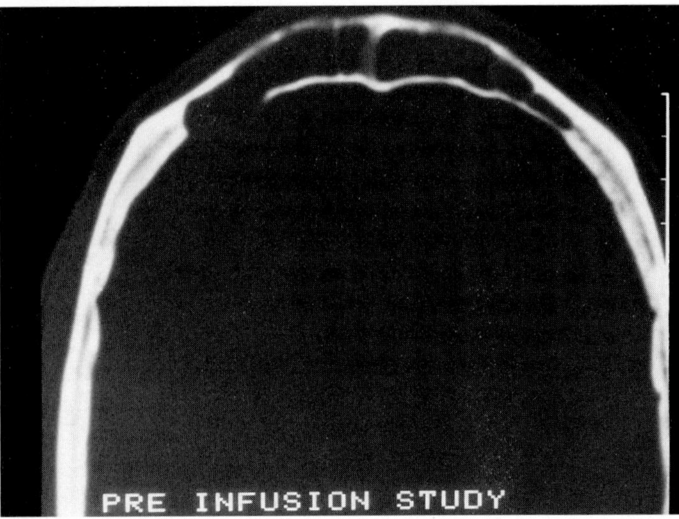

Fig. 8–4. Patient with extensive pansinusitis and polyposis with significant frontal sinus disease. It was only after an osteoplastic flap was made that nasal disease was controlled. **A,** Marked pansinusitis occulding all sinuses. **B,** Same patient as in *A* but with significant frontal sinusitis disease with opacification and posterior wall erosion.

Surgical Approach

The surgical approach for extensive massive polyposis and sinus disease has to be a marsupialization with widespread removal of disease. It is not functional![1] Safety is the key to any endoscopic approach to extensive disease. The same technique is followed for both first time and revision surgery.

Endoscopic polypectomy is performed initially, taking great pains to identify and preserve the middle turbinate. In most revision surgery for extensive polyps, the middle turbinate has been removed to some extent. It is still important to locate whatever remnant still exists as a reference point to the skull base.

If, as in most cases, the middle turbinate is full of polypoid disease posteriorly, part of the middle turbinate requires sacrifice. I try to do this at the end of surgery so I can preserve the landmark as long as possible. Once all polyps outside of the middle meatus have been removed endoscopically such that the choana is visible, attention is turned to the ethmoid sinus. In an unoperated extensive polyp case, the uncinate process is present and incised with removal of polypoid tissue in the infundibulum. The next goal is to locate the maxillary sinus ostia and perform a wide antrostomy. A Lusk probe is used to find the ostia, and then a curved suction is used to dilate the antrostomy. Under a 30 degree telescopic guidance, a wide antrostomy is created using a straight punch forceps, large right angle forceps, and a backward biting forceps. Marked obstructive intrasinus polypoid disease is removed to the extent that a wide unobstructed maxillary sinus drainage is created. This is especially helpful in the asthma patient. This new antrostomy helps locate the lamina papyracea, which is essential as a landmark in extensive cases. Polypoid disease is then cleaned through the bulla ethmoidalis to the basal lamella, which is measured at 6 cm in adults. Surgery should proceed straight back with minimal surgery to the upper ethmoids, which are attacked last to avoid nuisance bleeding and to permit initial identification of all landmarks. The posterior ethmoid is cleaned of all polypoid disease proceeding to the anterior wall of the sphenoid. The sphenoid sinus anterior wall is measured usually at 7 cm and then the surgeon probes for the sphenoid ostia. Usually the membranous part of the posterior middle turbinate where the posterior ethmoid sinus drains into the nose is easily removed, often along with posterior ethmoid polypoid disease. The sphenoid ostia can then be cannulated and opened with a Frazier suction, straight forceps, and sphenoid punch. A sphenoidotomy as wide as possible is created and obvious disease in the sinus is removed, whether it is polyp, fungus, or mucopurulent secretions, while great care is taken not to disturb the posterior sphenoid structures. Once the sphenoid is open, enough landmarks are present to remove superior disease safely. The sphenoid sets the skull base, the antrostomy, the lamina papyracea, the remnant of middle turbinate, the medial boarder of dissection. Superior disease is then removed from posterior to anterior as described by Wigand[6] (Fig. 8–5). Safe removal of posterior superior and anterior superior disease is enhanced using a small curved suction with a broad tip as a cell finder. Cells are probed beginning just outside the sphenoid, always working laterally away from the middle turbinate. Once probed and dissected, polypoid disease is resected. Care is taken to avoid overzealous removal of disease medially against the middle turbinate in the area of the anterior ethmoid artery. This is the thinnest part of the skull base and the most prone to CSF fistula.[7] Lastly, the frontal recess and agger nasi cells are probed and opened. Occasionally a prominent ethmoidal artery can be avulsed during dissection or tissue removal causing hemorrhage intranasally or intraorbitally. Suction cautery nicely controls the intranasal bleeding. Immediate proptosis and chemosis reflects intraorbital bleeding and requires decompression if medical treatment cannot reduce the hematoma. The eye should be watched closely when working in the superior lateral ethmoid sinus (fovea ethmoidalis). Only limited disease is removed against the middle turbinate around the anterior ethmoid artery to avoid entrance into the brain. The frontal recess is cleaned of disease as needed (see Chapter 3). A probe will help find the frontal sinus. Usually in massive disease the frontal recess is expanded and will admit a long curved suction that can be used to identify the frontal sinus and to introduce irrigation. If the frontal sinuses are large and totally opacified, especially in the revision case, surgery from below may not be successful. Revision cases, especially with frontal sinus erosion and purulence, should be considered for an osteoplastic flap. Giraffe frontal sinus forceps and Kuhn curette can help remove polypoid disease from the frontal recess, sometimes allowing for a wide frontal recess. A large frontal recess opening (>4 mm) is encouraged and will be less likely to close. Longstanding disease often causes thickened bone due to osteitis, and it may not be possible to open a large recess. Any small recess requires diligent postoperative debridement and dilation to ensure patency. However, in some patients the frontal recess is often obstructed, with recurrent polypoid disease but it is not problematic.

Small scarred frontal recesses, especially in revision cases, are difficult to open endoscopically and may require simultaneous trephination or further external surgery to control the disease if the patient is symptomatic (see Chapter 3). Nonetheless, intensive postoperative medical therapy may reduce frontal disease markedly once the bulk of disease is removed from the nose and lower sinuses. After the frontal sinuses are opened, the agger nasi cells are checked for anterior extent. Occasionally, they will extend superiorly into the frontal recess and cause a circuitous drainage from the frontal sinus. Part of the agger nasi will require removal superiorly or medially to establish frontal sinus discharge. On occasion, the agger nasi cells may extend anteriorly over the nasolacrimal duct and sac, requiring removal. Close attention to the orbit is necessary to avoid injury to these structures.

In first time surgeries of extensive polyp disease, the middle turbinate may be preserved if it is not involved with polyposis. However, there is usually polyposis posteriorly in the middle turbinate where the posterior ethmoid sinuses drain. After polyps are removed, the remainder of the middle turbinate may be flaccid and require removal. If not, spacers, adhesion to septum, or suture ties may be used to help keep the middle turbinate medial. In most longstanding or revision cases, the middle turbinate is compromised by disease and has to be removed. Cautery should be

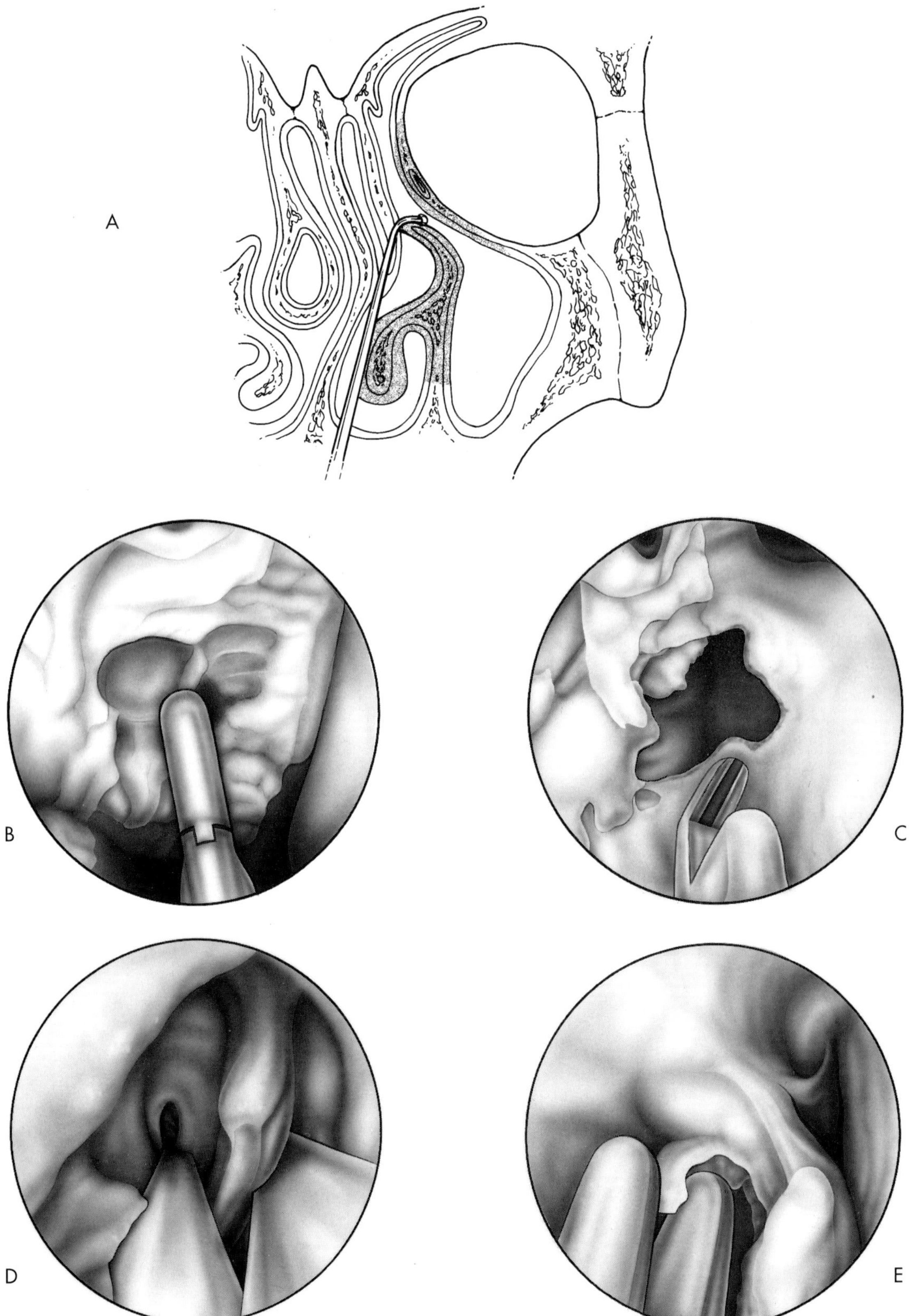

Fig. 8–5. Wigand or posterior to anterior approach for massive polyposis. **A**, Finding of the maxillary antrostomy to locate the lamina papyracea. **B**, Entrance directly into the posterior ethmoids. **C**, Entrance into the sphenoid sinus to define the skull base. **D**, Clearing of the posterior superior ethmoids after using a cell finder to locate cells. **E**, Frontal recess/agger nasi surgery is performed last.

used on all middle turbinate remnants and on the base of the sphenoid to avoid postoperative hemorrhage from the sphenopalatine vessels. Cautery should be performed 0 to 3 weeks after surgery. The anterior ethmoid artery can be likewise cauterized if bleeding. Unipolar cautery should not be used in or on the orbit or in the sphenoid sinus to avoid injury to the optic nerve or medial rectus muscle. I use a high middle meatal Merocel packing placed inside a piece of folded Telfa for hemostasis. The recovery room staff is alerted to observe for eye changes, decreased vision, and any change in mental status. A lower Telfa pack that had been placed in the inferior nose is removed after a few hours, prior to the patient's discharge, but the upper Telfa/Merocel pack is left in place. The patient is discharged on prednisone 40 to 60 mg/day for 3 to 4 days, saline spray, oxymetazoline decongestant, an antibiotic, and pain medication.

Postoperative Care

The patient is seen in the clinic 4 to 6 days after surgery, a topical anesthetic is then given, and the upper packing is removed. All loose clotted blood and debris are removed from the sinus area, and the sphenoid and maxillary sinuses are specifically suctioned clear (Fig. 8–6). Any fixed, hard clots

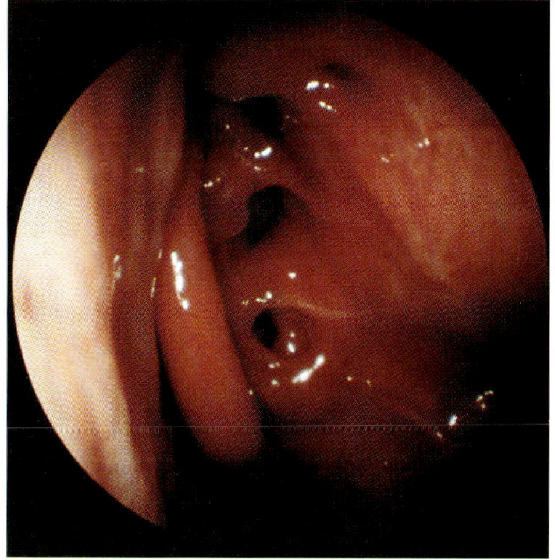

Fig. 8–6. Typical postoperative debris and opening after massive endoscopic marsupialization at 2 weeks.

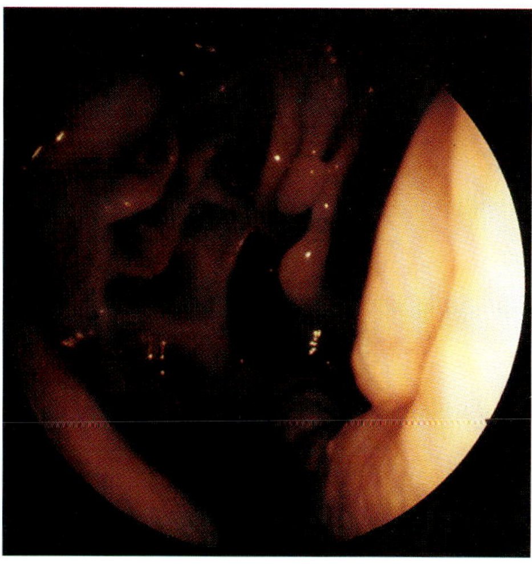

Fig. 8–7. Healed marsupialized endoscopic nasal sinus cavity at 8 weeks.

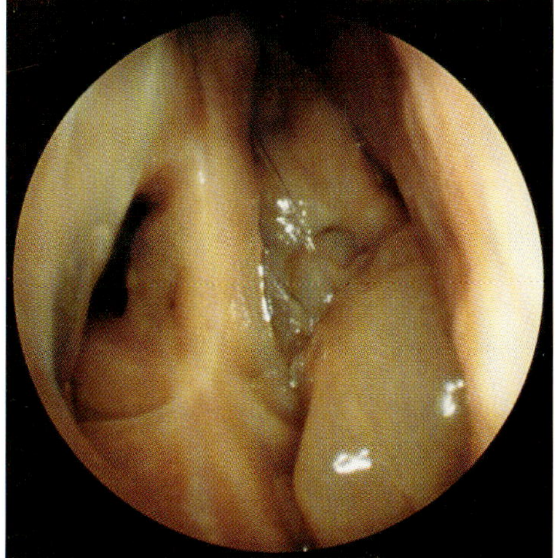

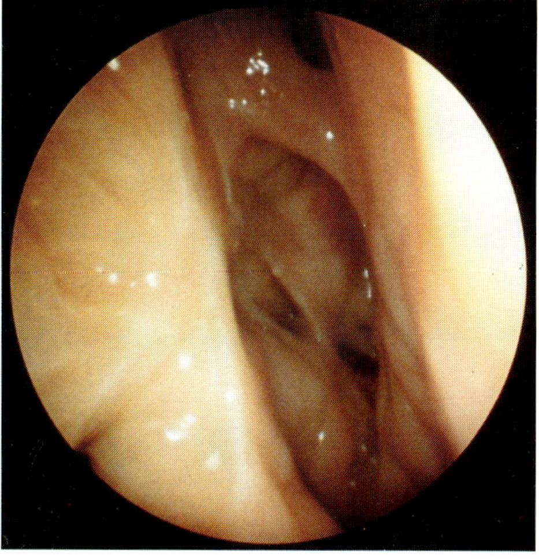

Fig. 8-8. Before and after views of postoperative cavity with recurrent polyposis and after the use of a prednisone burst followed by a daily topical and low dose (5 mg) long-term prednisone.

are left alone. Removing these clots any time before they loosen increases the risk of hemorrhage. All patients are started on self–irrigations. Antibiotics and pain medication are continued. Prednisone is decreased to 5 mg daily, which will be continued for 5 to 6 weeks and then decreased to 5 mg every other day indefinitely, especially if the patient has asthma or Samter's Triad. The patient is then seen weekly and endoscoped and debrided. Debridement is performed initially with the head mirror, forceps, and suction. A rigid 30 degree telescope is then used to debride and suction specific areas such as the maxillary, sphenoid, and frontal sinuses. After the first visit, the frontal sinus requires personal attention with gentle cannulation, dilation, and debridement. Whereas most of the ethmoid and sphenoid are healed by 4 weeks, the frontal sinus and the maxillary sinus (if markedly polypoid) may take 6 to 8 weeks or more to heal. It is not uncommon to see maxillary sinus retention cysts in the postoperative period; these can be opened and marsupialized in the clinic. Occasionally, a steroid burst and antibiotics are required 3 to 5 weeks postoperatively to assist healing and reduce polypoid regrowth (Fig. 8–7).

Medical therapy, which includes prednisone 5 mg every other day and a topical steroid inhaler aerosol (not AQ) is very important to control recurrent polyps (Fig. 8–8). Allergy identification and treatment are also necessary for best success.

Summary

Extensive sinus disease can be approached safely with near total removal of disease if a unified approach is developed.

REFERENCES

1. Hoffman DF, May M, Mester SJ. Functional endoscopic sinus surgery—experience with the initial 100 patients. *Amer J Rhinol.* 1990; 4:129–132.
2. Friedman WH, Katsontomis GP, Swore M, Kay S. Computed tomography staging of the paranasal sinuses in chronic hyperplastic rhinosinusitis. *Laryngoscope.* 1990; 100:1161–1165.
3. Stankiewicz JA. Complications in endoscopic intranasal ethmoidectomy: An update. *Laryngoscope.* 1989; 99:686–690.
4. Stankiewicz JA. Complications of endoscopic sinus surgery. *Otolaryngol Clin No Amer.* 1989; 22:749–758.
5. Stankiewicz JA. Greater palatine foramen injection made easy. *Laryngoscope.* 1988; 98:580–581.
6. Wigand ME. Transnasal ethmoidectomy under endoscopic control. *Rhinology (Eur).* 1981; 19:7–15.
7. Kainz J, Stammberger H. The roof of the anterior ethmoid. A place of least resistance in the skull base. *Am J Rhinol.* 1990; 3:191–199.

9

Fungal Sinusitis

David H. Henick and *David W. Kennedy*

The purpose of this chapter is to discuss the approach to the patient with chronic fungal sinusitis. The spectrum of this entity can be manifested by three distinct clinical forms: 1. allergic fungal sinusitis, 2. noninvasive disease, and 3. invasive disease in both the immunocompetent and immunocompromised patient (chronic invasive and acute fulminant fungal sinusitis). Pre- and postoperative considerations, as well as the surgical techniques employed during the operation, will be discussed.

Microbiology

Fungi belong to a taxonomic classification of plants known as Thallophyta. They represent a point in the spectrum of microorganisms between bacteria and protozoa. A true fungus lacks chlorophyll, does not require light to grow, and has a body made of branching intertwined elements or hyphae, which form a dense mat called a mycelium. Most fungi are not pathogenic in man, and fewer than a dozen are said to be capable of producing fatal infections.[1]

The spectrum of microorganisms responsible for producing chronic fungal sinusitis can be divided into four main categories based on appearance in tissue: 1. broad nonseptate hyphae (Fig. 9–1) (*Rhizopus, Conidiobolus, Basidiobolus, Absidia*), 2. narrower septate hyphae, or nonpigmented fungi (*Aspergillus, Pseudallescheria, Scedosporium*), 3. dematiaceous fungi, or pigmented fungi (*Bipolaris, Dreschslera, Curvularia, Alternaria, Cladosporium*, and 4. rounded forms (*Candida, Sporothrix, Rhinosporidium*). Although the principal fungal organisms causing chronic infections of the paranasal sinuses belong to the genii *Aspergillus* and *Zygomycetes*, any of the organisms listed above have the capacity to manifest clinically as either a noninvasive, invasive, or allergic fungal sinusitis. Therefore, it is the manifestation of the disease that is more important than the actual organism causing the infection. In contrast to yeast organisms, the hyphal forms are responsible for the majority of infections seen in humans.[2,3]

Aspergillus is an organism that is commonly associated with all forms of chronic fungal sinusitis in the immunocompetent patient. As a saphrophyte, aspergillus is typically found in soil, dust, decaying organic matter, fruits, and grains. All species of *Aspergillus* are septated hyphae structurally composed of six essential elements: 1. fungal cell, 2. base cell, 3. conidiophore, 4. vesicle, 5. sterigma, or phialides, and 6. conidia (Fig. 9–2). Conidiophores typically expand into large vesicles, which give rise to multiple sterigmata, which produce long chains of conidia. Species are identified on the basis of the size, color, and shape of the condiophore, sterigma, and conidia (see Table 9-1). Species of *Aspergillus* branch in a dichotomous fashion at 45° angles. A characteristic unique to aspergillosis is its round culture shape due to its centrifugal linear growth. This explains the concentric bulb-shaped appearance as it develops in the maxillary antrum. Each layer consists of a dense network of innumerable hyphae: mycelium.[4]

In the Sudan, aspergillosis is endemic; *Aspergillus* has been cultured from bedding, straw roofs, timber, and earth floors of Sudanese dwellings. Elsewhere in the world aspergillosis is less common. *A. fumigatus* is clearly the most commonly encountered species of *Aspergillus* in the United States. By contrast, *A. flavus* is the sole causative agent identified in the Sudan. Other species, such as *A. niger*, are rarely cultured from the nose and paranasal sinuses and may not be pathogenic (Table 9–2).[5,6]

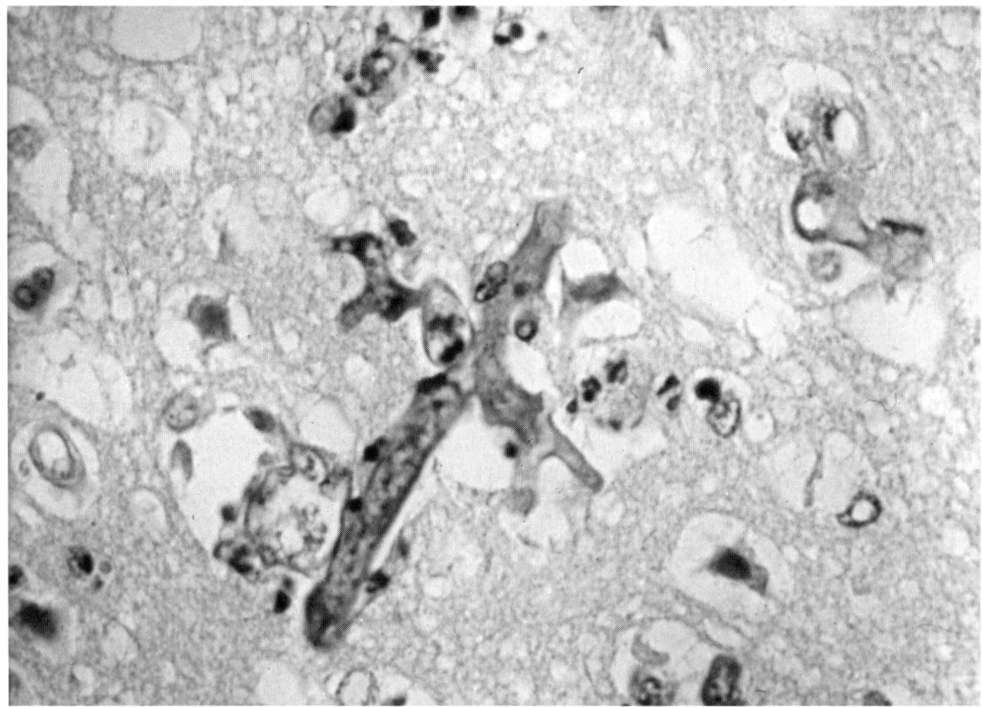

Fig. 9–1. Broad nonseptated hyphae are characteristic of mucormycosis.

Table 9–1 Colony and microscopic characteristics as found in Czapek-Dox Agar culture

Species	Conidiophore length	Vesicle width [μm]	Series of sterigmata	Conidia color	Conidia diameter [μm]
A. fumigatus	<300 μm	20–30	One	Gray/green/blue-green	2.5–3.0
A. flavus	<1 mm	25–45	One or two	Yellow/green	3.5–4.5
A. niger	1.5–3.0 mm	45–75	Two	Black	4.0–5.0

Clinical and Preoperative Considerations

ALLERGIC FUNGAL SINUSITIS

The term allergic fungal sinusitis[6–27] has been used synonymously with allergic *Aspergillus* sinusitis and, in many instances, has been shown to be analogous to the entity allergic bronchopulmonary aspergillosis (ABPA) based on similar serologic and histopathologic findings.[20–22,24] Patients with this condition exhibit a characteristic allergic mucin which, on light microscopy, reveals eosinophils, Charcot-Leyden crystals, and hyphae. Classically, these patients have a history of atopy with longstanding allergic rhinitis, asthma, nasal congestion, nasal polyposis, headaches, and, sometimes, visual disturbances.[16,26] The chronic sinusitis often leads to repeated sinus surgery over a period of months or years, and patients may have peripheral blood eosinophilia.

Diagnostic criteria of allergic fungal sinusitis have been proposed similar to those described for ABPA. These criteria include: 1. eosinophilia, 2. immediate skin reactivity for fungal antigens, 3. serum precipitin IgG antibodies against fungal antigens, 4. elevated total IgE, 5. nasal obstruction from mucosal edema and/or polyposis, 6. suggestive computed tomography (CT) findings include increased density of inspissated material (Fig. 9–3) and characteristic magnetic resonance imaging (MRI) findings include mucosal hypertrophy surrounding an area of signal loss seen on T2-weighed images, and 7. confirmatory pathology (allergic mucin with hyphae) with or without positive fungal cultures. A "definite" diagnosis exists if all seven criteria are fulfilled. Fulfillment of six criteria constitutes a probable diagnosis.[17,25]

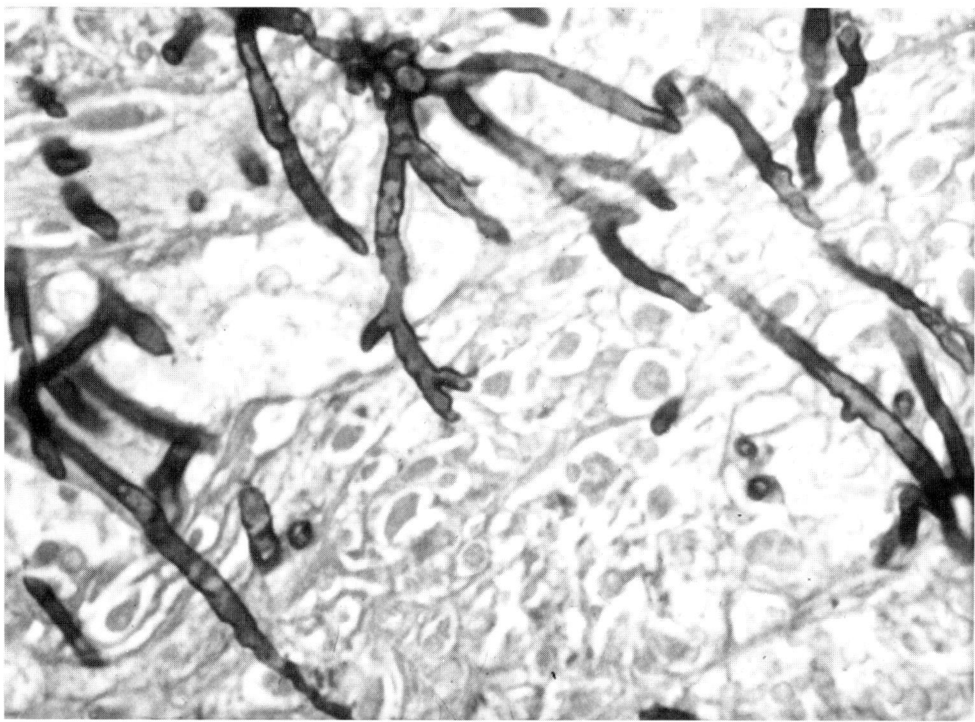

Fig. 9–2. Narrow septated branching hyphae at 45° angles are characteristic of aspergillosis.

Table 9–2 Types of aspergillosis sinusitis

Clinical forms	Pulmonary counterpart
Allergic aspergillosis sinusitis (AAS)	Allergic bronchopulmonary aspergillosis [ABPA]
Noninvasive colonization	Pulmonary aspergilloma
Invasive aspergillosis:	
Subacute or chronic invasive	Chronic necrotizing pulmonary aspergillosis
Disseminated	Invasive pulmonary aspergillosis

Due to the expansile nature of the disease, bony remodeling, likely due to pressure necrosis, is commonly observed and may produce clinical presentations similar to those seen in patients with chronic invasive fungal sinusitis, including proptosis, hypertelorism, and periorbital swelling. Despite the changes seen in the bony architecture, however, tissue invasion by hyphae is not a feature seen with allergic fungal sinusitis.

In contrast to noninvasive fungal sinusitis, allergic fungal sinusitis has a relative paucity of fungal hyphae. Noninvasive fungal sinusitis, on the other hand, lacks the significant eosinophil response seen in allergic fungal sinusitis. The unresolved issue in allergic fungal sinusitis is whether the hyphae are simply saprophytes growing on inspissated mucus of a poorly drained paranasal sinus or are antigens that are crucial in the allergic process.[2]

NONINVASIVE

Noninvasive fungal sinusitis[28–40] may be defined as the presence of a mycellal mass that remains confined to the lumen of the sinus cavity for months or years; typically in the maxillary antrum of an immunocompetent patient. Clinical features include unilateral nasal obstruction and congestion; pressure sensation without pain; occasional facial swelling; and a gelatinous gray-green, oily rhinorrhea. Due to a fungal concrement acting as a foreign body, a local inflammatory response may accompany the mass. The clinical course may be punctuated by exacerbations of pain and fever during episodes of superimposed acute bacterial

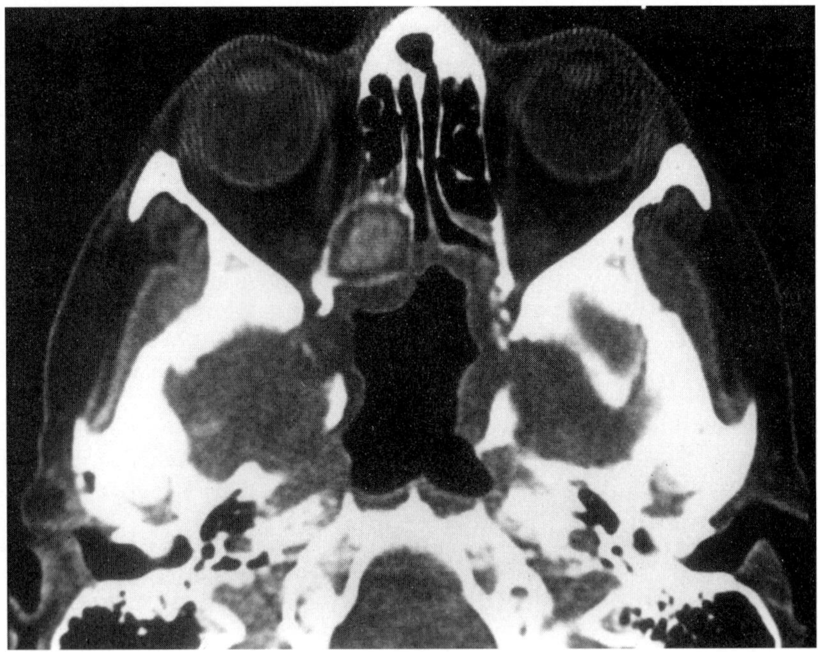

Fig. 9–3. This patient presented with unilateral periorbital headaches. This axial CT image demonstrates an enhancing allergic fungal mass involving a single right posterior ethmoid air cell.

sinusitis. The mechanism by which the mycelial mass predisposes to the intermittent episodes of bacterial sinusitis is probably obstruction of the natural sinus ostium.

Invasion is diagnosed by biopsy of the adjacent sinus mucosa. As with allergic fungal sinusitis, fungi do not invade the adjacent mucosa and bone; however, the presence of hyphae in superficial eptihelial layers may occur in noninvasive disease.

INVASIVE

Chronic invasive fungal sinusitis[41–67] is characterized by tissue invasion, often resulting in bone destruction with extension into the orbit or brain. Affected individuals may be immunocompetent, mildly immunocompromised (as by diabetes mellitus) or immunocompromised from other causes. Invasion can occur in immunologically normal individuals. However, this is rarely seen outside of the Sudan.[57] The course in these patients is not fulminant, as seen in the neutropenic host. The slowly progressive nature of this disease has been associated with chronic necrotizing pulmonary aspergillosis.[61]

The etiology of orbital and intracranial involvement are based on their anatomic proximity to the paranasal sinuses and the intrinsic ability of the fungus to cross local anatomic barriers. Fungi enter the sinuses initially through the nose. The maxillary sinus and the anterior ethmold are the most commonly involved areas. Less frequently, the mycotic process may extend to the posterior ethmoid, sphenoid, or even the frontal sinus.

Primary infection of the ethmoid labyrinth can erode laterally through the lamina, papyracea, displacing the eye, and resulting in either hyperteiorism or proptosis.[68] Extension of infection peripherally along the optic nerve posteriorly might give rise to an orbital apex syndrome,[2,45] a superior orbital fissure syndrome, or an orbital abscess.[45] Further extension through the superior orbital fissure may give rise to further complications involving the middle cranial fossa. Unlike acute bacterial sinusitis involving the orbit, subperiosteal abscesses are uncommon in fungal sinusitis. Superior extension from the ethmoid sinus can give rise to frontal lobe abscesses or cerebritis.

Primary infection of the maxillary may extend superiorly to involve the floor of the orbit giving rise to unilateral proptosis,[52,61] or extend inferiorly into the floor of the sinus into the hard palate.[48,62] It can extend laterally into the nasal turbinates and ethmoid sinuses. It may extend posteriorly into the pterygopalatine and, subsequently, into the infratemporal fossa.

In relation to the sphenoid sinus, erosion of the infection through its superior wall could lead to invasion of the sella turcica, whereas lateral wall invasion could result in unilateral blindness due to compression of the optic nerve or compression of the cavernous sinus and carotid artery leading to associated neurologic and vascular complications.[47,69] Posterior extension can involve the cilvus and brainstem as well.

Transversion of the chronic fungal infection through the posterior wall of the frontal sinus has initiated abscess formation in the frontal lobes.[41,43,68] Chronic fungal meningitis, an infection difficult to cure even with a prolonged course of amphotericin B, has resulted when meninges have been seeded by extension of fungal infection either from the frontal sinuses or from the sphenoid sinus.[2]

Aspergillus hyphae have been found to invade dura, blood vessel walls, and bone. Intracranial involvement can occur via several mechanisms: 1. thromboangiitis of the adjacent valveless veins by direct extension from the paranasal sinuses, 2. by a fungal aneurysm derived from hematogenous spread from infected sinuses, or, most commonly, 3. the fungus may involve the orbit, with subsequent extension into the intracranial cavity. *Aspergillus* may involve the internal carotid artery in its intracranial course, which may cause thrombosis or rupture with fatal hemorrhage.[67]

FULMINANT ASPERGILLUS SINUSITIS

Fulminant aspergillosis[68–84] proceeds as a rapidly progressive, gangrenous necrosis of the soft tissue and bony structures of the midface. Patients at risk are severely neutropenic, although occasionally steroid therapy or other causes of qualitative neutrophil dysfunction may be responsible. This illness often progresses rapidly and may not respond to aggressive medical and surgical interventions. Patients with immunoglobulin disorders are usually susceptible to fungal infections, but conditions causing neutropenia, or T-cell deficits, such as lymphomas and immunosuppressive therapy, AIDS, congenital immunodeficiencies, following bone marrow or solid organ transplants, recipients become predisposed to mucormycosis as well as to aspergillosis. These patients usually have defects in several components of their host defenses and are frequently hospitalized and treated with antibiotics and corticosteroids; therefore, they have an increased incidence of these infections.

The diagnosis of fulminant aspergillosis should be considered in any immunocompromised patient with nasal symptomatology. The earliest sign is spiking fevers associated with neutropenia. On physical examination, visual inspection of the face for erythema, edema, or discoloration is important. The eyes should be evaluated for proptosis, chemosis, oculomotor paresis, decreased visual acuity, and retinal engorgement. A hallmark feature identified upon nasal endoscopy is evidence of crusting, which may cover a paraesthetic region of gangrenous mucosa. Classically, these lesions have been described as initially involving the anterior aspect of the inferior turbinate; however, the location may vary considerably. The mouth should be evaluated as well for necrotic lesions of the hard palate.

A potassium hydroxide preparation from nasal crusts and biopsies of any underlying discoloration of the nasal mucous membrane may provide a rapid diagnosis. Antral irrigations are often unrewarding in either establishing a diagnosis or resolving an antral opacity found on radiographic examination.[69]

Antecedent antifungal therapy with amphotericin B does not preclude the development of aspergillus rhinosinusitis. The disease may be indolent for days or weeks, erupting only if the patient's neutrophil count fails to recover. In addition, fulminant sinusitis may resolve or occasionally remain as a chronically invasive disease, even when the patient becomes immunocompetent.[2]

Laboratory and Pathologic Findings

ALLERGIC FUNGAL SINUSITIS

In allergic aspergillosis sinusitis, immunologic assays—such as fungal antigen-specific IgE and IgG, total IgE, and precipitating antibodies—are useful to rule out other fungal diseases—such as fungus balls—and to document allergic fungal sinusitis. Patients with allergic aspergillosis sinusitis may demonstrate elevated serum IgE titers as well as a positive skin test with the *Aspergillus* antigen. In addition, serum IgE levels directed against *Aspergillus* are often elevated. Like the allergic bronchopulmonary aspergillosis patient, a hypersensitivity to the *Aspergillus* antigen, as shown by an immediate skin test reaction (type I) followed some hours later by an Arthus reaction (type III), occurs. The absolute eosinophil count is usually elevated. It should be noted that many fungi other than *Aspergillus,* such as *Cuevularia* and *Alternaria,* may also cause an allergic fungal sinusitis.[10]

Chest roentgenograms, pulmonary consultation, or both, may be indicated to rule out concurrent allergic bronchopulmonary fungal disease, although simultaneous allergic fungal disease of the sinuses and lungs is rare.[15] Finally, histopathologic examination of the tissues to look for allergic mucus (hyphae, eosinophils, Carcot-Leyden crystals), should be performed to rule out other fungal diseases.

NONINVASIVE

Although few immunologic studies have been performed on patients with fungus balls, repeated clinical observations documenting the lack of systemic or local abnormalities suggest that immunologic parameters are normal in patients with fungus balls. In spite of probable immunocompetence, there are often other predisposing factors, such as local tissue hypoxia or exposure of the host to a massive fungal load.[44]

The underlying problem in noninvasive and invasive fungal maxillary sinusitis may be obstruction within the narrow passages of the ostiomeatal complex as a result of chronic inflammation, allergy, or anatomic deformity. The fungal growth then begins on retained secretions within the affected sinus.

Endoscopic diagnosis of the affected sinus with noninvasive aspergillosis will typically reveal a buttery-soft to crumbly-hard fungal mass. At surgery, there can be severe inspissation of mucus that histologically resembles the mucoid impaction of allergic bronchopulmonary aspergillosis. Mycotic concretions may be encountered in the maxilloethmoid angle or in the ostium of the maxillary sinus. The mucous membrane lining the sinus may appear unremarkable if there is no inflammation, or it may demonstrate significant polypoid degeneration or acute superimposed bacterial inflammation.

Culture isolation from unfixed fungal material should be performed immediately to prevent excessive dehydration. Incubation at 37° C for 14 days on Sabouranud's agar with the use of an antibiotic to inhibit bacterial growth is performed. Culture results may be unreliable as hyphae are ubiquitous in the environment, including the clinical microbiology laboratory. Routine nasal and respiratory cultures of patients at risk may be helpful in establishing an early diagnosis of invasive aspergillosis. Blood cultures are invariably negative.

The only reliable means of confirming the diagnosis is the histologic demonstration of fungus in the inspissated material. In fixed tissue, hyphae can be seen readily with an hematoxylin and eosin (H & E) stain. Identification can also be made with silver stains: Gridley, PAS, and methemanine silver. *Aspergillus* can be identified by its smaller size, dichotomous branching and the 45° angle of the branches, and septated hyphae. Mucor is very rare in the noninvasive form of fungal sinusitis.[1]

INVASIVE

A number of different tests of immunologic function have been performed to assess abnormalities associated with chronic invasive fungal sinusitis, but the studies to date have failed to identify any consistent defects. The list of normal studies includes absolute neutrophil counts and monocyte counts, the percentage of mononuclear cells with positive staining for nonspecific esterase and myeloperoxidase, the phagocytic and fungicidal activity of peripheral blood monocytes against conidia, and such additional phagocyte functions as superoxide generation, chemiluminescence, nitroblue tetrazoolium reduction, and chemostaxis.[2,3,85,86]

In general, total lymphocyte counts and delayed-type hypersensitivity skin testing exhibit normal reactivity in these patients.[48,85,86] Serum concentration levels of immunoglobulin classes G, A, and M and complement studies have been normal, but total serum concentration of IgE may be elevated.[3,86] As of now, no definitive conclusion regarding the immunologic integrity of patients with chronic invasive fungal sinusitis has been made. However, the current literature seems to suggest that most patients with chronic invasive fungal sinusitis probably possess intact immunologic function.[3]

On gross pathologic examination, tissue invasion is a subjective finding of the involved soft tissue and bone at the time of surgery, usually characterized by hypertrophic or polypoid mucosa. The key diagnostic feature, however, is histopathologic identification of excised tissue showing hyphal fragments invading mucosa, submucosa, bone, or contiguous structures.[87,88] The number of invasive organisms may be extremely low, requiring a prolonged search for hyphae through numerous tissue sections stained with methenamine silver or periodic acid-Schiff. A Langhan's giant cell inflammatory response may be found adjacent to the infected soft tissue. Results of cultures performed without the inclusion of biopsied material may not be useful because heavy growth of a fungus from, for example, a sinus aspirate, may yield any airborne fungal contaminant.

Similar to noninvasive fungal sinusitis, one may find tenacious rubbery or putty-like material or greasy mucus in the sinus cavity. The material is usually brown or green and may be so thick and inspissated as to require curettage. It often has a foul odor, which may help to explain the cacosmia described by many patients. The surgeon may also find loss of bony integrity of the sinus wall, with softening detected by probing or friable bone noted during curettage.[87,88]

The differential diagnosis of invasive fungal sinusitis includes mucormycosis or lethal midline granuloma. Rhinocerebral mucormycosis may pursue a course almost identical with that of fulminant aspergillosis; however, it usually occurs in the clinical setting of diabetic acidosis and is characterized by the presence of broad nonseptate hyphae of phycomycetes in deep tissue stain. Other diseases to consider are neoplasms, chronic sinusitis with osteomyelitis, atrophic rhinitis, tuberculosis, lues, rhinoscleroma, and Wegener's granulomatosis.[38,53,56] Silver stains would differentiate these latter diagnostic categories from a fungal infection. Finally, the differential of bony erosion of the paranasal sinuses should include squamous cell carcinomas, inverting papillomas, meningiomas, schwannomas, and malignant melanomas.

Radiographic Findings

SINUS RADIOGRAPHS

Fungal sinus disease has been described as having nonspecific radiologic features of chronic maxillary sinusitis; i.e., nodular mucoperiosteal thickening, absence of air fluid levels, clouding of the ethmoid sinuses, as well as sinus wall destruction and focal increased attenuation on both plain radiolography and pluridirectional tomography. These characteristics, however, do not accurately differentiate between chronic sinusitis and neoplasia.[89]

Stammberger et al.[87,88] reported that increased attenuation seen on plain radiographs represents tertiary calcium phosphate and calcium sulfate deposits within necrotic areas of the mycelium. They reported that these focal areas of hyperattenuation were present on 50% of plain radiographs and pluridirectional tomographs. In half of these patients the increased attenuation was similar to that of a soft-tissue inflammatory mass; in the other half, discrete, very dense areas were observed.

CT

In allergic fungal sinusitis, rearrangement or erosion of bony barriers has been described, but histopathologic examination does not reveal tissue invasion. These bony changes are thought to reflect pressure remodeling, as may be seen with expansile mucoceles. Patchy areas of increased density, particularly in the presence of unilateral disease, is strongly suggestive of allergic fungal sinusitis. However, these focal areas are not uncommonly seen in patients with cystic fibrosis or patients with severe sinus disease associated with Samter's triad.

Noninvasive mycelial masses usually appear as an increased soft tissue density confined to one sinus. The maxillary sinus is most commonly involved; however, noninvasive fungal masses of the sphenoid sinus or frontal sinus have also been reported.[32,39] CT is more sensitive than standard radiography or pluridirectional tomography in depicting very dense opacities, which reflect calcium phosphate deposition in *Aspergillus* masses.[4]

CT is useful in delineating the extension of abnormal soft tissue densities into contiguous structures such as adjacent sinuses, orbit, brain, or sella tursica. Although this may suggest invasive disease, it may also represent an extension of an allergic fungal infection (see Fig. 9–3). There is no clear radiologic differentiating feature between noninvasive and invasive fungal disease on CT except with clear evidence of dural or periorbital involvement. In addition, the presence of multiple or diffuse areas of increased attenuation on an unenhanced CT scan strongly suggests invasive fungal involvement.

MRI

MRI imaging is even more sensitive than CT in identifying fungal disease. Preliminary studies by Zinreich et al.[89] have suggested that the ferromagnetic elements (iron, manganese, and calcium) within fungal concretions give a decreased signal intensity on T1 and very decreased signal intensity on T2-weighted MR images (Fig. 9–4). Occasionally a similar picture can be obtained from dense proteinacious inspissated secretions, although the MRI is a diagnostic adjunct to the CT. The inability of MRI to reveal bony details, however, has prevented this modality from replacing CT scanning for diagnostic imaging of fungal sinusitis.

In addition, MRI can provide crucial information in evaluating the extent of orbital involvement and in determining if intracranial masses are intradural or extradural. Contiguous extension of a primary process to the orbits, cavernous sinuses, infratemporal fossa, and pterygopalatine fossa and the brain can be more precisely delineated than with a CT scan.[3]

CT or MRI plays a critical role in the evaluation of *invasive* fungal sinusitis. In addition to providing information about the paranasal sinuses, these techniques reveal contiguous areas of critical importance, such as the orbits, the cavernous sinuses, and the brain. The results elucidate the extent of disease, help determine the best approach for diagnostic and/or therapeutic surgical intervention, and provide additional information regarding prognosis. It is important to realize, however, that neither the presence of bony erosion or bony expansion indicates invasion. Bone erosion may occur with noninvasive forms of fungal sinusitis, and the diagnosis of invasion can be made only with histologic evidence of fungus within the tissues. In cases where fungal disease is invasive

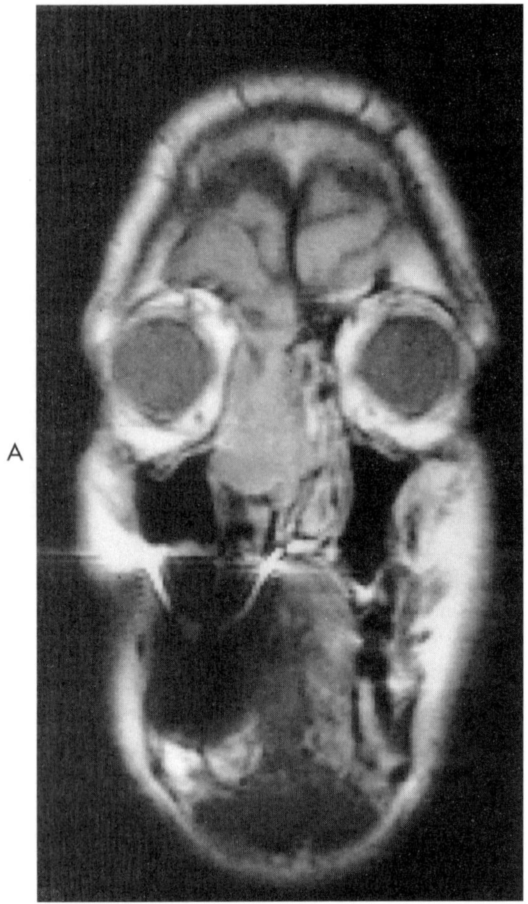

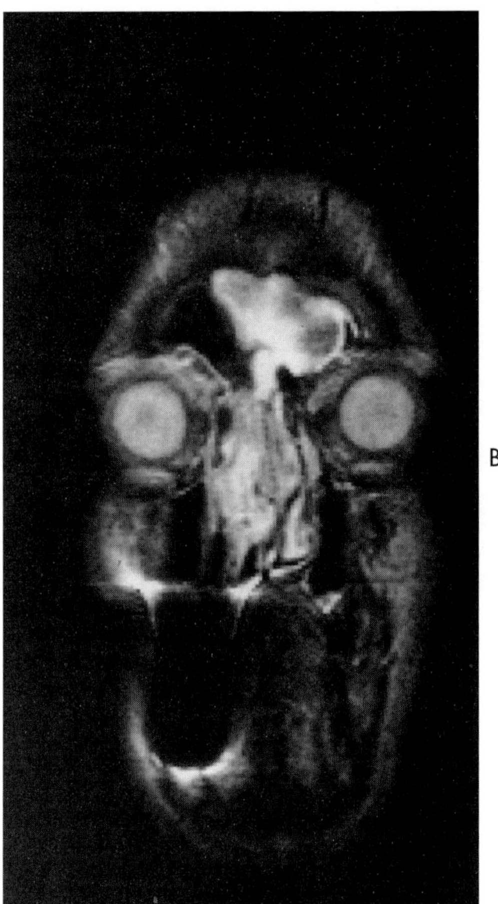

Fig. 9–4. **A,** This is a T1-weighted MRI scan of a 30-year-old woman with a chief complaint of right-sided nasal obstruction. Endoscopically, she had extensive right nasal polyps. This image demonstrates fungal involvement of the right frontal region. A low-intensity enhancement of the proteinaceous material of the fungal debris gives rise to the signal intensity seen on this image. **B,** A T2-weighted MRI scan for the same patient. Note that the fungal debris loses its signal intensity in the right frontal region to create a signal void. The nasal polys enhance in both T1 and T2 images.

or fulminant, it appears that bone offers a relatively poor barrier to the spread of disease and is frequently involved. However, dura and periorbita are more resistant to invasion. Thus, even when fungal disease is invasive, bony erosion of the skull base or lamina papyracea does not necessarily indicate significant dural involvement or involvement of the intraorbital contents.

Treatment

ALLERGIC FUNGAL SINUSITIS

Treatment of allergic fungal sinusitis requires the control of the polypoid disease with surgery; antibiotics; topical and, when necessary, systemic steroids. Surgical treatment consists of primary drainage and debridement of fungal debris and inspissated mucus to improve drainage of the involved sinuses with the use of the endoscopic technique. This also has the effect of reducing the antigenic fungal burden, which elicits the host response. Meticulous postoperative care with prolonged endoscopic follow-up is essential if the recurrence of disease is to be minimized.

Postoperative medical therapy with systemic steroids has been advocated by many authors.[8,9,16,26] Long-term topical nasal corticosteroids are a commonly employed treatment; however, recurrence rates are very high without the concomitant use of oral steroids, which are able to inhibit inflammatory antigen-antibody reactions and reduce sputum production. It is important to caution that steroid therapy can be confidently recommended only when vital structures such as the orbit and brain are not threatened and when careful histopathologic examination excludes the presence of tissue invasion.

There are no controlled studies that address the length of administration and dose necessary to achieve and maintain remission of disease. However, Allphin et al.[8] have achieved therapeutic success with prednisone 0.5 mg/kg for 2 weeks, followed by tapering dosages every other day for 3 months. Corey et al.[10] empirically derived a schedule that consists of prednisone 80 to 100 mg/day, tapered over several weeks to the lowest dose necessary to maintain a disease-free state, usually between 10 and 20 mg and as low as 2 to 5 mg. If possible, the dose is eventually tapered to an alternate day schedule. Patients should be evaluated closely during steroid therapy because there is a theoretical concern that even topical steroids could increase the likelihood of fungal invasion. Ideally, the steroids should be tapered and have the dosage adjusted based upon the endoscopic appearance of the ethmoid cavity.

Broad-spectrum antibiotic coverage may be required for a prolonged period following surgical intervention. It appears that there is frequently significant bony osteitis in this disorder, and it may take some time for residual inflammation to resolve. Because there is no evidence of colonization or tissue invasion, intravenous antifungal medications are not indicated.

Successful treatment should demonstrate a decrease in total and fungus-specific IgE, a decline in precipitin antibody levels, endoscopic resolution of sinonasal mucosal edema/polyps and fungal concretions, and an improvement in clinical symptoms.[17]

NONINVASIVE

Treatment of noninvasive fungal sinusitis is primarily accomplished with surgical debridement and adequate drainage. Neither systemic steroids nor local or systemic antifungal chemotherapy are required. Recurrence is infrequent, even during prolonged follow-up.[29–38,37–40]

Surgical management of the middle meatus is performed by standard endoscopic surgical techniques.[90] Operative findings may demonstrate complete fungal casts of the middle meatus, which have caused pressure necrosis of the natural ostium of the maxillary sinus. This may create a defect large enough to avoid any further surgical manipulation. A biopsy of the mycotic mass and the adjacent mucous membrane must always be obtained.[88] If the mycosis is noninvasive, the mucosa should be preserved. If there is evidence of osteitis, the patient should be placed on postoperative antibiotics.

The trocar, introduced through the canine fossa, offers several advantages in the management of maxillary sinus involvement. It can be used to break up hard masses or to manipulate fungal material from any antral wall. Biopsy forceps or the curved suction tip catheter can be used to remove mobilized debris directed toward the natural ostium. In addition, the trocar allows the use of variously angled endoscopes to provide full inspection of all corners of the sinus. Creating a wide middle meatal antrostomy may be necessary to remove completely the large casts of fungal debris. If removal of the fungal masses cannot be accomplished with this technique, or if there is reason to believe that fungal masses may be hiding behind polypoid hyperplastic mucosa, the maxillary sinus may occasionally have to be explored by a Caldwell-Luc procedure. Biopsy of the underlying mucosa is recommended if tissue invasion is a consideration. However, identification of fungus in only the superficial mucosal layers should not be taken as evidence of invasion.

Isolated fungal sinusitis of the sphenoid can be managed by removing its anterior wall and marsupializing the contents of the sphenoid anteriorly. There are limitations in the use of the endoscopic technique for the frontal sinus. If only the frontal recess and the area adjacent to the ostium is involved, it may be possible to remove fungal masses through the ostium. However, with more extensive involvement, i.e., lateral recesses of the frontal or total frontal sinus involvement as with invasive mycosis, an anterior external approach is indicated.[87,88]

INVASIVE

The treatment of invasive fungal sinusitis in both the immunocompromised and immunocompetent host is similar: surgery and antifungal agents. The distinction between invasive and fulminant disease is the occurrence of profound neutropenia, commonly associated with the latter entity, and the necessity for WBC transfusions. Due to the rapid morbidity associated with fulminant fungal sinusitis in the immunocompromised patient, aggressive treatment, using a high index of suspicion, must be instituted as soon as possible. No single modality has been proven adequate for patients with progressive fulminant fungal sinusitis during a persistent, severe neutropenia. Success depends upon both early treatment and recovery of adequate neutrophil counts.[51]

Wide surgical excision of bone and soft tissue in invasive and fulminant fungal sinusitis is required, especially if there is a delay in the reestablishment of functioning leukocytes in those patients with less than 500 cells/cu mm. All efforts should be made to preserve essential anatomic barriers, such as dura and orbital periosteum, if possible. These structures typically provide a good boundary to limit the further spread of infection, even when clinically involved with disease. After surgical debridement of diseased tissue, however, relapse may occur several times.[2] Surgical procedures become increasingly difficult due to distortion of normal anatomic landmarks by chronic infection or scar tissue, and some cases prohibit complete surgical resection. However, if an intracranial extension becomes well circumscribed and the location permits surgical removal, long-term cures can be achieved.[57]

Patients with greatly advanced disease may not be curable, and palliation may be the realistic goal in such cases. In those more fortunate patients whose diseased tissue can be surgically extirpated completely or almost completely and who receive a prolonged course of antifungal chemotherapy, a CT scan should be obtained approximately 1 month after surgery. The study should then be repeated every 3 or 4 months to look for early evidence of recurrence, such as new abnormal soft- tissue densities or loss of normal bony architecture.[2] This recommendation is based upon the suggestion that early intervention against small masses or recurrent disease is more effective than the later treatment of more extensive disease.

Several reported cases with careful long-term follow-up indicate patient relapse even after surgical debridement and prolonged courses of antifungal chemotherapy. These cases provide compelling evidence that a full course of amphotericin B, which is the present drug of choice in invasive aspergillosis, is indicated.

No thorough or prospective studies have been done relating dosage to outcome, and recommendations as to dosage are based mainly upon the ability of the patient to tolerate the drug. However, amphotericin is usually given as 2 to 4 gm IV over several weeks. The mechanism of action of amphotericin B on a molecular level is related to its combination with sterols in cell membranes, resulting in the leakage of potassium from susceptible cells. Subsequently, larger molecules, such as nucleic acids, are also lost, and the cells die. Cells need not be in the growing phase to be affected. Fisher[91] suggests that AmB does not greatly influence the course of aspergillosis in leukemia and that the outcome is related much more to granulocytopenia and underlying disease processes. Early diagnosis is essential in the hope of obtaining adequate control with AmB, perhaps even with the use of empirical therapy in neutropenic patients with later confirmation of the diagnosis.

Amphotericin B administration almost always causes toxicity. Thrombophlebitis, chills, fever, headache, and nausea and vomiting are frequent acute side effects. Long-term reactions include hypokalemia, nephrotoxicity, bone marrow suppression, and ototoxicity. Amphotericin B is probably fungistatic rather than fungicidal at the concentrations that can be safely obtained clinically. Because of the limitations imposed by the toxicity, efforts are under way to modify the polyene macrolides to retain the same effectiveness while reducing the side effects.[65] Ribosomal amophotericin is now available in Europe. The high risk of relapse has prompted clinicians to follow the initial intensive period of antifungal chemotherapy with a prolonged course of oral therapy with an agent such as ketoconazole or itraconazole. The long-term stability of several reported patients treated in this manner supports this approach.[2]

Use of white blood cell (WBC) transfusions in invasive aspergillosis in neutropenic patients has not been studied in a controlled fashion, but some data suggest their efficacy.[80,92] The rationale for WBC transfusion is reasonable, given the central role of quantitative and qualitative neutrophil disorders in the pathogenesis of invasive aspergillosis.[81] It acts as a holding strategy aimed at providing the patient's bone marrow with time to recover, at least partially. Without endogenous WBC production in adequate numbers, the patient's prognosis is bleak. However, transfusions are time-consuming, costly, and sometimes associated with adverse reactions, including noncardiogenic pulmonary edema in patients concurrently or subsequently starting AmB therapy. WBCs have at least some role in patients not responding to maximal antifungal therapy and aggressive surgery. However, transfusions should be instituted without delay, before the patient is beyond saving.[81]

The most realistic goal in some patients who fail to benefit from multiple therapeutic maneuvers is palliation. For those more fortunate patients whose diseased tissues can be removed completely or almost completely and who then receive a generous course of antifungal therapy, CT should be performed approximately 1 month after surgery as a baseline examination followed by repeat studies every 3 to 4 months to look for new soft-tissue densities, loss of bony architecture, or abnormal tissue in contiguous structures. Early reintervention directed against a small burden of infected tissue seems to exert more clinical impact than later measures aimed at more extensive disease.

REFERENCES

1. Haines JH, Salkin IF. The biology and identification of fungal aeroallergens. In: Settipane GA, ed. *Rhinitis,* 2nd ed. Rhode Island: OceanSide Publications; 1991 p 63–75.
2. Washburn RG, Kennedy DW, Begley MG, et al. Chronic fungal sinusitis in apparently normal hosts. *Medicine* 1988; 67(4):231–247.
3. Washburn RG. Chronic fungal sinusitis in the nonimmunocompromised host. In Sinusitis; p 205–226, 1994.
4. Stammberger H, Jakse R, Beaufort F. Aspergillosis of the paranasal sinuses. X-ray diagnosis, histopathology, and clinical aspects. *Ann Otol Rhinol Laryngol.* 1984: 93:251–256.
5. Johnson JT. Infections. In: Cummings CW, Fredrickson JM, Harder LA, Krause CJ, Schuller DE, eds. *Otolaryngology-Head and Neck Surgery,* 2nd ed., Mosby-Year Book; 1993: p 931.
6. Mahgoub ES. Mycosis of the Sudan. *Trans Soc Trop Med Hyg* 1977: 71:184–88.
7. Adam RD, Paquin ML, Petersen EA, et al. Phaeohyphomycosis caused by the fungal genera Bipolaris and Exserohilum: a report of nine cases and review of the literature. *Medicine.* 1986; 65:203–217.
8. Allphin AL, Strauss M, Abdul-Karim FW. Allergic fungal sinusitis: problems in diagnosis and treatment. *Laryngoscope.* 1991; 101:815–20.
9. Bartynski JM, McCaffrey TV, Frigas E. Allergic fungal sinusitis secondary to dematiaceous fungi—Curvularia lunata and Altrenaria. *Otolaryngol Head Neck Surg.* 1990;103:32–39.
10. Corey JP. Allergic fungal sinusitis, *Otol Clin No Am.* 1992, 25:225–230.
11. Friedman GC, Hartwick RW, Ro JY, et al. Allergic fungal sinusitis. Report of three cases associated with dematiaceous fungi. *Am J Clin Pathol.* 1991; 96:368–72.
12. Goldstein MF, Atkins PC, Cogen FC, et al. Allergic *Aspergillus* sinusitis. *J Allergy Clin Immunol.* 1985;76:515–24.
13. Gourley DS, Shisman BA, Jorgensen NL, et al. Allergic bipolaris sinusitis: clinical and immunopathologic characteristics. *J Allergy Clin Immunol* 1990;85:583–591.
14. Hartwick RW, Batsakis JG. Sinus aspergillosis and allergic fungal sinusitis. *Ann Otol Rhinol Laryngol.* 1991;100:427–430.
15. Jonathan D, Lund V, Milroy C. Allergic aspergillus sinusitis—an overlooked diagnosis? *J Laryngol Otol.* 1989;103:1181–1183.
16. Katzenstein AI, Sale SR, Greenberger PA. Allergic aspergillus sinusitis: a newly recognized form of sinusitis. *J Allergy Clin Immunol.* 1983;2:89.
17. Loury MC, Leopold DA, Schaefer SD. Allergic aspergillus sinusitis. *Arch Otolaryngol Head Neck Surg.* 1993;119:1042–1043.
18. Macmillan RH, Cooper PH, Body BA, Mills AS. Allergic fungal sinusitis due to Curvularia lunata. *Hum Pathol.* 1987;18:960–964.
19. Manning SC, Schaefer SD, Close LG, Vultcyh F. Culture-positive allergic fungal sinusitis. *Arch Otolaryngol Head Neck Surg.* 1991;117;174.
20. Shah A, Khan ZU, Chaturvedi S, et al. Concomitant allergic *Aspergillus* sinusitis and allergic bronchopulmonary aspergillosis associated with familial occurrence of allergic bronchopulmonary aspergillosis. *Ann Allergy* 1990;64: 507–512.
21. Sher TH, Schartz HJ. Allergic *Aspergillus* sinusitis with concurrent allergic bronchopulmonary *Aspergillus:* report of a case. *J Allergy Clin Immunol.* 1988;81:844–846.
22. Slavin RG, Bedrossian CS, Hutcheson PS, et al. A pathologic study of allergic bronchopulmonary aspergillosis. *J Allergy Clin Immunol.* 1988;81:178–125.
23. Sobol SM, Love RG, Stutman HR, Pysher TJ. Phaeohyphomycosis of the maxilloethmoid sinus caused by Drechsiera spicifera: a new fungal apthogen. *Laryngoscope.* 1984;94:620–627.
24. Ravis WD, Kwon-Chung KJ, Kleiner DE, et al. Unusual aspects of allergic bronchopulmonary fungal disease: Report of two cases due to Curvularia organisms associated with allergic fungal sinusitis. *Hum Pathol.* 1991;22:1240–1248.
25. Rosenberg M, Patterson R, Mintzer R, et al. Clinical and immunologic criteria for the diagnosis of allergic broncopulmonary aspergillosis *Ann Intern Med.* 1977;86:405–413.
26. Waxman JE, Spector JG, Sale SR, Katzenstein AA. Allergic *aspergillus* sinusitis: concepts in diagnosis and treatment of a new clinical entity. *Laryngoscope.* 1987;97:261–266.
27. Zieske LA, et al. Dematiaceous fungal sinusitis. *Otolaryngol Head Neck Surg.* 1991;104(4):567–577.
28. Axelsson H, Carisll B, Welbring J, Winblad B. Aspergillosis of the maxillary sinus. *Acta Otolaryngol.* 1978;86:303–308.
29. Catalano P, Lawon W, Bottone E, Lebenger J. Basidiomycetous (Muschroom) infection of the maxillary sinus. *Otolaryngol Head Neck Surg.* 1990:102:183–185.
30. Horton WD, Osguthorpe JD. CT findings in sphenoid sinus aspergillosis. *Otol Head Neck Surg.* 1989;100:606–609.
31. Kopp W, Fotter R, Steiner H, Aspergillosis of the paranasal sinuses. *Radiology* 1985;156:715–716.
32. Lavelle WG. Aspergillosis of the sphenoid sinus. *ENTJ* 1988;67:266–269.
33. Levine PA, Yanagisawa E. Aspergillosis of the maxillary sinus. *Arch Otolaryngol.* 1977;103:560–563.
34. McGinnis MR, Buck DL, Katz B. Paranasal aspergilloma caused by an albino variant of *Aspergillus* fumigatus. *So Med J.* 1977;70:886–888.
35. Nishioka G, Schwartz JG, Rinaldi MG, et al. Fungal maxillary sinusitis caused by Curvularia lunata. *Arch Otolaryngol Head Neck Surg.* 1987;113:665–666.
36. Pena CE. Aspergillus intranasal fungus ball. *Am J Clin Pathol.* 1975;64:343–344.
37. Rockhill RC, Klein MD. Paecliomyces illacinus as the cause of chronic maxillary sinusitis. *J Clin Microbiol.* 1980;11:737–739.
38. Rommet JUL, Newman RK. Aspergillosis of the nose and paransal sinuses. *Laryngoscope.* 1982;92:764–768.
39. Simmons BP, Johnson G, Abar RC. Fungus ball of the sphenoidal sinus in an immunocompetent host. *So Med J* 1982;75:762–764.
40. Stevens MH, Aspergillosis of the frontal sinus. *Arch Otolaryngol.* 1978;104:153–156.
41. Ahuja GK, Jain N, Vijayaraghoyan M, Roy S. Cerebral mycotic aneurysm of the fungal origin. *J Neurosurg.* 1978;49:107–110.
42. Bassloumy A, Maher A, Bucci TJ, et al. Noninvasive antromycosis. *J Laryngol Otol.* 1982;96:215–228.
43. Brown JW, Nadell J, Sanders CV, Sardenga L. Brain abscess caused by Cladosporium trichoids (Bantianum): A case with paranasal sinus involvement. *So Med J.* 1976;69:1519–1521.
44. Corey JP, Romberger CF, Shaw GY. Fungal diseases of the sinuses. *Otolaryngol Head Neck Surg.* 1990;103:1012–1015.

45. Crivelli G, Riviera LC. Unilateral blindness from aspergilloma at the right optic foramen. *J Neurosurg.* 1970;33:207–211.
46. Dykean ME, Biller J, Yuh WT, et al. Carotid-cavernous sinus thrombosis caused by *Aspergillus fumigatus:* magnetic resonance imaging with pathologic correlation—a case report, *J Vasc Dis.* 1990;652–656.
47. Fuchs HA, Evans RM, Gregg CR. Invasive aspergillosis of the sphenoid sinus manifested as a pituitary tumor. *So Med J.* 1985;78:1365—1367.
48. Garau J, Diamond RD, Lagrotteria LB, Kabins SA. Altemaria osteomyelitis. *Ann Intern Med.* 1977;86:747–748.
49. Green WR, Font RL, Zimmerman LE. Aspergillosis of the orbit. *Arch Ophthmal.* 1969;82:302–313.
50. Harpster WH, Gonzalez C, Opal SM. Pansinusitis caused by the fungus Dreschslera. *Otolaryngol Head and Neck Surg.* 1985;93:683–685.
51. Holt GR, Stadefer JA, Brown WE, Gates GA. Infectious diseases of the sphenoid sinus. *Laryngoscope.* 1984; 94:330–335.
52. Hora JF. Primary aspergillosis of the paranasal sinuses and associated areas. *Laryngoscope.* 1965;75:768–773.
53. Jahrsdoerer RA, Ejercito VS, Johns ME, et al. Aspergillosis of the nose and paranasal sinuses. *Am J Otol.* 1979;1:6–14.
54. Killingsworth SM, Wetmore SJ. Curvularia/Drechslera sinusitis. *Laryngoscope.* 1990;100:932–937.
55. Lew D, Southwick FS, Montgomery WW, et al. Sphenoid sinusitis. A review of 30 cases. *N Engl J Med.* 1983;309:1149–1154.
56. McGuirt WF, Harrill JA. Paranasal sinus aspergillosis. *Laryngoscope.* 1979;89:1563–1568.
57. Milosev B, Mahgoub ES, Aal OA, El Hassan AM. Primary aspergilloma of the paranasal sinuses in the Sudan. *Br J Surg.* 1969;56:132–137.
58. Morgan MA, Wilson WR, Neel B, Roberts GD. Fungal sinustis in healthy and innumocompromised individuals. *Am J Clin Pathol.* 1984;82:597–601.
59. Pingree TF, Holt R, Otto RA, Rinaldi MG. Bipolaris-caused fungal sinusitis. *Otolaryngol Head Neck Surg.* 1992;106:302–305.
60. Rolston KVI, Hopfer RL, Larson DL. Infections caused by Drechslera species. Case report and review of the literature. *Rev Inffect Dis.* 1985;7:525–529.
61. Sandison AT, Genties JC, Davidson CM, Branko M. Aspergilloma of the paranasal sinuses and the orbit in northern Sudanese. *Sabouraudia.* 1969;6:57–69.
62. Shuger MA, Montgomery WW, Hyslop NE. Alternarela sinusitis. *Ann Otol Rhinol Laryngol.* 1981;90:251–254.
63. Shugar MA. Mycotic infections of the nose and paranasal sinuses. In: Goldman JC, ed. *The Principles and Practice of Rhinology.* John Wiley and Sons; 1987:38–39, 717–734.
64. Stamm MA, Frable MA. Invasive sinusitis due to *Pseudallescheria boydii* in an immunocompetent host. *So Med J.* 1992;85:439–441.
65. Stevens MH. Primary fungal infections of the paranasal sinuses. *Am J Otolaryngol.* 1981;2:348–357.
66. Warder FR, Chikes PG, Hudson WR. Aspergillosis of the paranasal sinuses. *Arch Otolaryngol.* 1975;101:683–685.
67. Weinstein M, Theron J, Newton TH. Aspergillosis involving the sphenoid sinus. *Neuroradiology.* 1976;11:137–139.
68. Lowe J, Bradley J. Cerebral and orbital *Aspergillus* infection due to invasive aspergillosis of the ethmoid sinus. *J Clin Pathol.* 1986;39:774–778.
69. McGill TJ, Simpson G, Healy GB. Fulminant aspergillosis of the nose and paranasal sinuses: a new clinical entity. *Laryngoscope.* 90;748–754.
70. Berlinger NT. Sinusitis in immunodeficient and immunosuppressed patients. *Laryngoscope.* 1985;95:29–33.
71. Corey JP, et al. Otolaryngology problems in the immune compromised patient. An evolving natural history. *Otolaryngol Head Neck Surg.* 1991;104:196–203.
72. Couch L. Rhinocerebral mucomycosis with cerebral extension successfully treated with adjunctive hyperbaric oxygen therapy. *Arch Otolaryngol Head Neck Surg.* 1988;114:791–794.
73. Denning DW, Stevens DA. Antifungal and surgical treatment of invasive aspergillosis, *Rev Inf Dis.* 1990;12:1147–1201.
74. Dyken ME, Biller J, Yuh WT, et al. Carotid-cavernous sinus thrombosis caused by *Aspergillus fumigatus:* Magnetic resonance imaging with pathologic correlation—a case report. *J Vasc Dis.* 1990;652–656.
75. Eisenberg L, et al. Mucormycosis. *Laryngoscope.* 1977;87:347–356.
76. Finn DC, Farmer JC. Chronic mucomycosis. *Laryngoscope.* 1982;92:761–766.
77. Kavanagh KT, Parham DM, Hughes WT, Chanin LR. Fungal sinusitis in immunocompromised children with neoplasms. *Ann Otol Rhinol Laryngol.* 1991;100:331–336.
78. Ouchi JW, et al. rhinocerebral mucomycosis: Results of aggressive surgical debridement and amphotericin B. *Laryngoscope.* 1988;98:1339–1342.
79. Pames LS, et al. Mycotic sinusitis: A management protocol. *J Otol.* 1989;18:176–180.
80. Swerdlow B, Derensinski S. Development of *Aspergillus* sinusitis in a patient receiving amphotericin B. *Am J Med.* 1984;76:162–168.
81. Talbot GH, Huang A, Proencher M. Invasive *Aspergillus* rhinosinusitis in patients with acute leukemia. *Rev Infect Dis.* 1991;13:219–232.
82. Viollier AF, Peterson DE, DeJongh CA, et al. *Aspergillus* sinusitis in cancer patients. *Cancer.* 1986;58:366–371.
83. Weingarten JS, Crockett DM, Lusk RP. Fulminant aspergillosis: early cutaneous manifestation of the disease process in the immunocompromised host. *Otolaryngol Head Neck Surg.* 1987;97:495–499.
84. Wiatrak BJ, et al. Functional endoscopic sinus surgery in the immunocompromised child. *Otoloryngol Head Neck Surg.* 1991;105:818–825.
85. Berry AJ, Kerkering TM, Giordano AM, Chiancone J. Phaeohyphomycotic sinusitis. *Pediatr Infect Dis.* 1984;3:150–152.
86. Frenkel L, Kuhls TL, Nitta K, et al. Recurrent bipolaris sinusitis following surgical and antifungal therapy. *Pediatr Infect Dis J.* 1987;6:1130–1132.
87. Stammberger H. Endoscopic surgery for mycotic and chronic recurring sinusitis. *Ann Otol Rhinol Laryngol.* 1985;94(suppl 119):1–11.
88. Stammberger H. Special problems. In Stammberger H, BC Decker; ed. *Functional Endoscopic Sinus Surgery.* Philadelphia, 1991;398–427.
89. Zinreich SJ, Kennedy DW, Malat J, et al. Fungal sinusitis: diagnosis with CT and MR imaging. *Radiology.* 1988;169:439–444.
90. Kennedy DW. Functional endoscopic sinus surgery technique. *Arch Otolaryngol Head Neck Surg.* 1985;111:643–649.
91. Fisher BD, Armstrong D, Yu B, Gold JWM. Invasive aspergillosis. Progress in early diagnosis and treatment. *Am J Med.* 1981;71:571–577.
92. Goering P, Berlinger NT, Weisdorf DJ. Aggressive combined modality treatment of progressive sinonasal fungal infections in immunocompromised patients. *Am J Med.* 1988;85:619–623.

10

Cerebrospinal Fluid Fistula and Endoscopic Sinus Surgery

James A. Stankiewicz

Cerebrospinal fluid (CSF) fistula most commonly occurs as a result of trauma, either as an accident or after surgical intervention. It is much less common for CSF fistula to be congenital or spontaneous. The treatment of CSF fistula of the nose and paranasal sinuses is greatly enhanced utilizing endoscopic sinus surgery techniques.[1–6] Presented in this chapter is a systematic way of diagnosing and treating nasal and sinus CSF fistula.

Anatomic Considerations

The cribriform plate is lower and thicker than the fovea ethmoidalis and is perforated with small fissures through which the olfactory nerve endings pass. The middle turbinate separates the cribriform plate from the fovea ethmoidalis and, laterally, can often be continuous with the fovea ethmoidalis, especially in the area of the anterior and middle ethmoid. The anterior and middle lateral fovea ethmoidalis, which joins the orbital bone, slopes downward like one side of a peaked roof until it joins the middle turbinate medially. At this point the fovea ethmoidalis and upper middle turbinate are superior to the cribriform.

This anatomy must be understood, for its violation will result in a CSF fistula. The dura at this level is very adherent to the cribriform plate and fovea ethmoidalis. Therefore, if the bone is penetrated, chances are excellent that a CSF fistula will occur. The lateral cribriform plate is easily fractured and, in the area of the anterior ethmoid artery (AEA), has a tendency for chip fractures.[5] In fact, the point where the anterior ethmoidal artery leaves the ethmoid to enter the olfactory fossa is the place of least resistance in the entire anterior skull base. Note that this is medial to the middle turbinate. The admonishment that the traditional, microscopic, or endoscopic surgeon must not operate medial to the middle turbinate is well known and should be respected.

The surgeon must not operate superiorly and medially in the fovea ethmoidalis against or into the middle turbinate, especially anterior to and around the area of the anterior ethmoid artery. This area is likewise thin and easily perforated. Stammberger points out that the bone in this vicinity is 10 times thinner than the lateral fovea ethmoidalis.[7] Disease in this area is better left alone than tampered with unless the surgeon is exceptionally familiar with the anatomy (Fig. 10–1).

The anterior fossa starts from the posterior wall of the frontal sinus where the lateral fovea ethmoidalis is present after draining the frontal recess

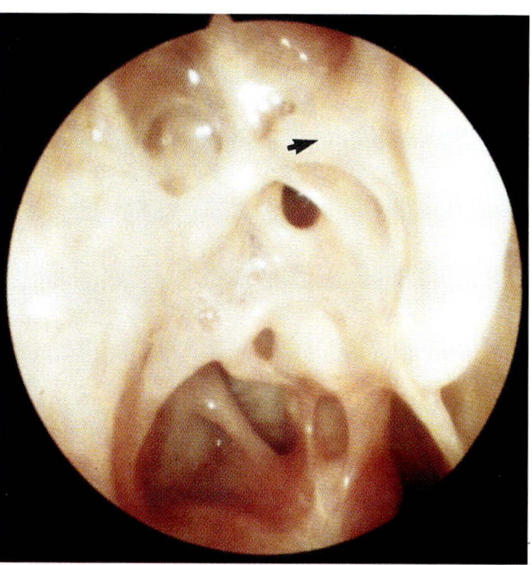

Fig. 10–1. Picture of skull base and anterior ethmoid artery adjacent to the middle turbinate where it is thinnest. (*arrow*)

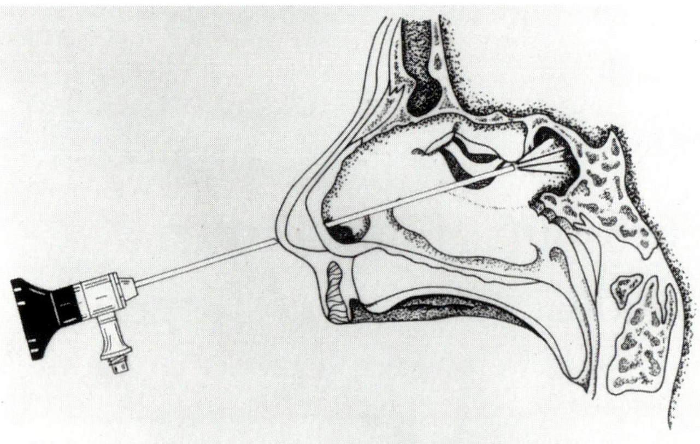

Fig. 10–2. Lateral skull drawing showing how skull base slopes downward the more posterior the surgeon operates. (From Stankiewicz JA: Cerebrospinal fluid fistula and endoscopic sinus surgery. *Laryngoscope*. 101:250–256, 1991. By permission.)

anteriorly. It is here just above the bulla ethmoidalis and sinus lateralis that the fovea is at its lowest point. It then gently slopes upward to meet with the skull base just above the sphenoid sinus. At its lowest point, injury to the ethmoid roof is possible and increases as the surgeon moves medially as described (Fig. 10–2).

The base of the skull just posterior to the AEA, especially medially, is a continuation of this area of weakness that may be further compromised by disease. In cases of extensive disease, especially with loss of landmarks, it is helpful to find first the sphenoid sinus, base of the skull, and dome of the ethmoid (moving posterior to anterior). The bone of the anterior sphenoid wall is usually very thin and is perforated easily. Hard bone is apparent just superior to this on the base of skull between the sphenoid opening and the anterior ethmoid artery.

If force is necessary to perforate what is felt to be the anterior sphenoid wall, chances are the surgeon is in the wrong place. As a general rule, the anterior sphenoid wall is found in a plane between the top of the inferior turbinate and the lower middle turbinate as one moves back posteriorly.

It is important to realize that all areas of anatomy may be compromised by the disease process, creating an even more treacherous situation.

The sphenoid sinus can be an area of CSF leak during endoscopic sinus surgery, especially if too much surgical effort is directed at the superior sphenoid sinus. Also as a result of neurosurgical procedures, such as hypophysectomy or skull base surgery, the sphenoid and posterior ethmoid sinuses can be the location of CSF fistula. It is important to note the posterior lateral position of the carotid artery and the superior lateral position of the optic nerve prior to any attempt at closure. In addition, the clivus sits just posterior to the sphenoid sinus, and clival lesions can be biopsied endoscopically with the potential for CSF fistula.

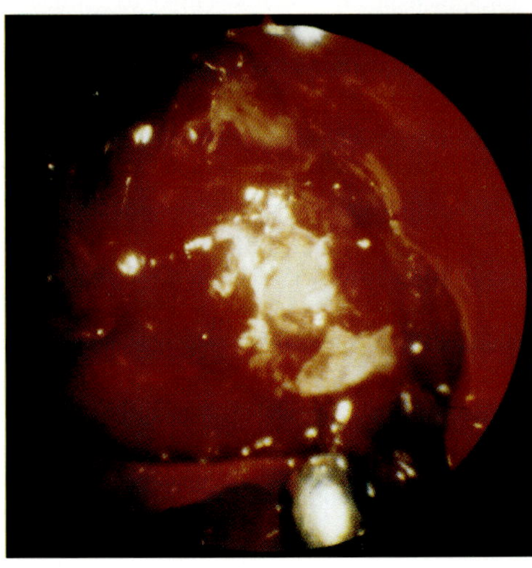

Fig. 10–3. A CSF leak as it occurred during surgery. Note the "Washout" sign with the dura clean of blood secondary to CSF.

Diagnosis

The diagnosis of CSF fistula is not difficult to make when it is seen during the course of nasal or sinus surgery (Fig. 10–3). Obviously microscopic or telescopic surgery is the best means of identifying the CSF fistula. CT scanning with intrathecal dye (omniopaque) is only of benefit if an active leak is present (Fig. 10–4). A slow or intermittent leak may not be located. Most cases of CSF fistula during sinus surgery occur under a general anesthetic due to loss of sensitivity and pain at the skull base. With skilled surgeons, these CSF fistu-

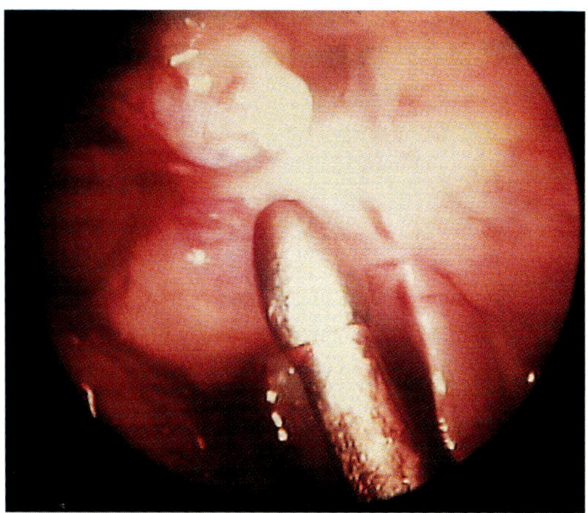

Fig. 10–4. CT scan of an active CSF fistula in the sphenoid sinus (just above suction tip).

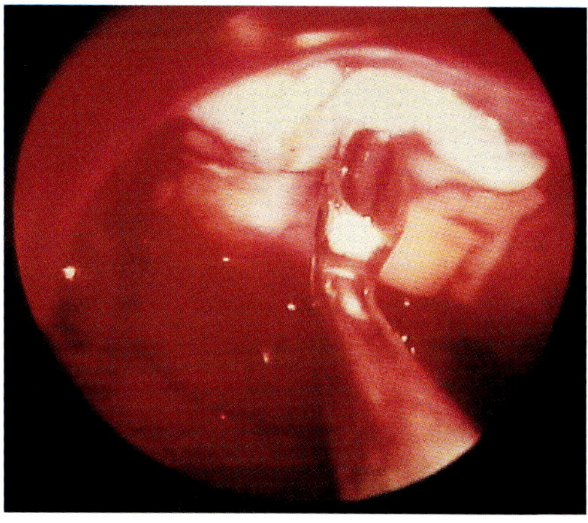

Fig. 10–5. Fluorescein dye just below an intrasphenoid CSF fistula. Note green color to either side of elevator instrument.

lae probably occur in about 1 in every 200 to 500 cases. General anesthesia, however, can aid in the diagnosis of immediate or delayed CSF fistula. When a small fistula barely leaks, its radiologic identification is difficult. Under general anesthesia, the anesthesiologist can valsalva the patient, creating increased CSF pressures and causing an increase in the CSF flow, thus allowing detection. If a lumbar tap or drain is in place, air or diluted fluorescein can be injected intrathecally permitting better endoscopic visualization of the fistula. Fluorescein is diluted by using 0.1 to 0.2 ml of 5% fluorescein for injection mixed with 5 to 10 ml of CSF. Intrathecal air will allow visualization of the leak almost immediately, whereas fluorescein may take 20 to 30 minutes (Fig. 10–5).

For delayed or spontaneous CSF fistula, endoscopic exam with or without fluorescein may greatly enhance isolation of the leak. It is important that not only the ethmoid and cribriform plate be visualized but also the sphenoethmoid recess and eustachian tube. Radiology studies such as MRI or CT scan with injection of omniopaque can help isolate the area of an active leak. The drainage area of the posterior ethmoid sinus laterally to the superior turbinate is not routinely viewed and could be a key area. Patients who have had extensive sinus or skull base surgery have most identifying landmarks removed but still require that the anatomy be viewed over and around scarring and recurrent disease.

Nuclear medicine scanning with pledgets inserted into all areas of potential leak may also be helpful. It should be noted that for these studies to be abnormal, readings should be impressively high. Borderline or slightly elevated readings are not reliable.

The timing of CSF leak is important. Intraoperative leaks should be repaired immediately. Delayed fistulae, if constant and unresponsive to conservative treatment, should be repaired within 1 to 2 weeks after diagnosis. Intermittent CSF fistulae, which persist despite conservative treatment, should be repaired within 3 to 4 weeks after diagnosis. Remember that leaks associated with sinus surgery occur in a contaminated area, and the risks of meningitis are greater than in a congenital or traumatic situation. Antibiotics can be helpful in patients with sinusitis and CSF leak to help prevent meningitis, though they are not recommended for a congenital or traumatic CSF fistulae to avoid resistant organisms.

Technique

GENERAL INFORMATION

The patient can have the fistula closed under a local or general anesthetic. In our series, all patients were under general anesthesia. The graft materials can include fascia lata, temporalis fascia, septal or turbinate mucosa, muscle, or fat. Hydroxyapatite, when available, may turn out to be the material of choice for closure. Appropriate preparation of an extra nasal graft site from which fascia, fat, and muscle can be taken is necessary. All removed graft material should be kept moist.

A lumbar drain is an option that should be considered. In general, a patient with a fresh fistula probably does not need a lumbar drain because no hypersecretion of CSF is present. A patient with a longstanding fistula has increased the amount of CSF produced to compensate for that which is lost. Unless a drain is used in this patient, an overabundance of CSF will be collected intranasally that will put pressure on any repair, increasing the risk of failure. Any lumbar drain has to be monitored extremely closely to avoid draining off too much CSF, which might be fatal. The physicians involved with the patient's immediate care should perform the drainage. Lumbar drains too aggressively drained may also result in a very uncomfortable headache with nausea and/or vomiting. A lumbar drain or spinal tap during the original repair of the fistulae may also allow for on-the-spot removal of as little as 30 cc of CSF, which can reduce brain herniation apparent through a large defect. This is absolutely necessary when closing a large defect or encephalocele from the nasal side. Fluorescein or air can be injected intrathecally, not only to aid in localization of a CSF fistula but also to allow assessment of the quality of closure.

Fibrin glue is made up by combining topical thrombin and 10% calcium chloride in a separate syringe and mixing this combination simultaneously with cryoprecipitate. This tissue glue nicely helps to hold the grafts in position.[3] An Avitene® slurry, Avitene® mixed with saline in a syringe, is also helpful for this purpose.[6]

CRIBRIFORM/FOVEA ETHMOIDALIS FISTULA

Cribriform plate fistulae are not as common as medial fovea ethmoidalis fistulae. Most CSF fistulae occur as a result of penetration of the skull base where the fovea ethmoidalis and middle turbinate merge. This area is higher than the cribriform plate and is associated with the anterior ethmoid artery. As mentioned before, the skull base, especially around the anterior ethmoid artery, is very thin and can be easily penetrated. The most important consideration of endoscopic CSF fistula repair is exposure. If the septum is deviated to such an extent that it compromises exposure, septoplasty is necessary. If the middle turbinate is large or prevents exposure, it should be removed as needed. The middle turbinate mucosa and bone can be stripped and used as a graft. In some instances, the remnant of the middle turbinate may be positioned as a flap to enhance closure, but is not necessary. Likewise, septal cartilage or bone may be useful in helping to correct a large defect with a fistula such as encephalocele. Angled telescopes are most helpful in visualizing the area of leak. Any debris or blood clot should be removed from the wound. The dura is usually very adherent to bone in this area and cannot be elevated. Dural elevation is best left alone to prevent further tearing or other CSF fistulae. Because of the adherence of the dura, it is difficult to tuck the graft between the skull base and dura, and, in most cases, this is not necessary. A large defect closure with brain herniation is enhanced with removal of CSF to allow the brain to shrink and to permit insertion of bone graft covered by mucosa. If the leak is a small one, a muscle or fat plug dipped in fibrin glue, if possible, is placed first to close the hole. The fibrin glue coated fascial patch is then placed over this plug. A second fascia, muscle, septal, or turbinate flap can then be placed to support the grafts. Gelfoam is layered in place. Lastly, a nasal trumpet is trimmed so it does not reach the oropharynx and is put into the nasal cavity as a bolster. A large defect or encephalocele defect created after removal should be bone grafted if possible. Then the closure proceeds in the same fashion as for smaller fistulae, as noted (Figs. 10–6 and 10–7).

A
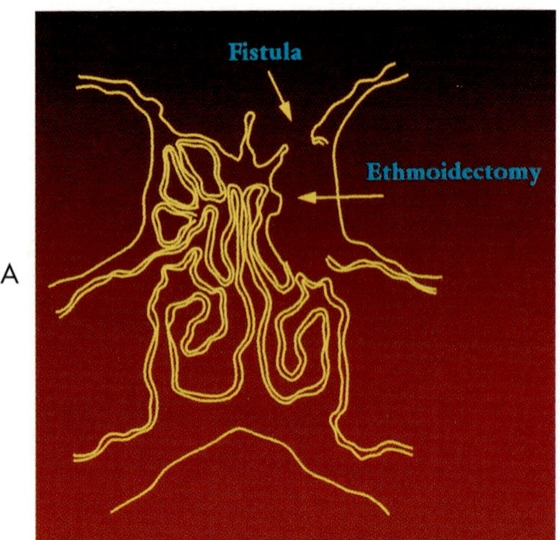

B
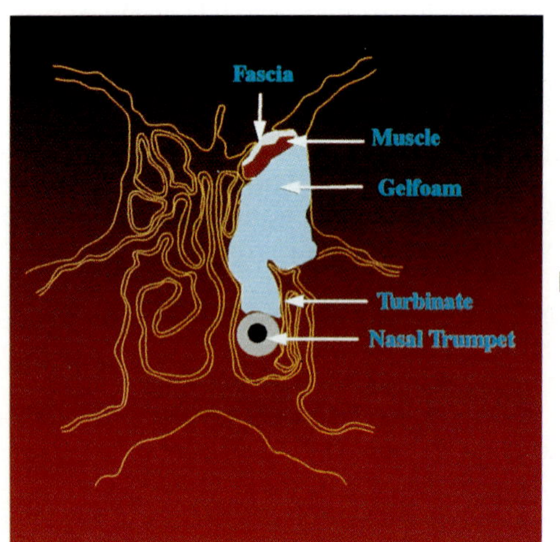

Fig. 10–6. **A,** Figure demonstrating CSF fistula in roof of ethmoid. **B,** Figure demonstrating layered repair of CSF fistula (From Stankiewicz JA: Cerebrospinal fluid fistula and endoscopic sinus surgery. *Laryngoscope* 101:250–256, 1991. By permission.)

SPHENOID SINUS CSF FISTULA

Sphenoid sinus CSF fistulae caused by sinus surgery are not seen nearly as commonly as fistulae due to neurosurgical procedures. Hypophysectomy is the most common cause, but any neurosurgical procedure entering into the sphenoid sinus can lead to a fistula. Repair is performed similarly to the fovea ethmoidalis or cribriform plate. The difference is that the repair is much more posterior, which increases the difficulty. Often, neurosurgical flaps or packing from above is encountered and need to be identified and debrided. A wide sphenoidotomy is created to give the best visualization and working area. The mucosal area immediately around the fistula should be debrided gently, but large scale removal of mucosa is not necessary. Successful control of the fistula involves plugging the opening with a muscle or fat plug over which is placed a fascial patch. A large defect may require a bone plug. All fascial grafts are dipped in fibrin glue. The fascial patch may be covered by muscle or fat, which temporarily obliterates the sphenoid sinus. An alternative is to fill the sphenoid only with fibrin glue, which does not work as well as fascial/muscle patching with fibrin glue. Intranasal packing is necessary to hold this sphenoid packing in place. I prefer Gelfoam packing. An alternative is to use gauze or Merocel® pack. Because the sphenoid is opened widely, it will stay open. When the fat or muscle packing atrophies or exits the sinus, the fascia covering the defect is all that remains (Fig. 10–8). As a result, mucosa in the sphenoid does not have to be widely removed, and the risk of mucocele is minimal. It is very difficult to rotate septal flaps into the sphenoid sinuses for coverage and, in general, they are not needed. Endoscopic exam nicely allows close follow-up.

POSTOPERATIVE CONSIDERATION

All patients are put on bed rest with the head elevated for 4 to 6 days. If a lumbar drain is present, it is monitored very closely. The nasal trumpet is removed after 5 days. Sneezing, coughing, and straining are discouraged. Stool softeners are used. The patient observes the same precautions against increasing CSF pressure at home. The sinus surgery traumatic CSF fistula patient is at risk for infection and possible meningitis, and coverage with an antibiotic is appropriate in this circumstance. The Gelfoam packing is left to disappear on its own. Endoscopic follow-up can begin in 2 to 3 weeks to determine repair success.

Clinical experience with 20 repaired CSF fistulae (8 ethmoid and 12 sphenoid) show excellent success with the above technique. All 20 patients have had their CSF fistulae controlled.

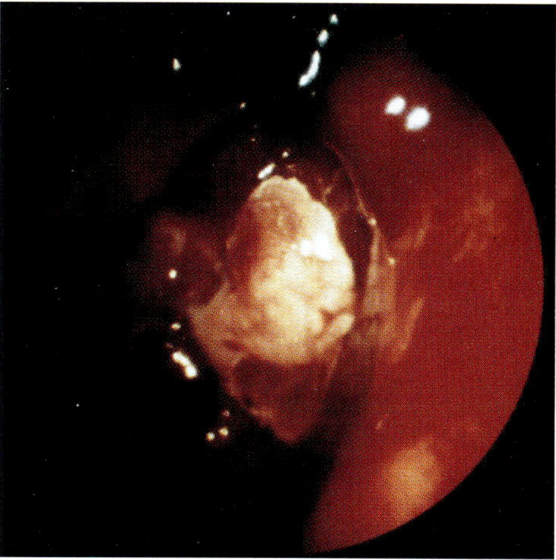

Fig. 10–7. Fascia graft in place over CSF fistula noted in Fig. 10–3.

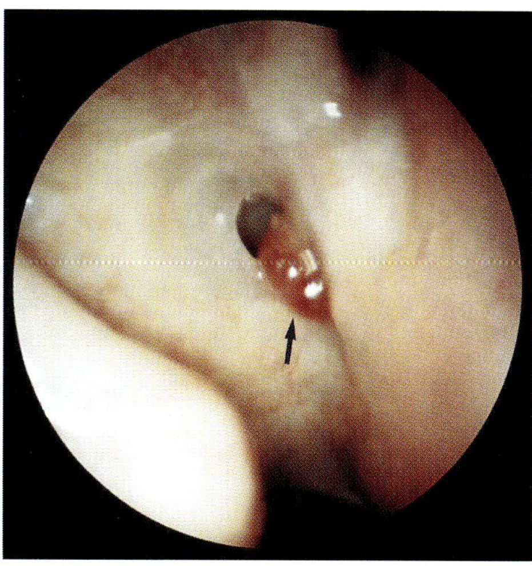

Fig. 10–8. Muscle remnant (arrow) of sphenoid packing with contracted opening of sphenoidotomy 3 months postsphenoid sinus CSF fistula repair.

Summary

CSF fistulae of a traumatic or spontaneous etiology that can be visually identified can be controlled using endoscopic techniques. Endoscopic intranasal closure is of major benefit, especially in the posterior skull base or sphenoid sinus, which can be a difficult area to get at neurosurgically.

REFERENCES

1. Mattox DE, Kennedy DW. Endoscopic management of cerebrospinal fluid leaks and cepholoceles. *Laryngoscope.* 1990; 100:857–862.
2. Papay F, Benningher M, Levine H. Transnasal transseptal endoscopic repair of sphenoidal cerebral spinal fluid fistula. *Otolaryngol Head Neck Surg.* 1989; 101:595–597.
3. Stankiewicz JA. Cerebrospinal fluid fistula and endoscopic sinus surgery. *Laryngoscope.* 1991; 101:250–256.
4. Papay F, Maggiano H. Dominguez S. Rigid endoscopic repair of paranasal sinus cerebrospinal fluid fistulas. *Laryngoscope.* 1989; 99:1195–1201.
5. Levine H, May M. *Endoscopic Sinus Surgery.* New York, NY: Thieme Medical Publishers, 1993. Chapter 7.
6. Stammber A. *Functional Endoscopic Sinus Surgery.* Philadelphia, PA: BC Decker, 1991. Chapter 11.
7. Kainz J. Stammberger H. The roof of the anterior ethmoid: A place of last resistance in the skull base. *Rhinology (USA).* 1990; 3:191–199.

11

Endoscopic Diagnosis and Treatment

Benign and Malignant Tumors

James A. Stankiewicz

The subject of endoscopic treatment of benign and malignant nasal sinus tumors is quite controversial. Indeed, the vast majority of these tumors should be treated in a traditional manner.[1–3] However, certain benign tumors and malignant tumors can be treated intranasally and endoscopically.[4–8] The treatment of malignant tumors is limited to traditional surgery and radiation failures. This chapter discusses an endoscopic approach to nasal and sinus tumors to define the role of endoscopic diagnosis and surgery in their treatment.

Endoscopic Diagnosis and Biopsy

Endoscopic diagnosis has revolutionized our ability to diagnose and perform follow-up after treatment of nasal and sinus tumors. Because of the endoscope, more tumors are diagnosed earlier, and difficult anatomic areas, previously unreachable, are able to be biopsied while avoiding the morbidity of an open procedure and, in some cases, a craniotomy. Rigid or flexible endoscopes should now be used routinely in adults and cooperative children to evaluate nasal and sinus complaints. Any suspicious nasal lesion, especially if unilateral, deserves biopsy after further radiologic evaluation localizes the extent of disease. Biopsy without radiologic backup is discouraged to avoid major catastrophes such as the well-known encephalocele biopsy with cerebrospinal fluid (CSF) leak and brain injury or massive hemorrhage from a vascular lesion when entering the carotid artery during biopsy (Fig. 11–1). In addition, a thorough

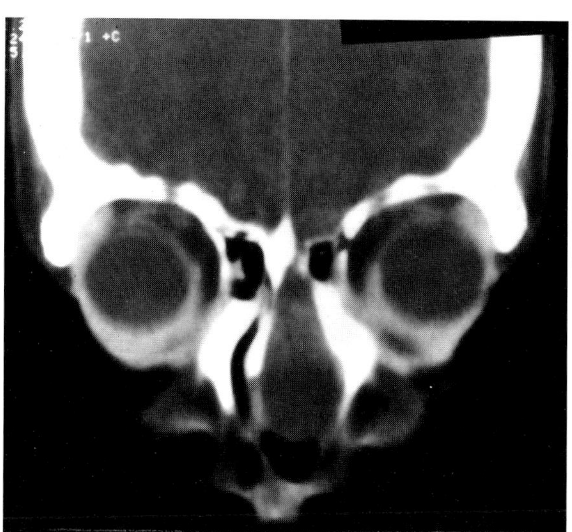

Fig. 11–1. Unilateral nasal lesion noted prior to definitive biopsy/repair on CT scan to be an encephalocele.

A 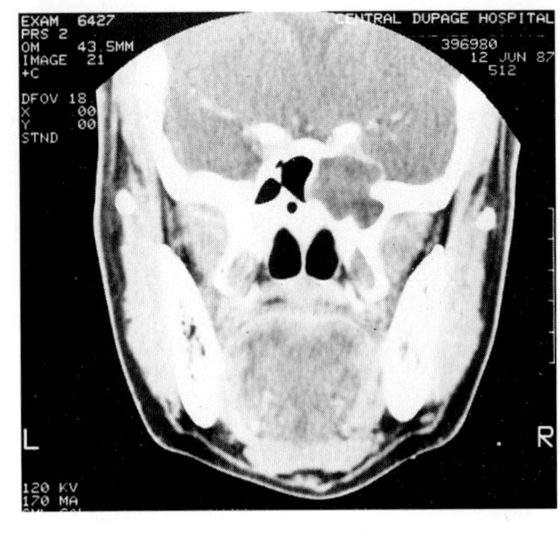

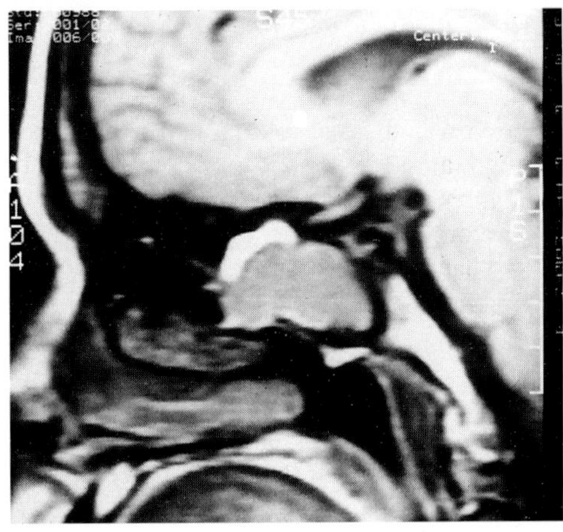 B

Fig. 11–2. CT scan and MRI indicating sphenoid that bled profusely at biopsy and on further work-up proved to be a renal cell carcinoma. **A**, CT scan; **B**, MRI

A 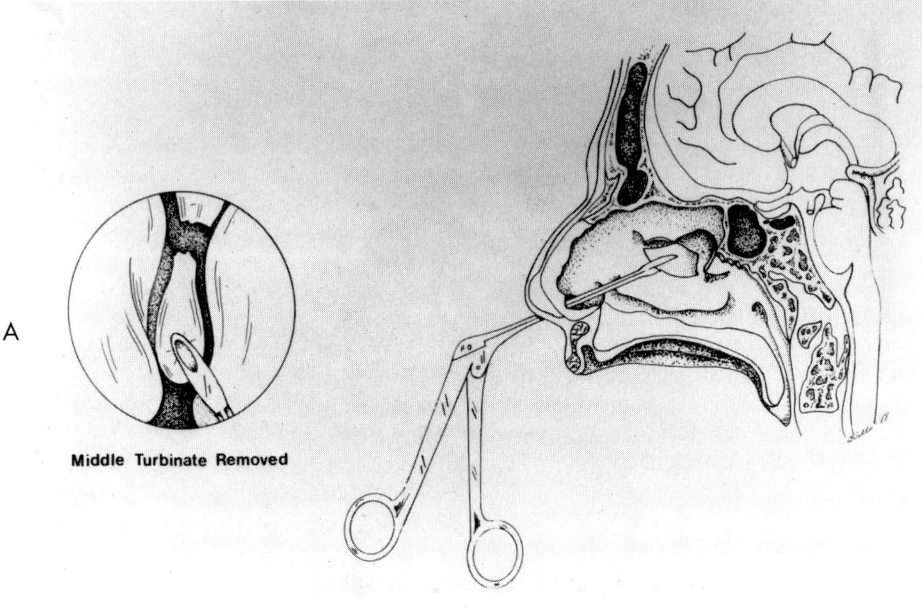

B 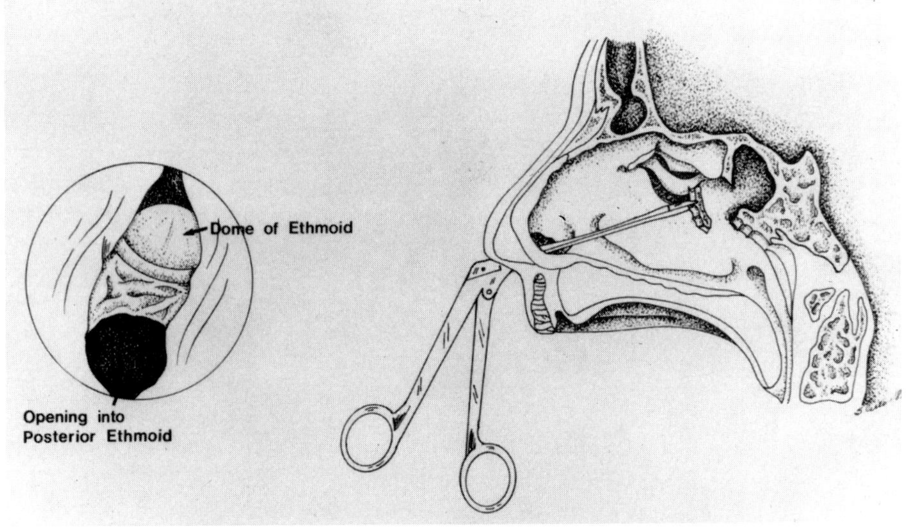

Fig. 11–3. **A**, Anterior superior and posterior inferior incision under endoscopic guidance into middle turbinate. **B**, Removal of anterior wall sphenoid sinus (From *Laryngoscope* 99:218-221, 1989).

systemic review of symptoms and a physical examination, along with appropriate blood and urine testing to rule out metastatic spread to the nose/sinuses from other anatomic areas, are important. A case that demonstrates the importance of the above occurred in our hospital just recently.

A 65-year-old gentleman was referred for biopsy of a right clivus and sphenoid sinus lesion present on CT scan and MRI. At surgery, marked hemorrhage occurred after passing a small Frazier suction into the sphenoid ostia. The nose was packed off and surgery was terminated. Upon closer inspection of his lab results, hematuria was present and a kidney ultrasound was positive for tumor effect. Renal biopsy indicated renal cell carcinoma with probable clival metastasis (Fig. 11–2).

Any area of the nose or sinuses is amenable to endoscopic biopsy. Maxillary sinus biopsy can be achieved through inferior and/or middle meatus with anterior endoscopic trocar sinusotomy if needed. We have performed six biopsies of sphenoid clival lesions. These lesions occurred in the clivus with or without extension into the sphenoid. The technique is straightforward. The sphenoid is approached after the lower part of the middle turbinate has been removed (Fig. 11–3). The posterior ethmoid cells are entered, and the anterior sphenoid wall is encountered, measured, and entered (see Chapter 4). A wide sphenoidotomy is performed and the lesion noted. Sphenoid lesions are then biopsied. In cases where the lesion is present in the clivus only without entrance into the sphenoid, the thin wall between sphenoid and clivus requires removal (Fig. 11–4). Great care is taken to stay near midline and inferiorly as the clivus is entered (Fig. 11–5). The main limitation to this approach at this time is instrumentation because endoscopic instruments in general are too short to reach the clivus. Laryngeal microinstruments or neurosurgical pituitary instruments are helpful. Enough tissue for biopsy is obtained, and nothing further is necessary unless a benign cyst is present, whereupon careful cyst wall marsupialization is curative.

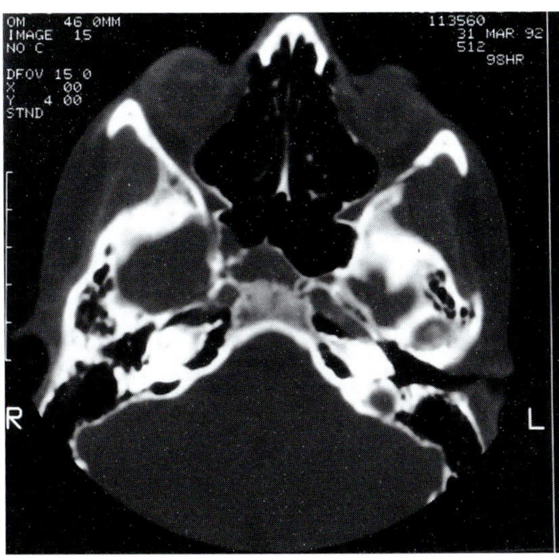

Fig. 11–4. Clival cyst in a 14-year-old with thin bony wall separating cyst from sphenoid which required removal. (Axial CT scan)

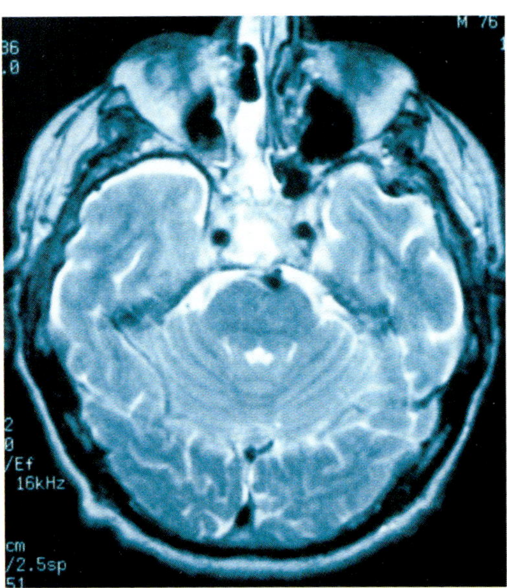

Fig. 11–5. Axial CT scan showing clival mass and position of carotid arteries relative to sphenoid and clivus.

In two instances, the endoscopic biopsy was curative—a 14-year-old with a benign cyst and with a history of headache and a pituitary cyst that caused ophthalmoplegia and vision loss had decompression biopsy that resolved the ophthalmoplegia and improved vision. Malignancies biopsied include squamous cell carcinoma, chordoma, and renal cell carcinoma (Fig. 11–6). Benign lesions include pituitary cyst, retention cyst, and fibrous dysplasia (Fig. 11–7).

Besides initial diagnosis and biopsy, endoscopy is extremely helpful in follow-up of nasal sinus lesions and also posttreatment skull base lesions. The ability of the endoscope to cover all areas is highlighted by a case of esthesioneuroblastoma treated with surgery and irradiation 5 years previously. The patient had been well, but developed mild epistaxis on the tumor side. Endoscopic exam and biopsy noted a small recurrent tumor right at the skull base (Fig. 11–8). Without endoscopic exam, localization of this tumor would have been impossible because both a follow-up CT scan and MRI did not show the lesion. This early diagnosis was very important in directing surgical

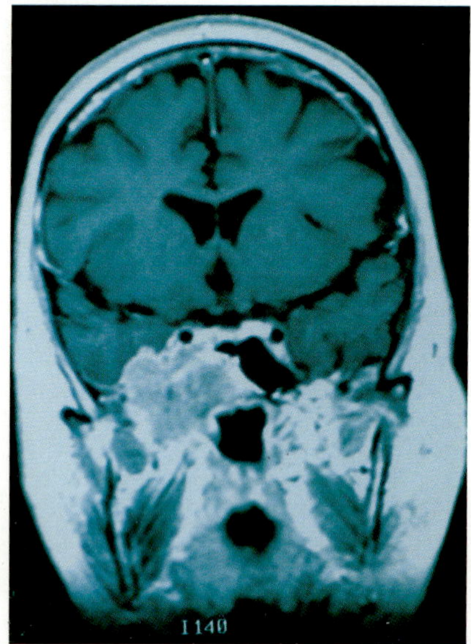

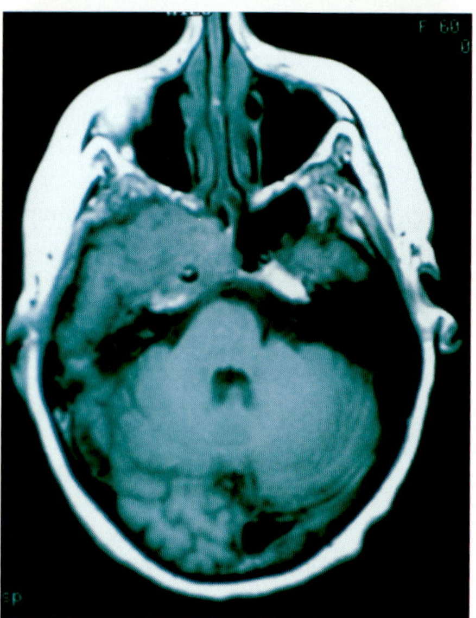

Fig. 11–6. MRI of patient with clival squamous cell carcinoma extending into sphenoid sinus.

planning and avoiding a future massive craniofacial resection.

Benign Lesions

The inverted papilloma is the most common benign tumor seen in the nose and sinuses requiring treatment. The best traditional treatment for inverted papilloma is medial maxillectomy with external ethmoidectomy if necessary. For inverted papilloma extending into the maxillary sinus away

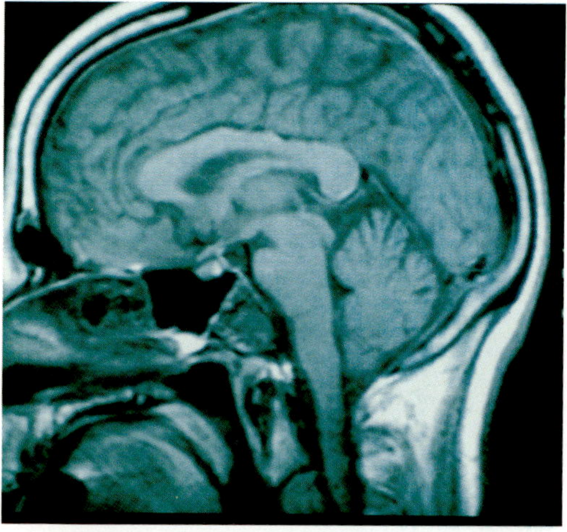

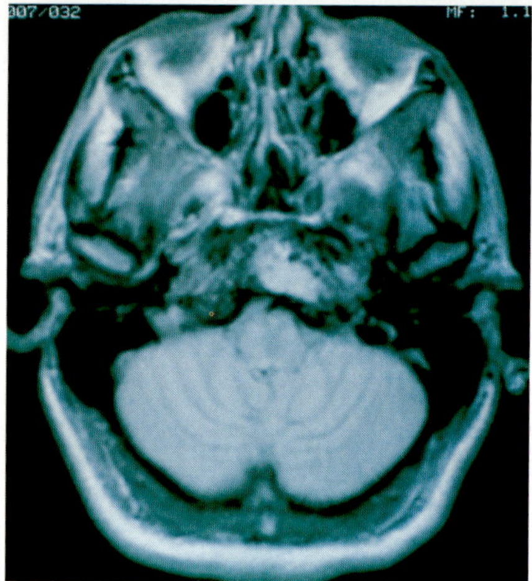

Fig. 11–7. MRI of clival mass in a 28-year-old found to be fibrous dysplasia at biopsy.

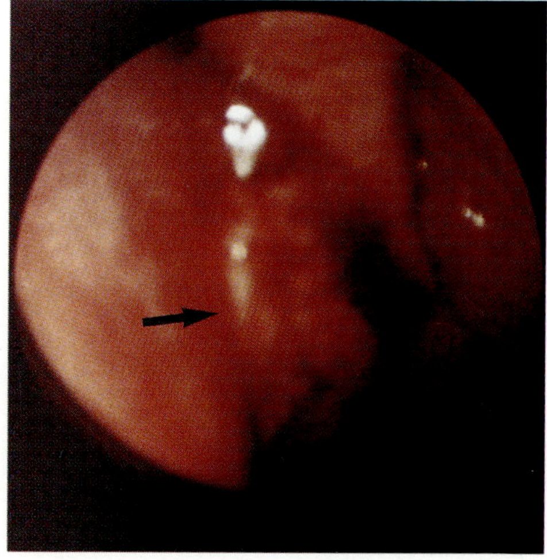

Fig. 11–8. Recurrent esthesioneuroblastoma diagnosed at endoscopy for symptoms of epistaxis (see arrow).

from the medial wall, medial maxillectomy is the procedure of choice.

For a benign tumor limited to the nasal cavity and medial wall of the maxillary sinus, however, endoscopic diagnosis and treatment is a consideration.[4–8] Fifteen patients with inverted papilloma have been treated primarily (10) or secondarily (5) with endoscopic sinus surgery.[5] Of the primary treated cases, one patient developed inverted papilloma 2 years after his initial surgery laterally in the maxillary sinus, requiring conversion to medial maxillectomy. In all cases, follow-up of at least 3 years shows no evidence of recurrent tumor. Five patients were treated secondarily after failure of traditional medial maxillectomy. Endoscopic debridement and sinus surgery have worked well for local control. In fact, one patient treated secondarily for small recurrences is now disease-free for 2 years (Fig. 11–9). One patient had a widespread inverted papilloma; and endoscopic diagnosis, debridement, and biopsy have helped to control tumor enlargement. Two patients had inverted papilloma spread to the frontal sinus and bilateral sphenoid sinuses, respectively. Endoscopic ethmoidectomy with a Lothrop procedure and osteoplastic flap followed by postoperative endoscopic observation helped control the frontal disease, and endoscopic bilateral ethmoidectomy/sphenoidotomy controlled the sphenoid disease (Fig. 11–10). Of interest, endoscopic examination in the latter case was diagnostic of inverted papilloma on the nonoperated side as it emerged out of the sphenoid into the posterior ethmoid.

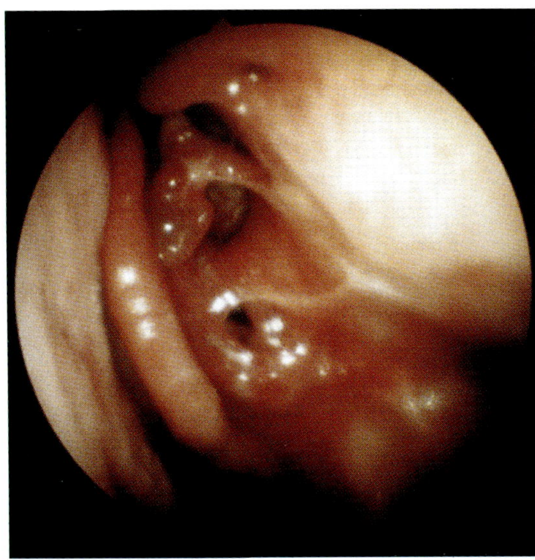

Fig. 11–9. Endoscopic view of secondarily controlled inverted papilloma with endoscopic sinus surgery.

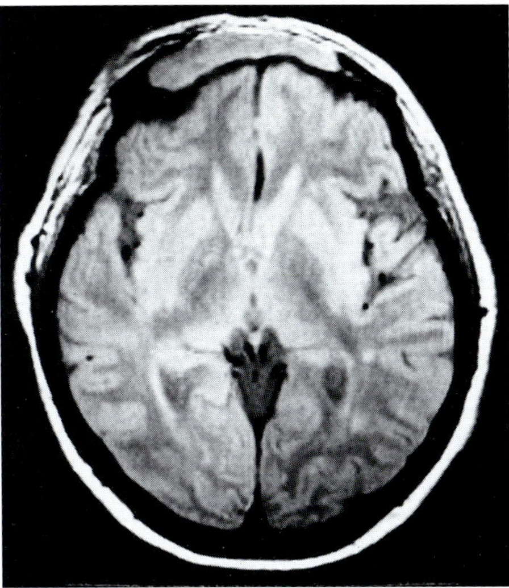

Fig. 11–10. Frontal sinus extension of inverted papilloma after failed external ethmoidectomy and medial maxillectomy. (MRI scan)

Similarly, other benign tumors, such as hemangioma, can be treated endoscopically.

Philosophy of Treatment

Benign tumors, especially inverted papilloma, are easily controlled endoscopically when limited to the septum, turbinates, and ethmoid/sphenoid sinuses. Complete removal, however, must be accomplished. Inverted papilloma has a tendency to spread to the nearest contiguous sinus, so it is always important to examine the next sinus to see if disease is present. In the case of inverted papilloma, this requires a wide antrostomy that allows telescopic examination intranasally and/or via canine fossa trocar puncture to assess tumor spread and perform appropriate biopsies. Any tumor spread beyond the medial wall requires mandatory medial maxillectomy. This philosophy is rigid and noncompromising.

Surgical Considerations

Lesions in the nose are approached surgically in the same way as endoscopic sinusitis surgery. Biopsy is performed in a controlled fashion in the operating room rather than in the clinic because some lesions are quite vascular and may present considerable problems (Fig. 11–2). If the lesion is not totally obstructive and limited to the septum, turbinates, ethmoid and nasal floor, or nasopharynx, excisional biopsy is often possible. I had one case of inverted papilloma hanging from the superior turbinate and a squamous cell carcinoma on a stalk in the nasopharynx that were removed completely endoscopically. Bulky lesions are more problematic as far as management because it is hard to assess the true spread of the tumor. With the aid of radiographic evaluation, disease in the sinuses can be judged tumor or infection. CT scan is helpful to define bone erosion and extent of overall disease. It will not define tumor versus sinusitis. Higher window resolution (2000 to 4000) will define disease extent. Low window setting (300 to 500) will define fungal lesions in sinusitis. MRI can show what is sinusitis and what is tumor. The difference becomes apparent in the T_2 image where inflammation is hyperintense and tumor is isointense. MRI can also define tumor spread into tissue barriers such as dura or periorbita. Frozen section diagnosis is necessary to localize disease and is problematic with bulky lesions. In general, however, large, bulky lesions are treated with medial maxillectomy, whereas if the maxillary sinus is virtually lesion-free, endoscopic surgery is acceptable.[6] Local control is the most important concern in most cases of benign tumor.[3] If disease remains after an endoscopic procedure, even a revision medial maxillectomy may not achieve control. Therefore, careful surgical planning is necessary and each tumor staged radiologically and endoscopically for extent of disease.

Typically with inverted papilloma, the lateral wall of the nose is involved, with the ethmoid and maxillary ostia as the target sites. All patients with a unilateral nasal sinus lesion should have an endoscopic nasal sinus examination and a CT scan for initial evaluation. If opacification of the sinus is present, an MRI can distinguish sinusitis from tumor. If disease is limited, endoscopic biopsy with disease removal should be considered with biopsy frozen section control. If disease is bulky and prominent in the maxillary sinus and nasal cavity, an endoscopic biopsy is performed for diagnosis and further, more aggressive treatment performed after results are known. If erosion is present on CT scan, malignancy has to be considered. MRI should be obtained to define tumor from sinusitis and to determine if tissue barriers, such as dura or periorbit, are involved. Any invasion of periorbita or dura other than mucocele is a contraindication to endoscopic nasal and/or sinus surgery.

Involved turbinates require partial or total removal depending upon disease extent. The ethmoid sinuses require marsupialization and, in some cases, endoscopic removal of the lamina papyracea if disease is adherent to it. Wigand uses an otologic drill to remove disease from the lamina papyracea.[4] All surgery must be done under strict biopsy control. Any area that is inaccessible to endoscopic biopsy needs an open procedure so that disease is appropriately evaluated and controlled. Benign lesions other than inverted papilloma do not require biopsy control and usually can be excised endoscopically from the septum or turbinates from which most arise. It is rare to find a benign noninverted papilloma tumor in the ethmoid, frontal, or maxillary sinus.

Malignant Tumors

Endoscopic diagnostic biopsy can localize nasal malignancy. For the most part, treatment for biopsy-positive malignant tumors requires open or external procedures. Exceptions occur in the rare instance of a malignancy attached to the nasal mucosa by a stalk such as in one case of squamous cell carcinoma attached to the nasal mucosa floor at the nasal/nasopharyngeal junction (Fig. 11–11). Any limited malignant tumor must be excised completely with consideration for post-removal radiation therapy if indicated. Esthesioneuroblastoma does present in the nose and can hang from a stalk on the cribriform plate (Fig. 11–12). Whereas the bulk of the tumor can surely be removed with the endoscope, great concern for spread through the cribriform plate intracranially is necessary. MRI scanning and CT scanning are necessary to determine intracranial spread through the cribriform plate. However, a recent case occurred where a limited recurrent esthesioneuroblastoma was present with no evidence of intracranial spread on CT scan and MRI. Craniofacial pathologic specimen review postoperatively did show involvement of the cribriform plate, but not dura. Thus, small esthesioneuroblastoma tumors may not be picked up in radiography. Because the tumor originates in the olfactory fibers as they come through the cribriform plate, the best treatment is an anterior craniofacial resection for definitive control. Endoscopic treatment should be considered only if craniofacial surgery is not an alternative. Drilling of the skull base must be done to make sure olfactory fibers are controlled.

The main value of the endoscope for malignancy is for postresection diagnostic follow-up allowing for the earliest localization of recurrence. One case, discussed above, of esthesioneuroblastoma 5-years postoperative resection and radiation therapy presented with a short history of intermittent epistaxis. Endoscopy showed a small recurrent lesion on the cribriform plate that was biopsy-positive. Further localized definitive surgery was accomplished with complete removal, perhaps

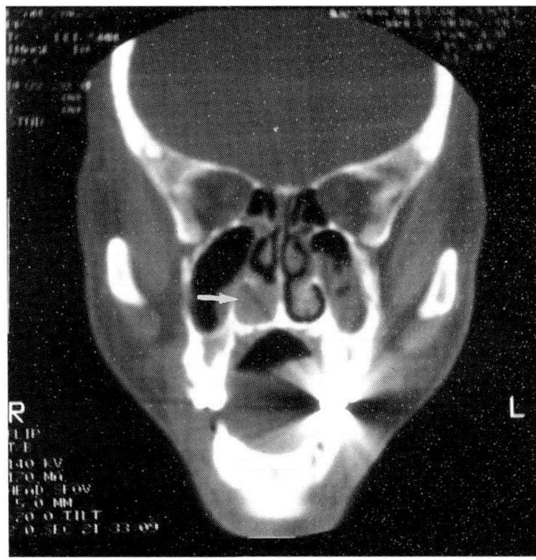

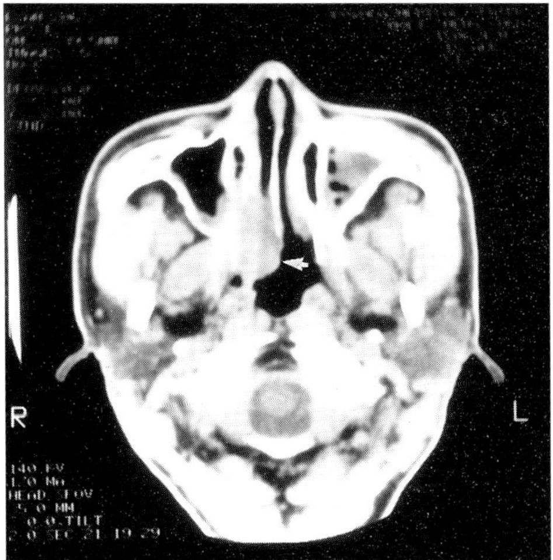

Fig. 11–11. Squamous carcinoma nose/nasopharynx on a stalk (coronal and axial views) (see arrows).

avoiding a much larger resection after delayed diagnosis.

Occasionally, extensive malignancies recur despite extensive surgery and radiation therapy. This is also the case for inverted papilloma with numerous surgeries failing to control tumor. Recurrent inverted papilloma is rarely radiated. Endoscopic sinus surgery can help debride the nose and sinuses of recurrent tumor and allow for biopsy control of failed surgical treatment of inverted papilloma to identify malignancy. Patients can breathe, and bleeding and crusting are controlled. Patients are a lot more comfortable with serial debridement and palliative endoscopic surgery.

Summary

Benign tumors limited to the nasal cavity and medial wall of the maxillary sinus can be con-

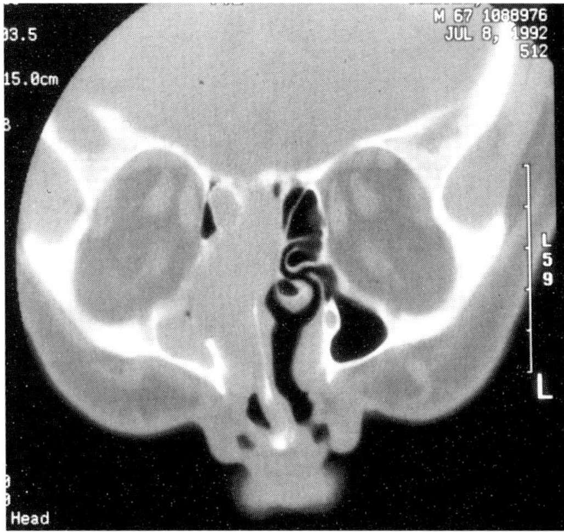

Fig. 11–12. Esthesioneuroblastoma, limited to nose, hanging from cribriform plate.

trolled with endoscopic sinus surgery. Any tumor that is bulky and extends past the medial wall of the maxillary sinus is not a candidate for endoscopic surgery. Malignant tumor can be diagnosed with endoscopic biopsy, but treatment, for the most part, requires external or open procedures. Endoscopic postoperative follow-up for diagnosis is the best way to localize early recurrence. Failed intensive surgery and/or radiation therapy for nasal malignancy does occur. Endoscopic palliative debridement can reduce morbidity. Failed surgery for inverted papilloma requires close endoscopic follow-up, debridement, and biopsy to identify any change, whether it is benign or malignant.

REFERENCES

1. Calcaterra T, Thompson T, Paglia B. Inverted papillomas of the nose and paranasal sinuses. *Laryngoscope.* 1980; 90:53–60.
2. Cummings C, Goodman M. Inverted papillomas of the nose and paranasal sinuses. *Arch Otolaryngol.* 1970; 92:445–449.
3. Lawson W, Benger J, Som P. Inverted papilloma: An analysis of 87 cases. *Laryngoscope.* 1989; 99:117–124.
4. Waits G, Wigand M. Results of endoscopic sinus surgery for the treatment of inverted papilloma. *Laryngoscope.* 1992; 917–922.
5. Stankiewicz JA, Girgis SJ. Endoscopic surgical treatment of nasal and paranasal sinus inverted papilloma. *Arch Otolaryngol Head Neck Surg.* 1993;109, 988–995.
6. Woodson J, Robbins K, Michaels L. Inverted papilloma. *Arch Otolaryngol.* 1985; 111:806–811.
7. Hoffman S, Stanziano G, Goodman D. Microscope rhinoscopy in the treatment inverted papilloma. *Laryngoscope.* 1984; 94:662–993.
8. Kamel R. Conservation endoscopic surgery in inverted papilloma. *Arch Otolaryngol Head Neck Surg.* 1992; 118:649–653.
9. Hyams V. Papillomas of the nasal cavity and paranasal sinuses: A clinicopathological study of 315 cases. *Am Otol Rhinol Laryngol.* 1971; 80:192–206.

12

Endoscopic Pituitary Surgery

Roger Jankowski

In the surgical treatment of diseases of the pituitary region, the transsphenoidal route has gathered widespread acceptance.[1–4] The number and variety of approaches described for reaching the pituitary fossa[5–10] indicate the difficulties inherent in this surgical procedure. Moreover, the number of incomplete tumor resections and the use of postoperative radiotherapy reflect the need for improving this technique.[11–13]

The nasal endoscope has provided increased visualization for the surgeon performing sinus surgery. This technology can now be advanced into areas beyond the sinuses, including hypophysectomy. We first described the *endonasal endoscopic approach* in 1992.[14] We also present here the *transseptal endoscopic approach* and the reasons why this may be the route of choice.

Preoperative Evaluation and Management

Endocrinologists select patients who are candidates for pituitary surgery. Today there remains considerable controversy as to indications for surgical intervention. As knowledge of pituitary endocrinology and pathophysiology continues to advance, recommendations for therapy may change.

The primary features considered by the surgeon are those related to the anatomy of the pituitary region. The size and pneumatization of the sphenoid sinuses may be a limiting factor. However more than 95% of pituitary adenomas are currently operated using the transsphenoidal route. The size and extensions of the tumor must be taken into account. Craniotomy may be considered if there is parasellar extension or if unusual intracranial extensions exist.

The choice of surgical approach is based on diagnostic imaging. Computed tomography (CT) scans give valuable information about the sphenoid sinuses and tumor extensions. Magnetic resonance imaging (MRI) also shows both the pituitary lesion and its relationship to a normal pituitary gland, and also shows the lesion in relation to the optic chiasm and carotid artery.

However, a number of lesions can mimic pituitary adenomas. Craniopharyngiomas often seem similar to pituitary adenomas. Because an aneurysm may mimic a pituitary adenoma, angiography should be considered when there is a suspicion that an aneurysm might be present. In addition, a meningioma may involve the sella and mimic a pituitary tumor. Each time there are questions about the nature of the pathology, a transcranial approach may be considered.

Preparation of the patient for surgery is guided by the results of the preoperative endocrine testing. Moreover, it remains customary to cover patients going into pituitary surgery with exogenous steroids during the course of the operation and during the immediate postoperative period, as their pituitary reserve of the pituitary adrenal axis may be impaired. Transient diabetes insipidus is seen postoperatively in 30% to 50% of patients and can be effectively managed with desmopressin. Perioperative prophylactic antibiotherapy is systematically given. Once the immediate postoperative period is over (usually 3 or 4 days), baseline pituitary hormone functions are again studied and appropriate replacement is initiated.

Sinusitis or rhinitis has to be treated before pituitary surgery and, if not healed, is a contraindication to the infrasellar approach. Antibiotherapy should be adapted to the pathogens found in the nose. Steroids are useful in curing edematous lesions. Endoscopic sinus surgery may help in some cases.

Endonasal Endoscopic Pituitary Surgery

The endonasal route provides rapid surgical access to the sphenoid and the pituitary fossa through the nasal cavities. An oral endotracheal tube is used for administering general anesthesia, and a pharyngeal pack is inserted. The patient is placed on the operating table in the semiseated position, with the head turned toward the surgeon. The midfacial area, including the nose and eyes, is prepared and draped, in a quadrangular fashion, with towels.

To reduce perioperative bleeding, all the local vascular pedicles around the nose (the end of the facial artery at the edge of the nasal ala, the angular artery, and the dorsal nasal artery), the mucous membrane of the septum, and the nasal floor and turbinates are injected with a 1% lidocaine solution with a 1:100,000 dilution of adrenaline. Nasal cavities are packed using gauze tampons saturated with 5% lidocaine and a 0.02% dilution of naphazoline hydrochloride.

The surgeon operates from the right side of the patient, his right hand working with the instruments and his left hand holding the telescopes. The assistant is positioned at the head of the table. Because video is used, the entire surgical team can take part in the different stages of the procedure (Fig. 12–1). CT scans and MRI documents are displayed in front of the surgeon. The Dessi self-washing pump (Micro-France®, Paris) is a useful tool that helps clean both the telescope and the operative field simultaneously without taking the telescope out of the nose (Xomed-Treace, Jacksonville, Fl).

A systematic nasal endoscopy is performed first, using either a 0 degree or 30 degree rigid Hopkins telescope. The operation can be carried out through one nostril or, if necessary, through both nostrils. The side is chosen on the basis of endoscopic and radiologic findings.

After recognition of both the arch of the choana and the end of the middle turbinate, identification of the anterior wall and ostium of the sphenoidal sinus is easy in those patients who do not have sinusitis. Careful resection of the middle concha with fine curved chisels allows a good view of the anterior sphenoidal wall. The posterior detachment of the middle turbinate can sometimes result in bleeding which can be treated easily with a Dessi bipolar cautery (Micro-France®, Paris).

The sphenoid sinus can be entered either through the natural ostium or by a puncture of the anterior wall, just above the arch of the choana and close to the midline. With the use of Kerrison forceps, the opening is enlarged down to the sphenoidal floor, as well as laterally to the sphenoethmoidal recess. However the surgeon must remember the anatomic variations in the relationship between the optic canal and the Onodi cell. In addition, the opening is enlarged medially to the sphenoidal rostrum. Enlarging the opening upward, above the ostium, has to be performed carefully because of the proximity of the cribiform plate. The ostium must be widened sufficiently to admit the simultaneous passage of a 4-mm telescope as well as other surgical instruments (Fig. 12–2).

At this point, when a unilateral approach offers only a narrow entry into the sphenoid sinus, it is necessary to remove the posterior and superior end of the vomer. A sickle knife is used to cross the

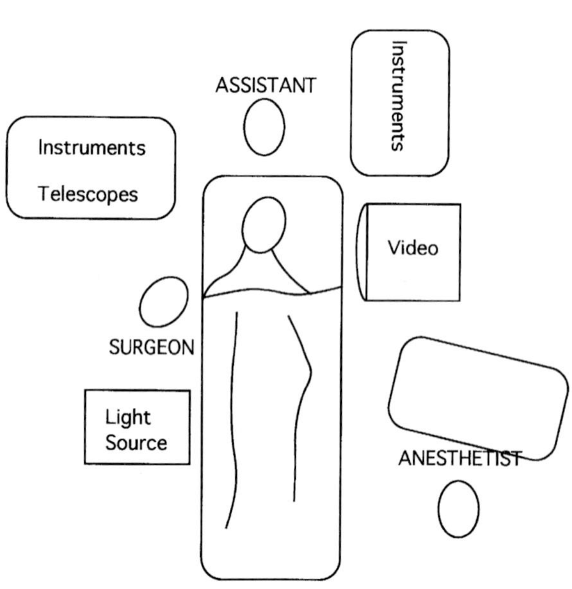

Fig. 12–1. Operating room arrangement for endoscopic pituitary surgery.

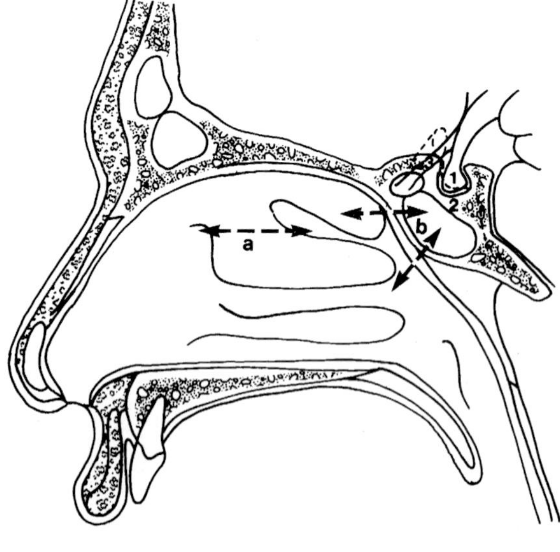

Fig. 12–2. The endoscopic endonasal route (**a,** resection of the middle turbinate; **b**, sphenoidotomy; **1**, pituitary gland; **2**, projection of the carotid artery on the lateral wall of the sphenoid sinus; **3**, projection of the optic canal).

posterior nasal septum 1 cm anterior to the sphenoid opening. Then the vomer as well as the sphenoid rostrum are removed with Blakesley forceps. The intersinus septum, which does not always stay in the midline, is resected. The sella turcica lies in direct view.

The sphenoid sinus is inspected with both the 0 degree lens and then the 30 degree lens to localize the dangerous landmarks. Removing the mucosa helps to identify the underlying structures. The area of the carotid artery is typically marked by a bulge in the lateral wall, and the optic canal can be identified superior to this bulge. The carotid artery is more often identified than the optic canal. Identification of these two structures is directly related to the extent of pneumatization of the sphenoid.

The bony floor of the sella turcica is then gently fractured with a sharp suction tube. A hook is brought in, and the dura is elevated away from the bone to allow its easy removal with Blakesley forceps. In this way, the pituitary dura can be sufficiently exposed, up to the roof of the sphenoid, down to the floor, and laterally from one cavernous sinus to the other. The surgeon must keep in mind the relief of each carotid artery canal, whose shape and bulge are often different from one side to the other (Figs. 12–3 and 12–4).

The dura mater is cauterized with a suction-cautery, with the intent of sealing any patent intercavernous venous sinuses. Needle aspiration of the sella is a safe procedure before opening the dura. This eliminates the possibility of an intrasellar aneurysm. Using a sickle knife, the dura is opened either in a cruciate fashion or in the form of an X (Fig. 12–5). A blunt hook serves for dissecting the subdural plane between the leaves of dura and the underlying gland. Cauterization of the leaves of dura causes them to shrivel and improves exposure of the pituitary gland. Dissection of the subdural planes is extended to mobilize the gland or the tumor, first inferiorly from the floor of the sella, then laterally from the walls of the cavernous sinuses, and finally superiorly away from the diaphragma sella. The adenoma is then resected using aspirators, dissectors, and appropri-

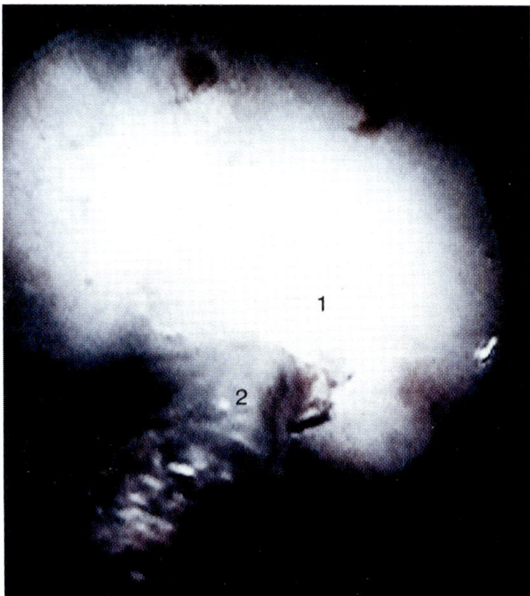

Fig. 12–3. The bony floor of the sella turcica (1) is gently fractured with a sharp suction tube (2) (right endonasal route, 0° lens).

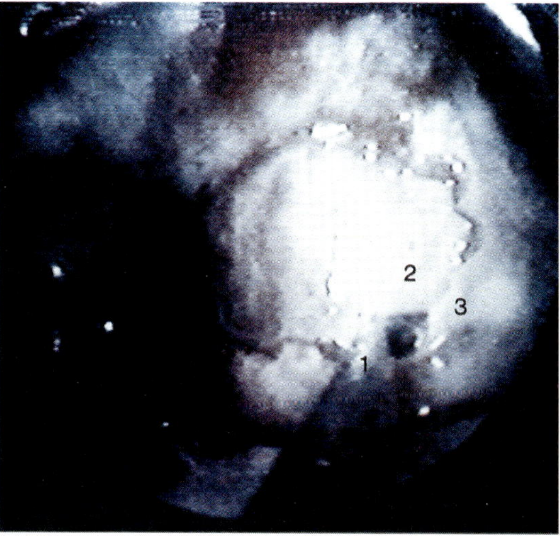

Fig. 12–4. A hook (1) is used to elevate the dura (2) away from the bone (3) (right endonasal route, 0° lens).

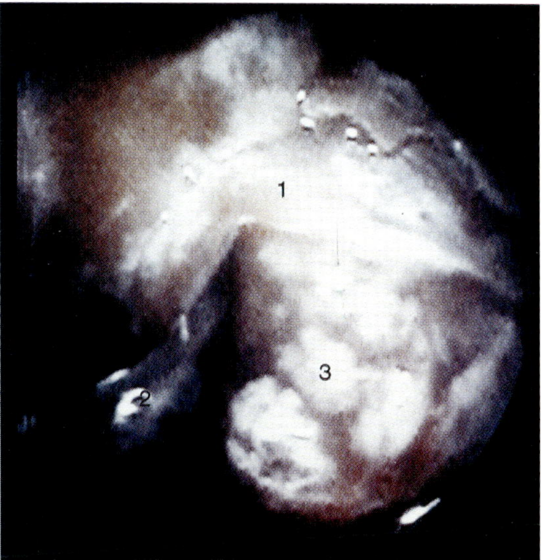

Fig. 12–5. The dura (1) is opened with a sickle knife (2) in a cruciate fashion. The tumor (3) bulges in the shenoid cavity (right endonasal route, 0° lens).

ate curettes (Fig. 12–6). Angled telescopes are particularly useful at this stage because they allow tumor resection under visual guidance.

The sella is plugged with muscle or fat only in the case of cerebrospinal fluid (CSF) leakage or bleeding. In the other cases, the tumor cavity is filled with Gelfoam®. Antibiotic-covered gauze strips are placed in one or both nasal cavities and are removed on the second day after surgery.

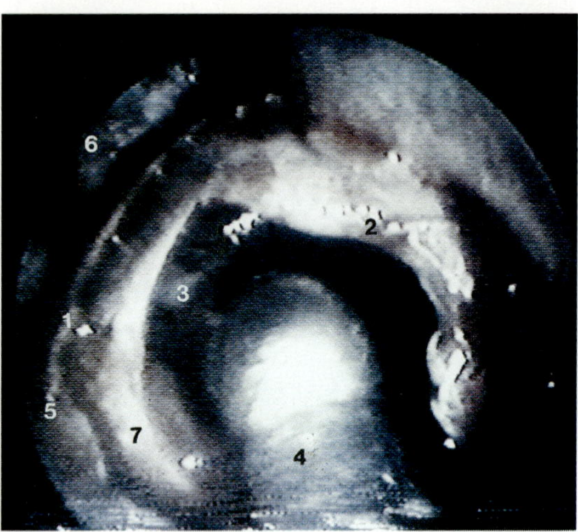

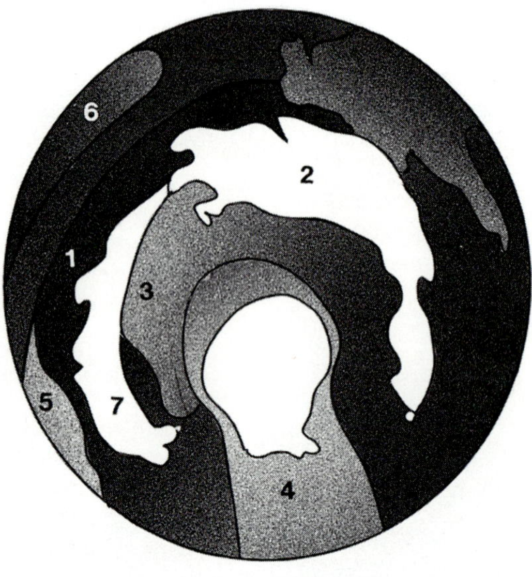

Fig. 12–6. Endoscopic view inside the right sphenoidal sinus during hypophysectomy (30° lens) (**1**, sella turcica; **2**, dura mater; **3**, pituitary fossa; **4**, suction tube; **5**, prominence of the carotid artery canal; **6**, prominence of the optic canal; **7**, sphenoidal cavity).

Transseptal Endoscopic Pituitary Surgery

Operating room arrangement and preparation of the patient are the same as in Figure 12–1. A right-sided hemitransfixion incision is made over the caudal end of the nasal septum. With a Cottle knife, the perichondrium is elevated from the cartilage on the right of the cartilaginous septum. The perichondrium is detached from the caudal end of the septum and then dissected on the left of the cartilaginous septum. A columella pocket is created between the medial crura by means of Knapp scissors. The "magic plane" is undermined with slightly curved blunt scissors, allowing elevation of the periostum over the pyriform aperture on both sides and the anterior nasal spine. Septum and nasal floor tunnels are easily created using, alternatively, a Guillen aspirator-elevator or a Cottle elevator, and are then connected by sharp dissection. The articulations of the cartilaginous septum with the spine, premaxilla, and maxilla ridge, and the perpendicular plate of the ethmoid, are dissected free so that the septum can be displaced to the left ("swinging door technique").

A long nasal speculum is then placed along the bony septum, and dissection of both mucosal flaps continues until the rostrum of the sphenoid is encountered. The bony septum is then removed with a rongeur, and the anterior face of the sphenoid with the sinus ostia on each side of the rostrum is exposed (Fig. 12–7).

At this point, if either one of the pieces removed from the bony septum is large enough, it will be kept for reconstruction of the sella floor. Alternatively, a piece of cartilage can be removed for the same purpose. In patients without septal deviation, a Beaver swivel knife is inserted to remove a portion of the cartilage, leaving an L-shaped strut for support of the external nose. However, as cartilage sometimes must be removed to correct a deviated septum, this cartilage can be used for the same purpose.

A self-retaining speculum is then positioned in the midline. Here, the telescopes are used for the first time to check the position of the self-retaining speculum and to achieve correct dissection and exposure of the face of the sphenoid. Rongeurs are used to resect the anterior wall and the intersinus septum. This route offers the widest entry into the sphenoid. Most often the 0 degree lens is sufficient to give a panoramic view over both sinuses and the main landmarks. The sella turcica is in front. Slight modifications of the view angle of the telescope offer, alternatively, good visualization of both the right and left carotid artery canal. All the walls of the sphenoid sinuses can easily be inspected. The 30 degree lens is sometimes needed

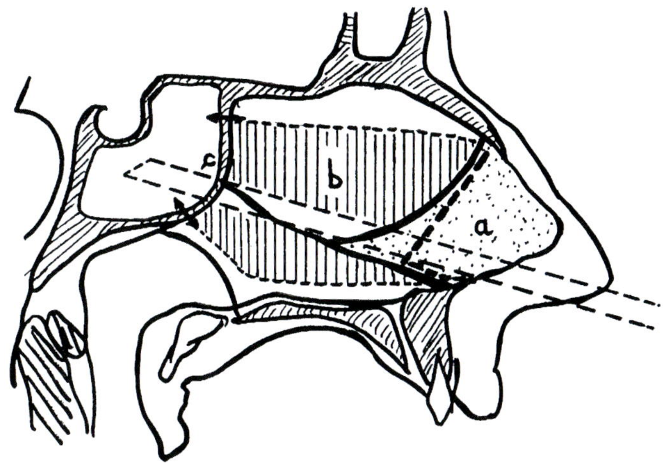

Fig. 12–7. The endoscopic transseptal route (**a**, the cartilaginous septum is dissected free and displaced to the left (swinging door technique); **b**, the bony septum is removed; **c**, the sphenoid rostrum and anterior wall is resected).

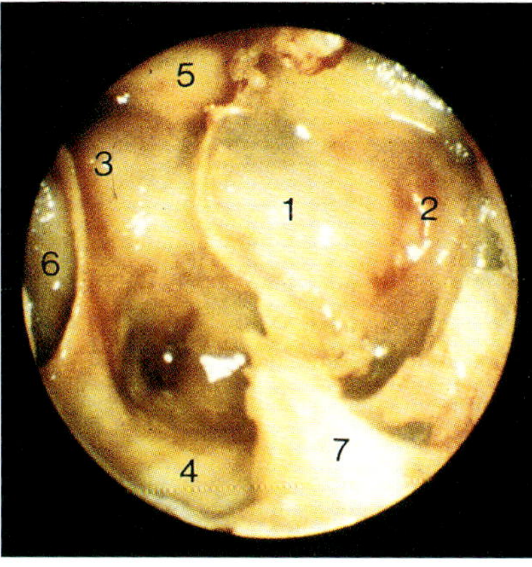

Fig. 12–8. Zero degree lens panoramic view over both sphenoid sinuses (endoscopic transseptal route) (**1**, sella turcica; **2**, left carotid artery canal; **3**, right carotid artery canal and intersinus septum; **4**, floor of the sphenoid sinus; **5**, roof of the sphenoid sinus; **6**, pneumatization of the lateral walls; **7**, sphenoid rostrum).

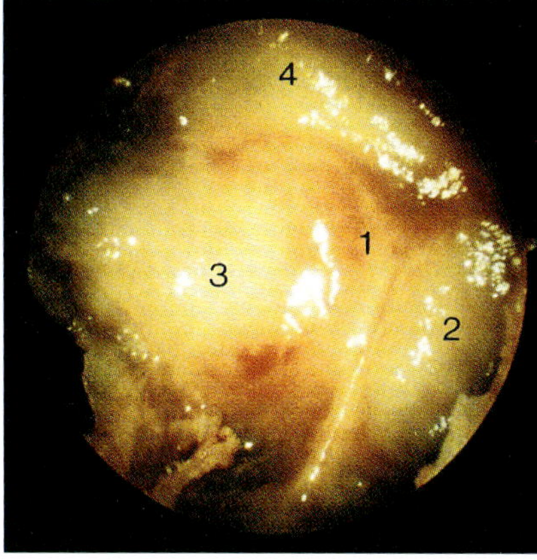

Fig. 12–9. Focus on the left carotid artery canal (**1**). Note that pneumatization of the sphenoid extends laterally (**2**) to the carotid canal (**3**, sella turcica; **4**, roof of the sphenoid sinus).

to appreciate the extent of pneumatization of the lateral walls (Figs. 12–8 and 12–9).

The telescope is connected to a camera, and the operation is conducted on a screen. We use a two-surgeon technique with the assistant holding the endoscope and the surgeon using two hands to hold the instruments.

The lining mucosa is carefully stripped from the posterior wall to expose the bony sella, and good hemostasis is achieved. The floor of the sella is usually thin enough to be lifted off with forceps or a small nerve hook. When the bone is thicker, it can be drilled away with a small diamond burr or removed with bone punches. The self-washing pump is very useful for keeping the lens clean. Wide lateral bony exposure of the sella is possible with reference to the course of the carotid artery. Bone is carefully removed superiorly to avoid damage to the circular sinus connecting the cavernous sinuses. In this region, dural adhesions to the tuberculum sella may rupture, producing sinus bleeding or a CSF leak (Fig. 12–10). Once the dura is exposed, a fine needle is inserted to eliminate an intrasellar aneurysm.

The dura is then cauterized and opened with a cruciate or transverse incision. The dural leaves are cauterized to cause further dural retraction and to prevent separation of the two dural layers. Dissection between the two layers can lead to inadvertent entry into the cavernous sinus.

If the tumor is cystic or soft, it is suctioned out. If the tumor is solid, a well-defined plane may exist around a microadenoma, which allows an easy resection. Identification of the normal pituitary gland may be difficult during removal of a large tumor. Angled telescopes are particularly useful in controlling suprasellar extensions (Figs. 12-11, 12-12, 12-13). Removal of tumors laterally must be carefully performed, as the tumor may be adherent to the cavernous sinus or may invade it. If the tumor is dense and fibrous and is not

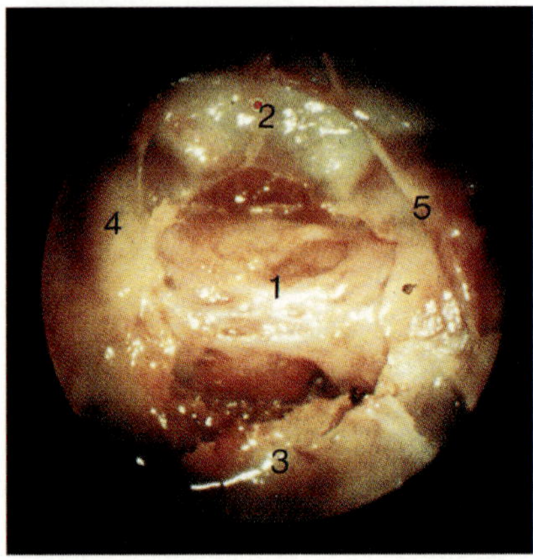

Fig. 12–10. The pituitary dura (**1**) is exposed up to the roof (**2**), down to the floor (**3**), and laterally from one carotid artery (**4**) to the other (**5**) (endoscopic transseptal route, 0° lens).

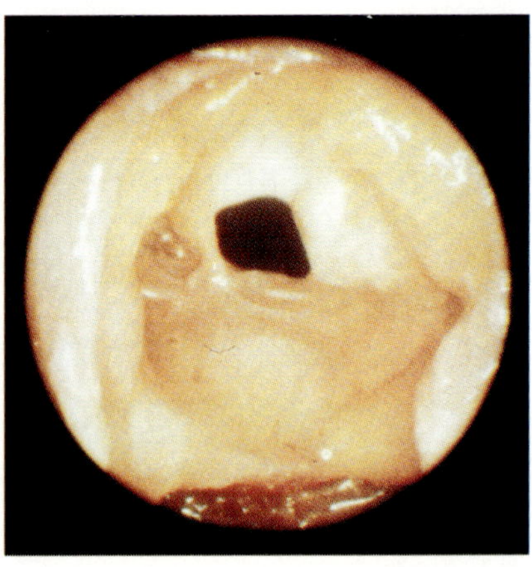

Fig. 12–12. Thirty degree lens endoscopic view inside the pituitary fossa after removal of the gland (transseptal route).

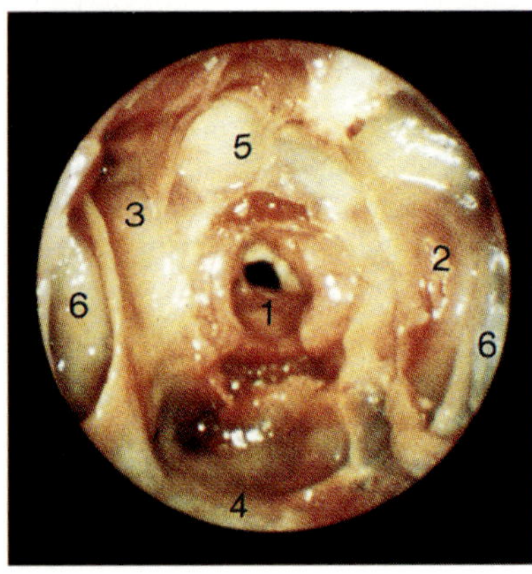

Fig. 12–11. Zero degree lens endoscopic view of the pituitary fossa after removal of the gland (transseptal route) (**1**, pituitary fossa; **2**, left carotid artery canal; **3**, right carotid artery canal and intersinus septum; **4**, floor of the sphenoid sinus; **5**, roof of the sphenoid sinus; **6**, pneumatization of the lateral walls).

easily removed by suction or by curettage, it is necessary to bite away the tumor with pituitary rongeurs of different shapes and sizes. Great care must be taken not to grasp and tear the capsule and surrounding arachnoid.

The diaphragm sellae and the capsule are left intact to avoid a CSF leak. When a CSF leak is seen intraoperatively, the sella is packed with autograft muscle or fat taken from the thigh or abdomen. This is also done when the prolapse of adjacent structures into the enlarged sella occurs. It is imperative that meticulous hemostasis be achieved before closure. The floor of the sella is then closed with a piece of cartilage or bone taken from the removed portion of the septum.

After closure of the sella, the self-retaining speculum is removed and septal reconstruction is undertaken. Actually, a septoplasty is performed in all patients who also had a former deviated septum to avoid postoperative nasal obstructive complaints. All deviated structures have to be removed. Guide sutures are used to attach the repositioned cartilage through the skin. The columella pocket keeps the cartilaginous septum in the midline. The septal skeleton is reconstructed by reimplantation of several pieces of crushed cartilage or plates of bone. The nostrils are packed with antibiotic-impregnated gauze around catheters that allow nasal breathing.

Postoperative Care

The advantage of the transsphenoid route is the relative lack of postoperative complications. Most patients are allowed fluids the day following surgery and are out of bed by the second day. The nasal packing is removed over a 2-day period. The patient is usually referred on the fourth day for postoperative evaluation, including full endocrinologic testing.

Discussion

ENDONASAL VERSUS TRANSSEPTAL ENDOSCOPIC APPROACH

The endonasal route has many disadvantages compared with transseptal route. Noninfected noses

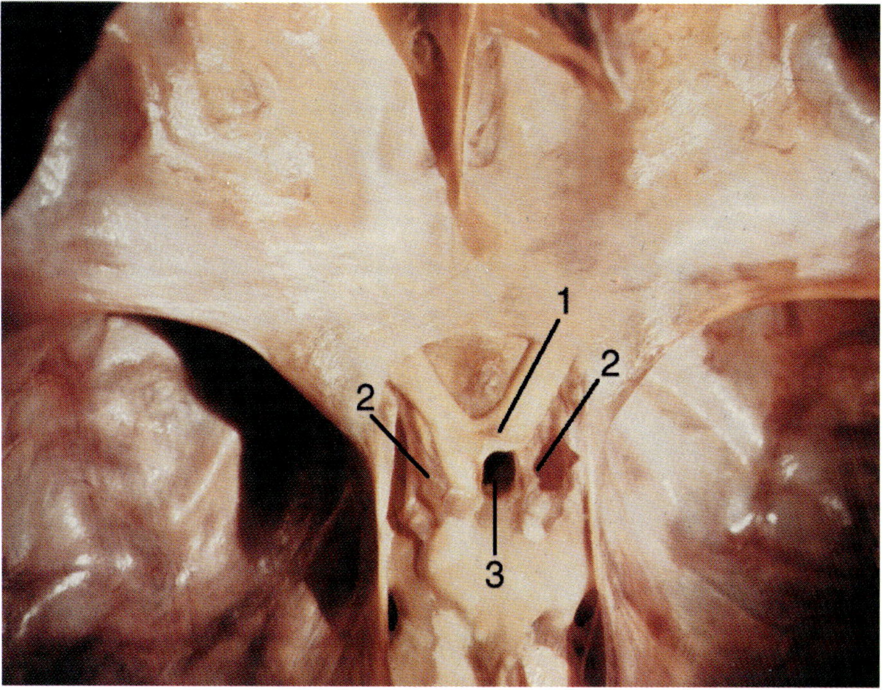

Fig. 12–13. Endocranial view of the hypophyseal region (**1**, optic chiasm; **2**, cavernous sinus; **3**, pituitary fossa).

always carry potential pathogens. Deviated septum is also common in symptom-free patients, and may make access to the sphenoid difficult. The endonasal route is narrow, even after resection of the middle turbinate and the dorsal end of the septum. These resections lead to crust formation and increase the risk of postoperative infection.

The transseptal route offers a more sterile access to the sphenoid. Exposure of the sella turcica is large and in direct vision. Once the self-retaining speculum is in place, moving the endoscope in and out the sphenoid sinus is easy.

ENDOSCOPIC SURGERY VERSUS MICROSURGERY

The telescope gives the surgeon the ability to have one eye on the sphenoid sinus, while the microscope allows the surgeon to view the outside of the nose. The main advantage of the endoscopic approach is the panoramic view it gives inside the sphenoid sinus and inside the pituitary fossa.

The endoscopic approach is achieved through a limited hemitransfixiant incision of the septal mucosa. The microscope approach needs either a sublabial incision or complementary incisions in the nose (alotomy, external approach) which can lead to functional or esthetic disability.[15]

However, whatever theoretical advantage this technique has, proof of its ability to improve tumor removal, especially in macroadenomas, remains to be seen.

REFERENCES

1. Laws ERJ. Pituitary surgery. *Endocrinol Metab Clin.* 1987;16(3):647–665.
2. Codaccioni JC. Résultats à moyen et long terme de l'adénectomie sélective hypophysaire. *Annales d'Endocrinologie.* (Paris) 1985;46:313–323.
3. Welbourn RB. The evolution of transsphenoidal pituitary microsurgery. *Surgery.* 1986;100(6):1185–1189.
4. Black PM, Zervas NT, Candia G. Incidence and management of complications of transsphenoidal operation for pituitary adenomas. *Neurosurgery.* 1987;20(6):920–924.
5. El-Fatih Baraka M. A modified incision for the transseptal trans-sphenoidal approach to the pituitary. *J Laryngol Otol.* 1989;103:670–671.
6. Anand J, Siddartha G, Thomas J. Transseptal fracture displacement approach for treatment of pituitary lesion. *Arch Otolaryngol Head Neck Surg.* 1991;117:340–341.
7. Stevens MH, Apfelbaum RI. Transnasal pituitary tumor surgery. *Laryngoscope.* 1990;100:427–429.
8. Peters GE, Zitsch RP. Columellar flap for transseptal transsphenoidal hypophysectomy. *Laryngoscope.* 1988; 98:897–899.
9. Wilson WR, Khan A, Laws ERJ. Transseptal approaches for pituitary surgery. *Laryngoscope.* 1990;100:817–819.
10. Lekas MD. The nasal gateway for pituitary surgery. *Am J Rhinol.* 1988;2:193–200.

11. Shone GR, Richards SH, Hourihan MD, et al. Nonsecretory adenomas of the pituitary treated by transethmoidal sellotomy. *J Royal Soc Med.* 1991;84:140–143.
12. Guidetti B, Fraioli B, Canore GP. Results of surgical management of 319 pituitary adenomas. *Acta Neurochir.* 1987;85:117–124.
13. Kennedy DW, Cohn ES, Papel ID, Holliday MJ. Transsphenoidal approach to the sella: the Johns Hopkins experience. *Laryngoscope.* 1984;94:1066–1074.
14. Jankowski R, Auque J, Simon C, et al. Endoscopic pituitary tumor surgery. *Laryngoscope.* 1992;102(2):198–202.
15. Nabe-Nielsen J. Nasal complication after transsphenoidal surgery for pituitary pathologies. *Acta Neurochir.* 1989;96:122–125.

13

Endoscopic Orbital Decompression–Graves' Disease

David H. Henick** and **David W. Kennedy

Dysthyroid orbitopathy—also known as Graves' disease or Graves' exophthalmopathy—is an autoimmune disorder. Its pathogenesis is believed to result from the development of antithyroglobulin immune complexes that bind to the membranes of extraocular muscles.[1] The ophthalmopathy of Graves' disease is characterized by an inflammatory infiltrate of the orbital contents, except for the globe, with lymphocytes, mast cells, and plasma cells. The orbital musculature is mainly involved and is often enlarged, especially the inferior rectus muscle. This increased volume of the orbital contents is responsible for the proptosis. In addition, muscle fibers show degeneration and loss of striations, with the ultimate development of fibrosis.[2]

Clinical signs of Graves' ophthalmopathy can be divided into two aspects. The first component is limited to lid retraction and a characteristic stare with widened palpebral fissures, infrequent blinking, lid lag, and failure to wrinkle the brow on upward gaze. These signs result from sympathetic overstimulation and usually subside when the thyrotoxicosis is corrected. This component is to be distinguished from infiltrative ophthalmopathy, which includes proptosis of varying degrees with ophthalmoplegia (Fig. 13–1). In addition, there is a congestive oculopathy characterized by chemosis, conjunctivitis, periorbital swelling, conjunctival ulcerations, exposure keratopathy, diplopia, and, most severely, optic neuritis or optic atrophy with visual loss. Malignant exophthalmos refers to the rapid progression of the disease, and exophthalmic ophthalmoplegia refers to the ocular muscle weakness that commonly accompanies this disorder and results in strabismus with varying degrees of diplopia. Exophthalmos may be unilateral early in the course of the disorder but usually progresses to bilateral involvement.[2]

The manifestations of Graves' disease can occur at any age, but most often appear in patients between 30 and 50 years of age. The optic neuropathy, however, is more likely to occur in patients over the age of 50. The female/male ratio is 3:1. The onset is rarely acute; typically, it is chronic and insidious, with a foreign body sensation and lid fullness evolving over weeks or even months. The process invariably becomes quiescent in 6 months to 3 years; however, the changes caused by fibrosis are permanent. Only 1% to 3% of patients develop severe malignant exophthalmos with loss of visual acuity—the consequence of severe corneal exposure or compression of the optic nerve at the orbital apex by thickened extraocular muscles. Interestingly, at least 10% of patients with dysthyroid ophthalmoplegia have no abnormality of any endocrine function either in the past, present, or future. Some authors have even suggested that the orbital process is not related to the thyroid disease and is a separate, organ-specific, autoimmune disorder. Therefore, thyroid function tests cannot always be used to prove the diagnosis because a normal result cannot exclude the diagnosis.[3] Furthermore, in those patients who are both hyperthyroid and have exophthalmos, the type and timing of treatment used does not appear to affect the severity of the orbital component.[4–6]

Proptosis in dysthyroid orbitopathy results from an increased intraorbital pressure due to the inflammatory edema and fibrosis of the extraocular muscles and fat. An inflammatory response of the immune complexes created by the accumulation of T lymphocytes sensitized to antigens of the extraocular muscles, fat, and orbital fibroblasts has been suggested.[7,8] Fibroblasts deposit hydropexic mucopolysaccharrides, which exacerbate the ex-

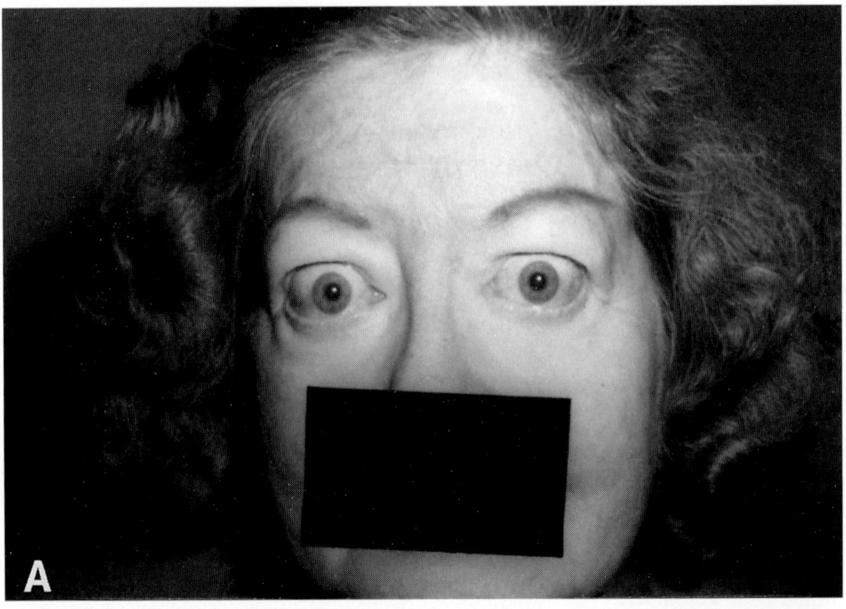

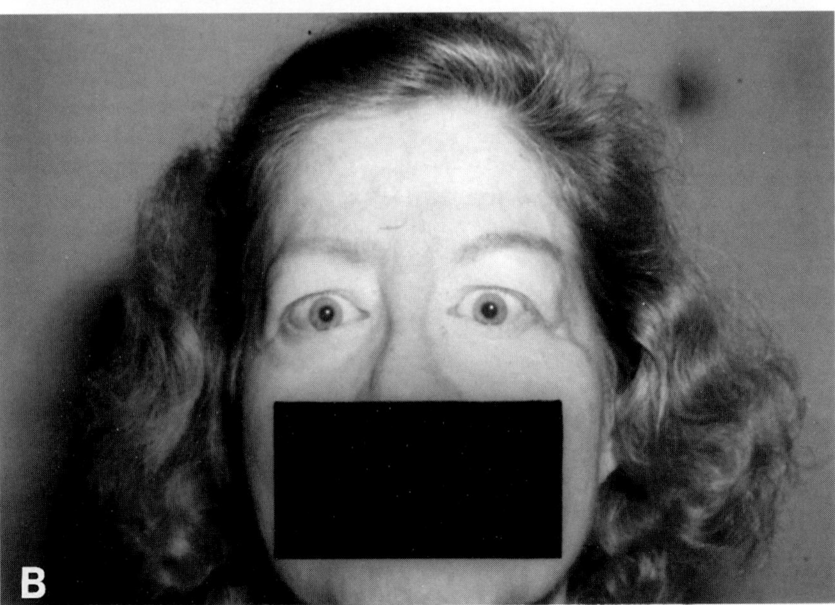

Fig. 13–1. Photographs of a patient who underwent bilateral endoscopic transnasal orbital decompressions and bilateral lateral orbitotomies taken preoperatively (**A**) and 3 months postoperatively (**B**). (From Kennedy DW, Matthew GL, Miller NR, Zinreich J: Arch Otolaryngol Head Neck Surg 116:275–282, 1990. By permission.)

pansion of the extraocular contents.[8] The following visual impairments may develop: 1) fibrosis of the levator palpebrae superioris may lead to exposure keratopathy due to an inability to close the eyelids,[9] 2) swelling or fibrosis of the extraocular muscles may lead to diplopia due to an asymmetric alteration of muscle function,[10,11] and, 3) compression of the optic nerve or vasculature may lead to optic neuropathy due to the enlarging extraocular muscles.[9,10,12] Progressive loss of visual acuity, decreased color vision, and central scotomas may result.

The most definitive treatment for Graves' ophthalmopathy remains surgical decompression. However, medical therapy for the systemic treatment of hyperthyroidism is best managed by an internist or endocrinologist. Propylthiouracil and methimazole inhibit the synthesis of thyroid hormones within the gland itself. Radioactive iodine (iodine 131) accumulates in the thyroid gland and emits ionizing β irradiation that destroys functioning thyroid cells. Propranolol suppresses some of the symptoms of hyperthyroidism, including tachycardia, palpitations, tremors, nervousness, hyperhidrosis, and spasticity. Systemic corticosteroids are the initial primary treatment for congestive symptoms and signs. Corticosteroids may be efficacious, but frequently provide only short-term benefit. Prednisone in doses of 60 to 100 mg may be useful for patients with lid edema, conjunctival chemosis and injection, and tearing and in some cases of myopathy, proptosis, or optic neuropathy associated with congestion. Concomitant use of a diuretic, such as hydrochlorothiazide 50 mg a day, may help reduce orbital edema. In general, steroids should demonstrate an effect within 2 weeks if they are going to be useful; otherwise, they should be rapidly tapered and discontinued.[3,13–17]

In general, congestive symptoms are first treated with corticosteroids. Radiation therapy is reserved for patients with contraindications to steroid therapy or for those who are dependent on steroids, but suffer side effects. In addition, rare cases of diplopia caused by acute congestion may also benefit from radiation. External beam radiation in doses of 20 Gy are delivered to the orbit in 10 fractions. Steroids are continued after completion of the radiation, because the radiation will commonly induce an exacerbation of inflammatory and congestive symptoms. As a rule, patients who do not respond to steroids or who are in a fibrotic, noncongestive stage of the disease process will not respond to radiation therapy.[3] In addition, external-beam irradiation is effective in the treatment of dysthyroid optic neuropathy, but it does not significantly improve proptosis in the majority of cases.[18–21]

The use of the immunosuppressive agents, such as cytoxan and cyclosporin, remains experimental and may be accompanied by potentially serious side effects.[4,19] Plasmapheresis in combination with immunosuppressive agents has been advocated for acute vision-threatening processes.[23–25] Orbital decompression remains the mainstay of therapy, which is aimed at the protection of the patient's vision.

Surgical intervention is reserved for those patients who have sustained the long-term effects of progressive enlargement and fibrosis of the extraocular muscle with an increase in the quantity of orbital fat. Orbital decompression is helpful in reducing exposure keratopathy secondary to proptosis. However, perhaps even more importantly, it can reverse the changes due to optic nerve compression, and the visual improvement can be dramatic. Extensive decompression of the orbital apex area is felt to be the most crucial aspect of the procedure.[23] Other surgical procedures include strabismus repair for diplopia and eyelid surgery for lid retraction. These surgical options, however, should be considered only after a complete and extensive orbital decompression has been accomplished.[23,26]

Various approaches to surgically decompressing the orbit have been performed. The following chart outlines the historical approaches to orbital decompression.

Year	Surgeon	Procedure
1911	Dollinger[27]	Lateral wall decompression via Kronlein approach
1931	Naffziger[28]	Superior orbital decompression into anterior cranial fossa
1936	Sewall[29]	Medial orbital wall decompression via external ethmoidectomy approach
1950	Hirsch[30]	Orbital floor decompression via Caldwell-Luc approach
1957	Walsh and Ogura[31]	Extend Hirsch's operation to include a medial wall decompression
1990	Kennedy[23]	Endoscopic transnasal orbital decompression of medial and orbital floor

Prior to the development of the endoscopic technique, the Walsh-Ogura[31] transantral decompression with a lateral orbitotomy was the preferred procedure to provide maximal overall orbital decompression. Orbital apex decompression was often best performed through an external ethmoidectomy approach. However, experience with endoscopic sinus surgery has allowed the otolaryngologist to perform a more extensive orbital decompression through the nose with excellent visualization and without the need for an external incision. Perhaps most importantly, performing the surgery with a transnasal endoscopic technique provides optimal orbital apex decompression; the key area for the prevention of visual loss due to optic neuropathy.

Radiographic Evaluation

Coronal computed tomography (CT) is essential for preoperative evaluation for possible orbital decompression. It provides information regarding the degree of ethmoid pneumatization and position of the skull base and medial orbital wall. Coronal cuts permit evaluation of the thickness of the orbital floor; a thick floor would be difficult to remove endoscopically through a middle meatal antrostomy with currently available instruments and represents a relative contraindication to this approach. Other anatomic variations that should be considered include the integrity and slope of the ethmoid roof as well as the medial orbital wall. In addition, it is important to assess the height of the posterior ethmoid and its relationship with the roof of the maxillary sinus, and to determine if the posterior ethmoids pneumatize posteriorly and superiorly to involve the optic nerve and/or the internal carotid artery. Axial plane CT scans are useful in demonstrating the relationship between posterior ethmoid cells, optic nerve, and orbital apex. They also clarify the relationship between the internal carotid artery and sphenoid and the relationship of the intersinus septae to these vessels.

Surgical Technique

There are several key elements to consider when performing an orbital decompression: 1) there must be meticulous skeletonization of the medial orbital wall during the ethmoidectomy, 2) removal of the orbital wall should be performed without entering the periosteum. Subsequently, the incision of the periosteum should be performed in a controlled fashion from posterior to anterior beginning laterally in the maxillary sinus, then superiorly in the ethmoid and working inferomedially, 3) the maxillary antrostomy should be made larger than expected due to the prolapse of the orbital contents, 4) bone should not be removed or the periosteum incised in the frontal recess region, and 5) in the early postoperative period, the eyes should be followed for increasing swelling and for visual changes.

Unlike endoscopic sinus surgery for inflammatory sinus disease, general anesthesia is typically employed due to the sensitivity of the periorbital structures. Local vasoconstriction with topical cocaine applied to nasal mucosa with topical applicators is performed, and the lateral nasal wall is injected with lidocaine 1% with 1/100,000 dilution of epinephrine under endoscopic visualization. A sphenopalatine block employed through the transoral route via the greater palatine foramen may help diminish the amount of bleeding.

A standard total sphenoethmoidectomy should be performed in an atraumatic fashion.[32,33] An infundibulotomy is performed by cutting the attachment of the uncinate process through mucosa and bone. The latter is subluxed medially and carefully removed. The bulla ethmoidalis is infractured and removed, exposing the medial orbital wall, an essential early landmark for the dissection. The ground lamella is opened posterior to the bulla, and the posterior ethmoid cells are then entered. After removing the cells of the posterior ethmoid, the bulge of sphenoid may be seen inferiomedially. The sphenoid sinus is entered by infracturing it medially and inferiorly, adjacent to the natural ostium. The mucosal lumen is identified, and further removal of the anterior wall is performed. The bulge of the carotid canal and optic nerve can be visualized frequently posterior and lateral within the sphenoid sinus.

The skull base is carefully skeletonized by removing residual intercellular partitions attached to the ethmoid roof, working in a posterior to anterior direction. With a curved suction, the roof of the ethmoid is further identified anteriorly. The anterior ethmoid artery usually lies immediately below the skull base. The slope of the roof of the ethmoid should be considered when dissection is performed in this area.

The 0° telescope is then changed to 30° angled telescope so that the frontal recess can be visualized. If the area of the sinus is not diseased and the mucosa looks normal, it should not be opened further. When possible, one should preserve the bony partitions (remnants of the agger nasi cells) in the region of the frontal recess.

The natural ostium of the maxillary sinus is identified by reflecting the remnant of the uncinate process inferiorly with a J-currette. Scissors are used to enlarge the opening posteriorly into the posterior fontanelle. The infraorbital nerve can be visualized in its canal along the roof of the maxillary sinus. This represents the lateral limit for bone removal. A very generous middle meatal antrostomy is performed, creating an opening which extends posteriorly to the posterior limit of the sinus and inferiorly into the root of the inferior turbinate. Back-biting forceps are used to enlarge the antrostomy anteriorly to the posterior margin of the nasolacrimal duct. The back-biting forceps may also be helpful in removing some of the medial orbital wall anteriorly or for removing some of the orbital floor in this area. This large middle meatal antrostomy is not only necessary for adequate exposure to the orbital floor, it compensates for the herniated orbital contents that will eventually compromise the patency of the natural opening.

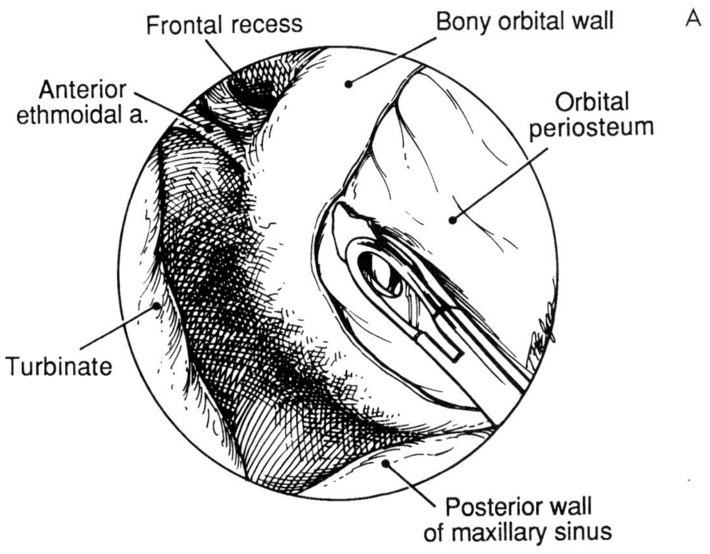

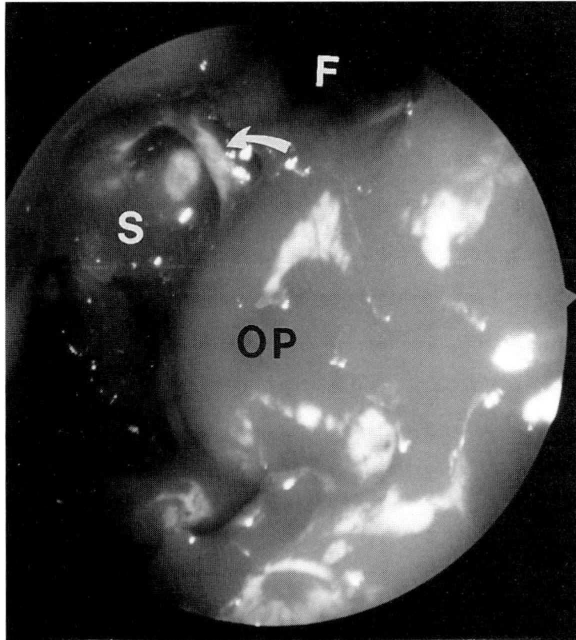

Fig. 13–2. Removal of the left medial orbital wall. **A,** Artist's rendition of removal of the medial orbital wall with Blakesley forceps under endoscopic visualization. **B,** Endoscopic photograph following removal of the medial orbital wall (30° wide angle telescope directed laterally). Superiorly, the skull base(s), the anterior ethmoid artery (curved arrow), and the frontal sinus (F) are seen. OP = orbital periosteum. (From Kennedy DW, Matthew GL, Miller NR, Zinreich J: Arch Otolaryngol Head Neck Surg 116:275–282, 1990. By permission.)

At this point, the skeletonized medial orbital wall is gently removed with an angled spoon. A blunt nerve hook or fine Blakesley forceps can also be used. Care is taken not to violate the orbital periosteum at this stage of the operation. A protrusion of orbital fat would obscure visualization for the remainder of the dissection. If a small defect in the orbital periosteum were to occur, however, bipolar cautery can be effective in decompressing the herniated fat.

The removal of the orbital wall is continued posteriorly towards the orbital apex (Fig. 13–2). Anteriorly, the medial orbital wall in the region of the frontal sinus is preserved to avoid the possibility of stenosis and subsequent frontal sinus obstruction. Posteriorly, a small rim of bone is preserved around the optic nerve. The orbital floor is downfractured with a J-currette or frontal recess currette. It may also be removed with 90° Blakesley forceps or 70° or 120° Giraffe forceps.

To incise orbital periosteum as far laterally as possible, a Beaver sickle knife is bent in a curved fashion to almost 90°. A 30° telescope is used and directed laterally as a linear incision in the periorbita is made from posterior to anterior (Fig. 13–3). Successive incisions are then made medially

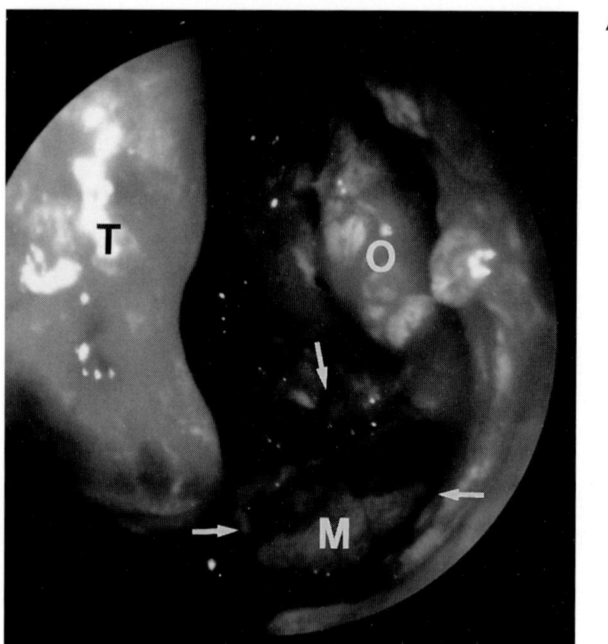

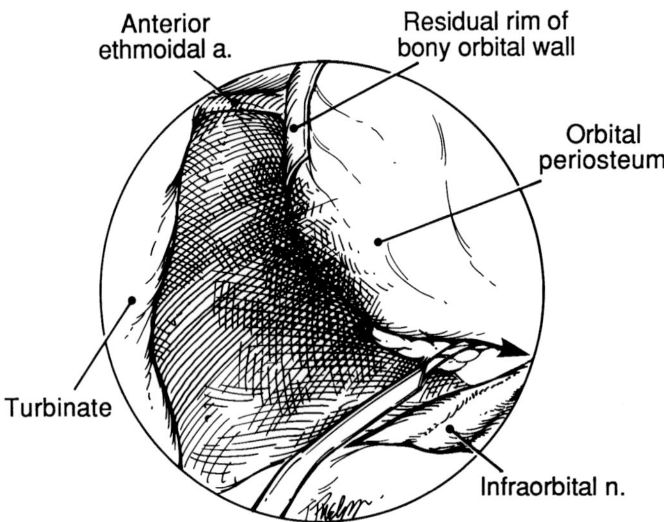

Fig. 13–3. Removal of the left orbital floor and incision of orbital periosteum. **A,** Endoscopic photograph showing maxillary sinus (M) and widened middle meatal antrostomy (arrows) with exposure of the orbital floor (30° wide angle telescope directed laterally). **B,** Artist's rendition shows incision of inferior orbital periosteum with an angled sickle knife. (From Kennedy DW, Matthew GL, Miller NR, Zinreich J: Arch Otolaryngol Head Neck Surg 116:275–282, 1990. By permission.)

within the maxillary sinus. The aim is to avoid obstruction of the surgeon's vision due to the herniation of the intraorbital contents while the incisions are made. Incisions are then made high on the medial orbital wall with a straight sickle Beaver knife or a #12 Bard Parker blade (Fig. 13–4). This allows for full herniation of orbital contents into the sinuses. Great care is used to incise only periosteum, and to avoid the rectus muscles. The immediate extent of decompression is then assessed by gently palpating the orbit and endoscopically viewing the transmission of the palpations to the herniated orbital contents.

If maximal eye regression is required, a lateral orbitotomy may then be performed. This procedure will enhance the orbital decompression by approximately 1 to 2 mm. It is also possible that this procedure may decrease any tendency towards postoperative diplopia by balancing the globe decompression medially and laterally. At the end of the operation, a rolled piece of Gelfilm coated in antibiotic ointment is inserted between the herniated orbital fat and the lateral aspect of the middle turbinate. Packing, if required, should only be performed loosely. Broad spectrum antibiotics are started postoperatively typically using a β-lactamase-resistant cephalosporin.

During postoperative care, the maxillary sinus is suctioned free of blood under endoscopic visualization. The Gelfilm can be removed after 1 week.

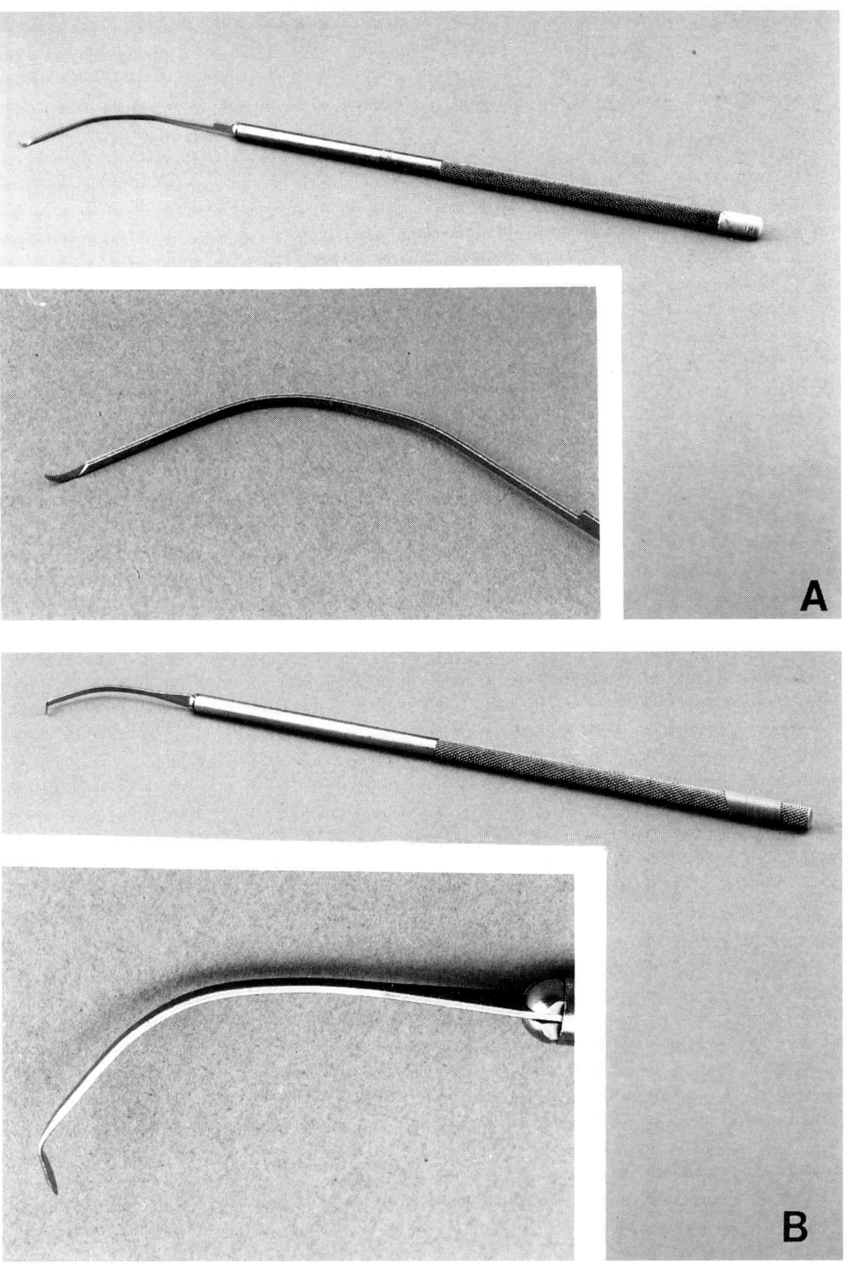

Fig. 13–4. A Beaver (Rudolph Beaver Inc, Waltham, MA) sickle knife (**A**) and Rosen knife (**B**) bent to allow incision of the periorbita within the right maxillary sinus. (From Kennedy DW, Matthew GL, Miller NR, Zinreich J: Arch Otolaryngol Head Neck Surg 116:275–282, 1990. By permission.)

Some regression of the eyes is observed even at the end of the operation, and further decompression continues to occur in the postoperative period.

Results

The advent of the intranasal endoscopes has significantly improved the anatomic visualization of the nose and paranasal sinuses. This has facilitated the transnasal decompression approach to the medial and inferior orbital walls that compares well with traditional methods. Warren and colleagues,[9] in a review of 305 patients undergoing Walsh-Ogura decompressions, noted an average ocular recession of 4 mm. Desanto and associates[34] reported an average recession of 5.5 mm in 200 patients who underwent transantral decompression. Kennedy and colleagues,[23] in a report on their initial endoscopic decompressions, reported a 4.7 mm mean decompression with the transnasal endoscopic approach alone (5 orbits); and 5.7 mm as a mean decompression with the transnasal endoscopic technique combined with a lateral orbitomy (8 orbits). These results compared favorably with traditional methods. Michel and coworkers[35] obtained a 3- to 4-mm reduction in proptosis for endoscopic decompression performed on 12 orbits. Metson and associates[36] reduced proptosis an average of 3.2 mm with the endoscopic approach alone (6 orbits), and 5.6 mm as a mean decompression with the transnasal endoscopic technique combined with a lateral orbitomy (16 orbits). Endoscopes permit a maximal posterior orbital decompression at the orbital apex, an area often not fully accessible via the external or transantral routes (Fig. 13–5). This provides optimal decompression of the optic nerve in cases of optic neuropathy. Endoscopic visualization of the medial orbital wall is superior to either the

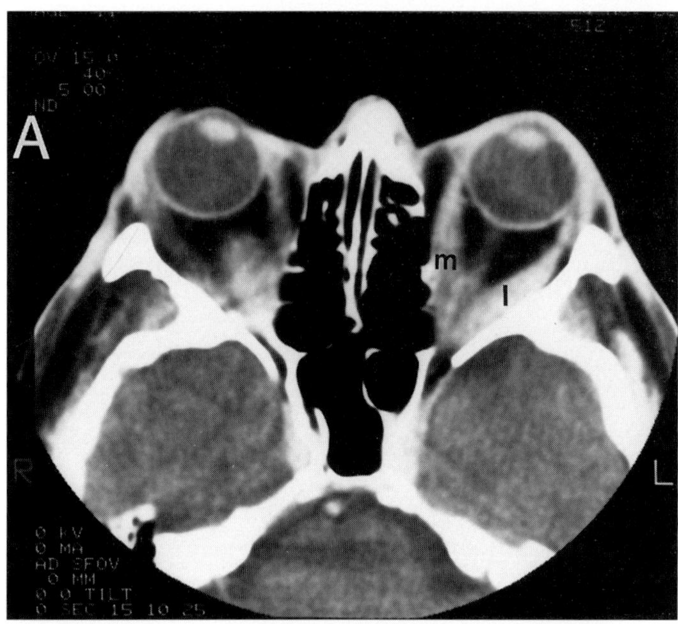

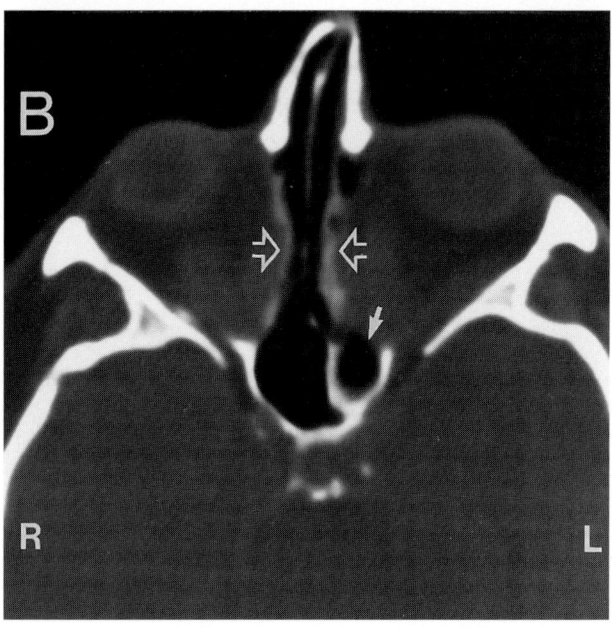

Fig. 13–5. Pre- and postorbital decompression CT scans of a patient with Graves' exophthalmos. **A,** Preoperative axial CT scan shows enlarged medial (m) and lateral (l) rectus muscles with compression of the orbital apex bilaterally. **B,** Postoperative axial CT scan shows left (L) sphenoidotomy (solid arrow), allowing medial expansion of orbital soft tissue to the middle turbinate with resultant increase in orbital apex space. (From Kennedy DW, Matthew GL, Miller NR, Zinreich J: Arch Otolaryngol Head Neck Surg 116:275–282, 1990. By permission.)

transantral or external ethmoid approaches, thus permitting a more complete medial orbital decompression.

In the authors' hands, transnasal orbital decompression has been a safe procedure accompanied by a minimum of morbidity. The scar of an external ethmoidectomy and the morbidity of a Caldwell-Luc antrostomy are avoided. As with other procedures for orbital decompression, diplopia may develop or worsen postoperatively. DeSanto[34] found an increase in diplopia from 54% preoperatively to 79% postoperatively with a standard transantral decompression. McCord[17] similarly described new diplopia in 5.7% of patients after a lateral transconjunctival decompression and in 40% of patients after a transantral decompression. Metson and colleagues[36] had 3 patients with preoperative strabismus develop worsened diplopia after surgery. Both Kennedy and associates[23] and Michel and co-workers[35] noted a deterioration in the postoperative diplopia in 2 of their patients.

The onset or progression of diplopia may not reflect a complication of surgery so much as the sequela of a good decompression, because new onset diplopia is more common in patients undergoing more extensive decompressions.[26] In the swollen orbit, there is usually considerable restriction of eye movement in all directions. This results from both proptosis and swelling or from fibrosis of the extraocular muscles. When the external restriction of proptosis is relieved by decompression, the less affected muscles are able to function, but the more swollen and fibrotic muscles (most commonly the medial recus, inferior rectus, or both) are not. The net result is an asymmetric limitation of eye movement instead of the preexisting symmetric limitation. Consequently, the patient may develop new or worsening diplopia that requires correction with prisms or extraocular muscle surgery. In general, patients with diplopia should undergo decompression before muscle surgery, because the extent of muscle correction that will be required may be significantly affected by the decompression.

Some surgeons strongly recommend maintaining some bone of the orbital wall inferomedially, as this decreases the risk of postoperative diplopia. Maintenance of bone posteriorly and inferomedially, in the portion of the orbital wall adjacent to the pterygoid plate, is felt to be particularly important. Partial, and possibly complete, reduction in the diplopia may be related to this anatomic region. However, we suggest that the preservation of this bone may have a significant, adverse effect on the extent of the globe regression potentially obtained from the surgical decompression.

A potential complication that we have not encountered is acute visual loss. As with all optical surgery, vision loss can occur from direct trauma to the optic nerve or its vasculature.[26] This risk is minimized through careful anatomic visualization and dissection by an experienced endoscopic surgeon. Because the surgery is performed under general anesthesia, it is technically more difficult, and the usual feedback provided by an awake patient when vital structures are manipulated is not available. The surgeon must be well versed in the normal anatomic landmarks and their extensive variations. This highlights the need for a high-quality preoperative CT scan, with both coronal and axial views, to serve as a "road map" during the decompression.

Advantages and Disadvantages of an Endoscopic Decompression

Endoscopic decompression permits maximal posterior orbital decompression of the orbital apex. This is especially important in cases of optic neuropathy where decompression of the optic nerve is essential. Although this degree of orbital apex decompression would be possible with an external ethmoidectomy approach, it would not be possible to perform a simultaneous decompression of the orbital floor through the same incision. Additionally, performing the operation intranasally avoids a medial canthal scar.

The extent of medial and apical orbital decompression is greater than in the Ogura-Walsh technique; and the morbidity of a Caldwell-Luc is avoided (Fig. 13–6). However, removal of the anterior orbital floor is not as complete as with a transantral approach—at the end of the procedure, a small triangular area of inferior orbital floor is left anteriorly, medially to the infraorbital nerve. A lateral orbitotomy maximizes the amount of decompression obtained.

In addition to a limited access to the anterior aspect to the medial orbital floor, decompression of the orbital floor lateral to the infraorbital nerve is not possible due to the anatomic constraints of the widened middle meatal antrotomy. However, it appears that these limitations are compensated for by the excellent extent of medial and posterior floor decompression. It has been suggested that the more limited decompression of the orbital floor laterally may prevent subsequent hypophthalmia and vertical gaze diplopia.[37] If every possible millimeter of regression is required, a simultaneous transconjunctival decompression of the anterior floor medial and lateral to the optic nerve is also possible.

Summary

In the hands of an experienced sinus endoscopist, transnasal orbital decompression is a procedure that can be performed with a minimum of morbid-

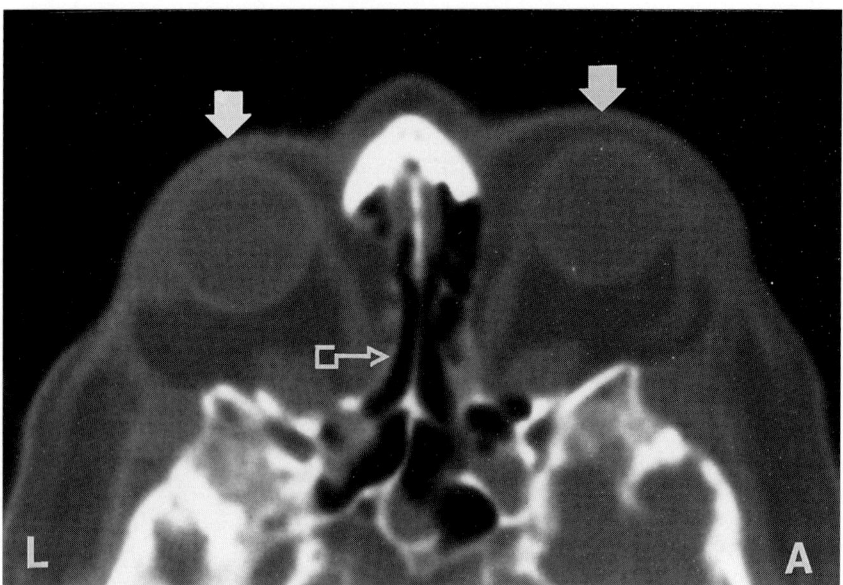

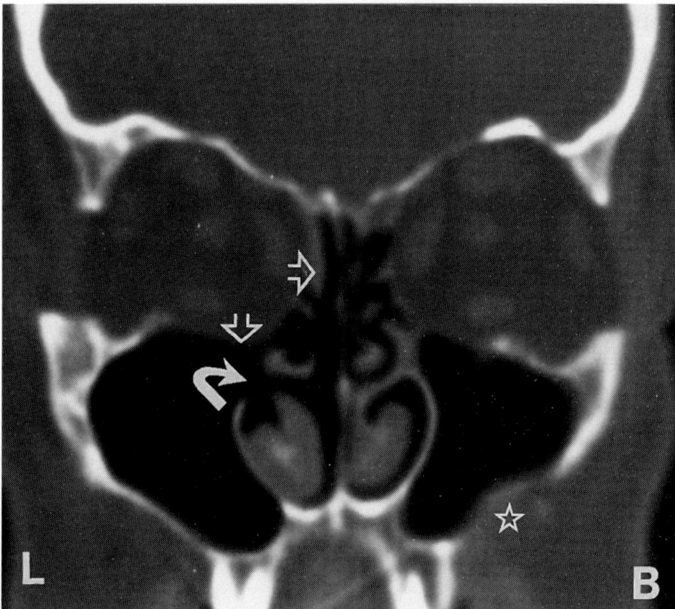

Fig. 13–6. Postoperative axial **(A)** and coronal **(B)** CT scans of a patient who underwent endoscopic decompression on the left and transantral decompression on the right. There is a greater degree of orbital decompression on the endoscopic (L) side than on the opposite (transantral) side. **A,** There is less proptosis on the endoscopic side (solid arrows) with a more extensive medial decompression to the level of the middle turbinate (open arrow). **B,** An increased medial and a comparable inferior decompression is observed on the endoscopic (L) side. Bilateral lateral orbitotomies were performed. There is a wide middle meatal antrostomy on the left (curved arrow) and evidence of a Caldwell-Luc procedure on the right (star). (From Kennedy DW, Matthew GL, Miller NR, Zinreich J: Arch Otolaryngol Head Neck Surg 116:275–282, 1990. By permission.)

ity. The necessity that the surgeon has extensive endoscopic experience to perform safely the transnasal approach cannot be overemphasized.

REFERENCES

1. Konishi J, Herman MM, Kriss JP. Binding of thyroiglobulin and thyroglobulin-antithyroglobulin immune complex to extraocular muscle menbrane. *Endocrinology.* 1974; 95:434–446.
2. Ingbar SH. *Diseases of the Thyroid.* In: *Harrison's Principles of Internal Medicine.* New York, McGraw-Hill; 1987:1743–1747.
3. Kortvelesy JS, Kennerdell JS, Van Dyk HJL. *Orbital Graves' Disease.* In: *Current Ocular Therapy 3.* Philadelphia, W.B. Saunders; 1990:643–646.
4. Hedges TR Jr, Rose E. Hyperophthalmopathic Graves' disease. *Arch Ophthalmol.* 1953;50:479–490.
5. Calcaterra TC, Thompson JW. Antral-ethmoidal decompression of the orbit in Graves' disease; ten-year experience. *Laryngoscope.* 1980;90:1941–1949.
6. Barbosa J, Wong E, Doe RP. Ophthalmopathy of Graves' disease. *Arch Intern Med.* 1972;130:111–113.
7. Weetman AP. Thyroid-associated eye disease: pathophysiology. *Lancet.* 1991;338:25–28.
8. Riley FC. Orbital pathology in Graves' disease. *Mayo Clin Proc.* 1972;47:975–979.

9. Warren JD, Spector JG, Burde R. Long-term follow up and recent observations on 305 cases of orbital decompression for dysthyroid orbitopathy. *Laryngoscope.* 1989;99:35–40.
10. Trobe JD, Glaser JS. Laflamme P. Dysthyroid optic neuropathy. *Arch Ophthalmol.* 1978;96:1199–1209.
11. Hodes BL, Shoch DE. Thyroid ocular myopathy. *Trans Am Ophthalmol Soc.* 1979;77:80–103.
12. Calcaterra TC. Management of exophthalmos. In: Cummings CS, Fredrickson JM, Harker LA, Krause CJ, Schuller DE, eds. *Otolaryngology-Head & Neck Surgery.* St. Louis, MO. CV Mosby; 1986:2543–2551.
13. Burde RM. *The orbit.* In: Lessell S. van Dalen JTW, eds. *Neuro-ophthalmology.* Amsterdam, Excerpta Medica; 1982:vol 2:272–279.
14. Kennerdell JS, Maroon JC, Buerger GF. Comprehensive surgical management of proptosis in dysthyroid orbitopathy. *Orbit.* 1987;6:153–179.
15. Putterman AM. Surgical treatment of thyroid-related upper eyelid retraction. *Ophthalmology.* 1981;88:507–512.
16. Rootman J. Graves' Orbitopathy. In: Rootman J, ed. Diseases of the orbit. Philadelphia, JB Lippincott; 1988:241–280.
17. McCord CD Jr. Current trends in orbital decompression. *Ophthalmology.* 1985;92:21–33.
18. Hurbli T, Char DH, Harris J, et al. Radiation therapy for thyroid eye diseases. *Am J Ophthalmol.* 1985;99:633–637.
19. Leone CR Jr. The management of ophthalmic Graves' disease. *Ophthalmology.* 1984;91:770–779.
20. Brennan MW, Leone CR Jr, Janaki L. Radiation therapy for Graves' disease. *Am J Ophthalmol.* 1983;96:195–199.
21. Threlkeld A, Miller NR, Wharam M. The efficacy of supervoltage radiation therapy in the treatment of dysthyroid optic neuropathy. *Orbit.*
22. Wall JR, Strakosch CR, Fang SL, et al. Thyroid binding antibodies and other immunological abnormalities in patients with Graves' ophthalmopathy: effects of treatment with cyclophosphamide, *Clin Endocrinol.* 1979;10:70–91.
23. Kennedy DW, Goodstein ML, Miller NR, Zinreich SJ. Endoscopic transnasal orbital decompression. *Arch Otolaryngol Head Neck Surg,* 1990;116:275–282.
24. Glinoer D, Etienne-Decert J, Schrooyen M, et al. Beneficial effects of intensive plasma exchange followed by immunosuppressive therapy in severe Graves' ophthalmopathy. *Acta Endocrinol.* 1986;111:30–38.
25. Dadona P, Marshall NJ, Bidey SP, et al. Successful treatment of exophthalmos and pretibial myxoedema with plasmapheresis. *Br Med J.* 1979;1:374–376.
26. Goodstein ML, Kennedy DW. An endoscopic approach for orbital decompression in dysthyroid orbitopathy. *Op Techn Otolaryngol-Head Neck Surg.* 1990;1:117–125.
27. Dollinger J. Die drickentlastlung der Augenhokie durch entfurnung der aussern Orbitalwand bei hochgradigen Exophthalmos aund Koneskutwer Hornhauterkronkung. *Dtsch Med Wochenschr.* 1911;37:1888–1890.
28. Naffziger HC. Progressive exophthalmos following thyroidectomy; its pathology and treatment. *Ann Surg.* 1931;94:582–586.
29. Sewall EC. Operative control of progressive exophthalmos. *Arch Otolaryngol Head Neck Surg.* 1936;24:621–624.
30. Hirsch O. Surgical decompression of exophthalmos. *Arch Otolaryngol Head Neck Surg.* 1950;51:325–331.
31. Walsh TE, Ogura JH. Transantral orbital decompression for malignant exophthalmos. *Laryngoscope.* 1957;67:544–549.
32. Kennedy DW. Functional endoscopic sinus surgery technique. *Arch Otolaryngol Head Neck Surg.* 1985; 111:643–649.
33. Kennedy DW, Zinreich SJ, Kuhn F, et al. Endoscopic middle meatal antrostomy: theory, technique, and patency. *Laryngoscope.* 1987;97(suppl 43):1–9.
34. DeSanto LW. The total rehabilitation of Graves' ophthalmopathy. *Laryngoscope.* 1980;90:1652–1678.
35. Michel O. Bresgen K, Russmann W, et al. Endoskopish knotrollierts endonasale Orbitadekompression beim malignan Ophthalmus. *KLaryngorhinootologie.* 1991;70:656–662.
36. Metson R, Dallow RL, Shore JW. Endoscopic orbital decompression, *Laryngoscope.* In press.
37. Leone CR Jr, Piest KL, Newman RJ. Medial and lateral wall decompression for thyroid ophthalmopathy. *Am J Ophthalmol.* 1989;108:160–166.

14

Endoscopic Optic Nerve Decompression for the Treatment of Traumatic Optic Neuropathy

Seth J. Silberman** and **James M. Chow

Traumatic acute loss of vision is one of the most serious non-life threatening sequelae in patients who survive closed head injury. It is estimated that approximately 2% of patients presenting with craniofacial injury each year are permanently blind as a result of the traumatic insult. The treatment of these patients is undertaken by the otolaryngologist, ophthalmologist, and neurosurgeon and is aimed at halting or reversing the progressive axonal degeneration that can lead to permanent blindness. This approach is primarily empirical and may involve observation, administration of megadose systemic steroids, and/or extracranial or intracranial decompression of the optic nerve. The application of endoscopic sinus techniques to optic nerve decompression is discussed as an alternative approach in the treatment of these patients.

Pathophysiology of Traumatic Blindness

The pathophysiology of acute or delayed axonal degeneration of the optic nerve has remained unclear since Hippocrates' initial observation that "dimness of vision occurs in the injuries to the brow, and is less noticeable the more recent the wound, but as the scar becomes old so the dimness increases."[1] Centuries later, Walsh and Lindbergh provided insight into the specific nature of these lesions based upon their histopathologic studies of optic nerves in human autopsy specimens.[2] They described three primary injuries that were thought to be responsible for the visual loss. Hemorrhage from the microvascular blood supply in the substance of the nerve and its vaginal sheaths was prevalent in their specimens. They also observed tears and contusion necrosis of the nerve from direct trauma, and edema and necrosis from systemic and localized vascular insufficiency (Fig. 14–1). Other contributing factors included vasospasm and extrinsic compression of the axially arranged nutrient vessels in the pia mater that originate from the central retinal artery and the ophthalmic artery.[3]

Surgical decompression is based upon the premise that anatomic disruption of the intracanalicular portion of the optic nerve or its supporting structures may be altered favorably by relieving the pressure on the optic nerve or by the removal of bony fragments impinging on the nerve. When performed within a critical period, it is believed that this can lead to the reversal of the resultant neuropraxia and functional stabilization or improvement of visual status. Radius and Anderson have shown experimentally that optic nerve axons in monkeys can survive pressure-induced interruption of axonal transport for approximately 8 hours and even total ischemia for up to 2 hours.[4]

However, the rationale for optic nerve decompression has not been established by scientific studies.[5–12] Table 14–1 shows the results of prior published clinical studies, the majority of which were uncontrolled retrospective series, dealing with various methods of treatment of traumatic optic neuropathy.[13] These data suggest a general trend favoring surgery combined with systemic steroids. Surgical decompression is more advantageous than observation alone but may not be superior to systemic steroids. In the National Spinal Cord Injury Study, a statistically significant improvement in overall outcome with respect to motor function was demonstrated for

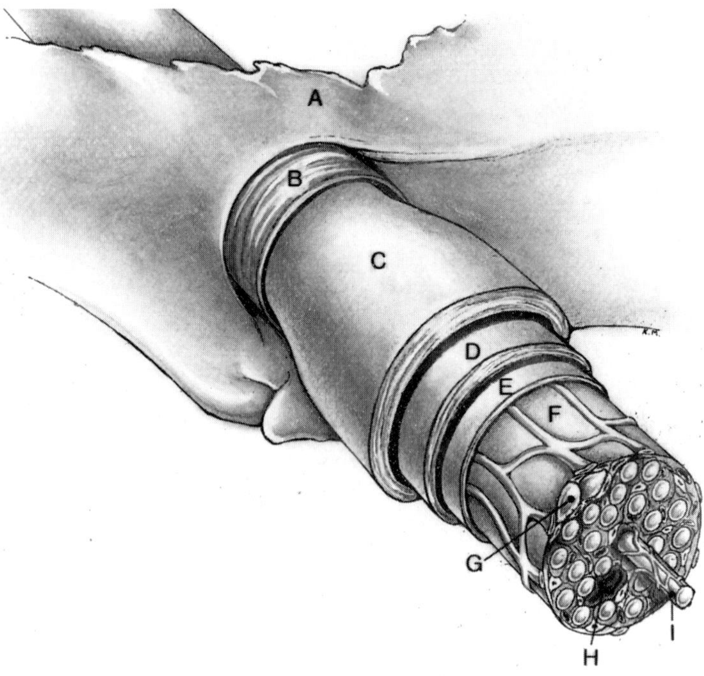

Fig. 14–1. Ultrastructure of optic nerve and associated injury. (A) Falciform crest; (B) annulus of Zinn; (C) dura; (D) arachnoid; (E) pia mater; (F) nutrient vessels from central retinal and ophthalmic arteries; (G) edema of epineurium, endoneurium and axons; (H) hematoma of interneuronal space caused by disruption of 7–20 micrometer nutrient capillaries in pial plexus (I).

Table 14–1. Results of Published Series: Treatment of Optic Nerve Trauma

Treatment	Subjects	Improve	Fail
Steroids	146	78 (53%)	68 (47%)
Surgical Decompression	383	200 (52%)	183 (48%)
Surgery & Steroids	42	29 (69%)	13 (31%)
No Treatment	257	89 (34%)	168 (66%)

the group receiving megadose methylprednisolone versus placebo effect in patients with an acute spinal cord injury.[14] After taking into account the similarities in the neurovascular arrangement between the spinal cord and the optic nerve, one could infer that a similar outcome would be expected from a well-controlled study for optic nerve injury. Whether medical or surgical intervention can impact upon the clinical outcome of these patients deserves close scrutiny in future studies. Nevertheless, in the absence of formal clinical studies, optic nerve decompression may have a role in selected patients with the goal of stabilizing or improving the visual status in a generally irreversible injury that results in severely compromised visual acuity or blindness.

Development of Optic Nerve Decompression

The endoscopic approach to optic nerve decompression is an adaptation of the transethmoid extracranial approach to the optic nerve which was originally described by Edward Cecil Sewall in 1926.[15] This operation has been popularized by Niho and others.[16–18] Fujitani published his results of endonasal microscopic optic nerve decompression and showed improvement in 48% of the surgically treated group versus 44% of the nonsurgical subjects.[19] Takahashi showed improvement in four of five patients using this technique.[20] In 1991, Aurbach published his report on endoscopic optic nerve decompression in the German literature.[21] We have performed this procedure on selected patients and present the technique for the experienced endoscopic sinus surgeon.

Anatomy

The successful endoscopic approach to the optic nerve requires familiarity with the anatomy of the optic canal in relation to the paranasal sinuses. This osseous canal is bounded by the roots of the lesser wing of the sphenoid bone and is quite variable in its dimensions, measuring 5.5 to 11.5 mm in length and 4.0 to 9.5 mm in diameter.[22] Proximally, the canal is elliptical in configuration, with the greatest dimension in the horizontal axis. A dural reflection, known as the falciform crest, forms the roof of the tunnel, marking the transition from the intracranial to the intracanalicular segment. The pia and arachnoid membranes comprise the other layers of the vaginal sheath and are continuous with the intracranial space and cerebrospinal fluid (Fig. 14–1). The bone which covers the optic nerve becomes progressively thicker and more dense as the nerve makes its course from the intracranial segment to the optic ring. The canal wall may be as thin as 0.21 mm proximally, while the bone can attain thicknesses as great as 0.75 mm at the optic ring, which is variably located at the junction of the posterior ethmoid and sphenoid sinuses.[22] The surgeon must be cognizant of the various anatomic configurations of this region as the nerve is approached. The ethmoid cells may extend posteriorly into the sphenoid sinus when Onodi cells are present, thereby completely surrounding much of the intracanalicular portion of the nerve (11.7% to 25% of subjects).[23] The sphenoid sinus may be hypoplastic, exhibiting a presellar (24%) or conchal configuration, with the development of the latter limited by the age of the patient.[24] In 4% of subjects the nerve may be covered by mucosa only, thereby rendering the fibers extremely susceptible to iatrogenic injury.[24] The canal is narrowest at the optic ring, in part due to the adherence of the dura, periosteum, annulus of Zinn, and the origins of the superior and medial rectus muscles. This relationship of the fixed adnexa and the relative elasticity of the optic nerve in its canal is thought to play a role in the transference of translational energy and resultant injury to the nerve or its blood supply.[25] Decompression traditionally includes removal of 180 to 270 degrees of the bony canal and opening the vaginal sheath, which must be performed with extreme care in this region to prevent further trauma to the nerve.

Within the sphenoid sinus, the optic nerve is usually found at the superior aspect of the lateral wall of the sinus, appearing as a mucosal prominence that follows the orientation of the optic cone (Fig. 14–2). Approximately 25% of the time this characteristic landmark will not be seen endoscopically and the surgeon must rely upon the position of the internal carotid artery to aid in proper identification and localization of the nerve.[24] The posterior ethmoid artery can usually be seen coursing superior and anterior to the nerve (Fig. 14–3) approximately 73.0 mm (range 70.0 to 75.0 mm) from the anterior maxillary spine. The annulus of Zinn and the anterior and posterior limits of the decompressed segment of the optic nerve are located 84.0, 81.1, and 89.6 mm, respectively, from the anterior maxillary spine.[26]

The internal carotid artery is the most medial structure in the lateral wall of the sphenoid sinus, located in the carotid sulcus of the lateral surface of the body of the sphenoid bone. Aurbach and colleagues demonstrated that the distance between the optic nerve and internal carotid artery ranges from 2.39 to 10.04 mm.[27] Extreme care must be taken to prevent injury to the internal carotid artery. The bone is 0.5 mm in thickness over the vessel, with approximately 8% of subjects possessing only a mucosal covering.[24]

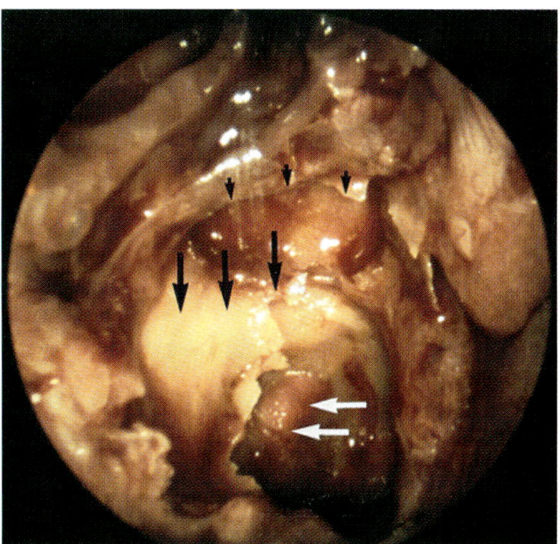

Fig. 14–2. Endoscopic view of lateral wall of right sphenoid sinus. Prominence of the optic canal (black arrows) and carotid canal (white arrows). Remaining portion of anterior wall of sphenoid sinus following its removal (small black arrows).

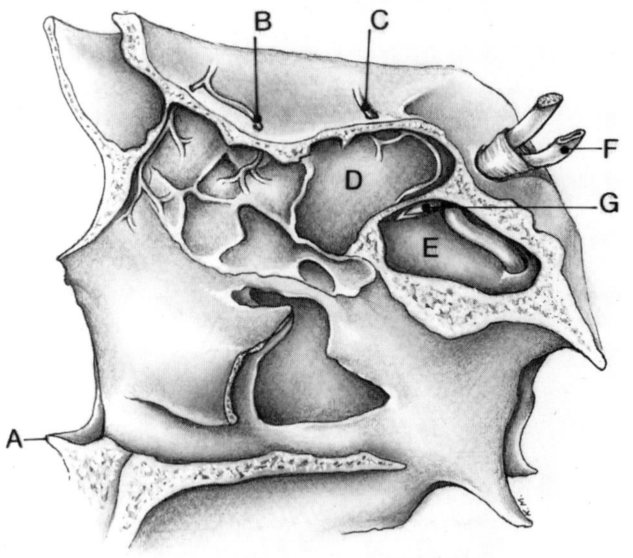

Fig. 14–3. Anatomical landmarks observed during endoscopic approach to the optic nerve. (A) Anterior maxillary spine used as reference point (see text for measurements); (B) anterior ethmoidal artery; (C) posterior ethmoidal artery; (D) posterior ethmoid sinus; (E) sphenoid sinus; (F) internal carotid artery; (G) optic nerve.

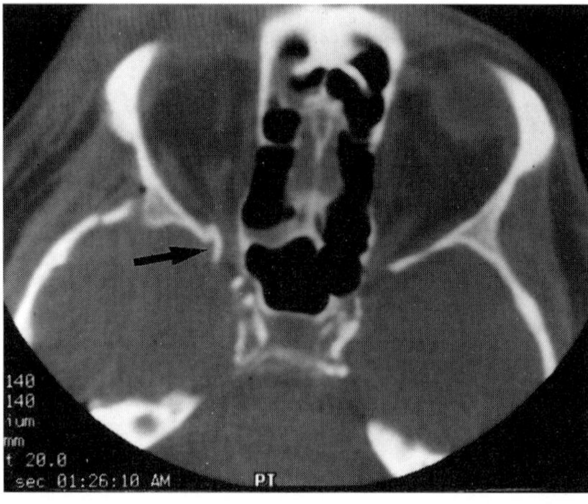

Fig. 14–4. Preoperative axial CT scan demonstrating fracture of the right anterior clinoid process with impingement of the optic canal (arrow).

Preoperative Considerations

Axial and coronal CT scans of the paranasal sinuses, including 1.5-mm axial sections of the orbit, are obtained at the initial evaluation of all persons being evaluated for traumatic vision loss. Precise imaging is essential to determine the nature, extent, and location of the injury so that an appropriate initial management plan can be formulated (Fig. 14–4). Information such as the presence of Onodi cells, the characteristics of the bone covering the optic nerve and internal carotid artery, as well as the degree of aeration of the sphenoid sinus, which is of particular importance in pediatric patients, can be used for surgical planning. Representative sections should be displayed in the operating suite during the procedure.

Ophthalmologic consultation will confirm the presence of optic neuropathy and exclude other causes of immediate or delayed visual deterioration such as hyphema, retinal detachment, or vitreous hemorrhage. Injury to the globe including scleral lacerations or corneal subluxation can preclude or delay any surgical manipulation of the orbit or its adnexal structures. Neurosurgical evaluation may obviate the need for optic nerve decompression from any of the extracranial approaches. Significant fractures of the anterior skull base associated with intracranial bleeding, cerebrospinal fluid fistula, foreign body, severe frontal sinus fractures involving the posterior table, or traumatic encephalocele are indications for an intracranial approach to the optic canal and the associated intracranial pathology.

Patients who present with immediate documented loss of vision and radiographic evidence of injury to the nerve should be considered for immediate endoscopic nerve decompression if there are no supervening contraindications.[16] If visual deterioration is delayed or if significant radiographic findings are absent, treatment consisting of observation versus steroids and/or decompression should be discussed with the patient. Unfortunately, there are no current data in the literature to support one particular method of treatment. Endoscopic optic nerve decompression may be considered when a 48-hour trial of megadose systemic steroids fails to improve vision in a final effort to reverse the various factors leading to compromise of neuronal function.[28]

Operative Technique

The patient is placed under general anesthesia and prepped and draped in the usual manner for endoscopic sinus surgery. The eyelids are taped closed over the lateral aspect of the upper lid and the orbital region should remain exposed to permit examination of the pupils and palpation of the globes intraoperatively. A mixture of tetracaine hydrochloride (8 cc of 2% solution) and ephedrine (2 cc of 5% solution) is sprayed into the nasal cavities, followed by placement of cotton pledgets containing the mixture. The remainder is utilized during the procedure in an aerosolized form to aid in hemostasis. Following this, the middle turbinate, ethmoid bulla, and uncinate process are infiltrated with lidocaine hydrochloride 1% and epinephrine 1:100,000 under direct endoscopic visualization. A septoplasty with or without alatomy may be required for simultaneous access of the endoscope and microdrill. The procedure consists of removal of all sinus structures medial to the optic cone and proceeds in an anterior to posterior direction. First, an infundibulotomy and complete middle ethmoidectomy are performed. Subsequently, the posterior ethmoid cells are entered and the middle turbinate is removed, thus permitting access to the entire anterior wall of the sphenoid sinus. The sphenoid ostium is located using a beaded probe and should be used as a reference point to determine the transition of the posterior ethmoid cells to the sphenoid sinus in the region adjacent to the orbit. Although the ostium is invariably located approximately 7.0 to 7.5 cm from the anterior maxillary spine, the Onodi cells adjacent to the optic cone may extend posterior to this point, potentially exposing the optic nerve to inadvertent instrumentation. Dissection too far superiorly to the sphenoid ostium can lead to penetration of the roof of the ethmoid sinus and entrance into the cranial cavity.

The sphenoid sinus is then entered through the anterior wall, and the anterior wall of the sinus is removed using various forceps. In some instances, the anterior wall of the sphenoid sinus may need to be drilled down to facilitate entry. The posterior ethmoidal artery is located proximal to this area and should be left undisturbed; active bleeding from the posterior septal rami of the sphenopalatine artery may be encountered just above the choana. Bipolar cautery should be utilized in this region to prevent conduction to the optic nerve via the inferior orbital fissure. After a wide sphenoidotomy is performed, the structures of the lateral wall of the sphenoid sinus are visualized using the 0 degree and 30 degree nasal telescopes. (Model #7200A and #27108BS—Karl Storz, Germany). The optic nerve is usually visualized in the superolateral portion of the sphenoid sinus and the internal carotid artery is seen coursing inferior and posterior to the nerve. Palpation using a blunt instrument may be carefully performed to locate any dehiscent portions of the optic nerve. Decompression is initiated utilizing an appropriate neurosurgical drill fitted with a 3- or 4-mm diamond burr. Drilling should commence just posterior to the optic ring area where the bone is of greatest thickness (Fig. 14–5). Frequent irrigation is needed so that the operative field does not become desiccated, resulting in thermal injury to the nerve and devitalization of the surrounding bone. Exposure of the nerve should approach or exceed 180 degrees of the circumference. As the dissection proceeds posteriorly, the bone may be removed with a small curette or otologic instrument of sufficient length. Proximal removal of the more dense bone at the optic ring is facilitated with the drill until the medial rectus fibers are visualized marking the anterior limit of the decompression. Distally, the optic nerve is traced until the posterior extent of the sphenoid sinus is reached or proximity to the internal carotid artery prevents safe access to the nerve. At this distance, special skull base instrumentation, such as the Fisch forceps (Xomed-Treace, Jacksonville, Fl) may be required to complete the dissection.

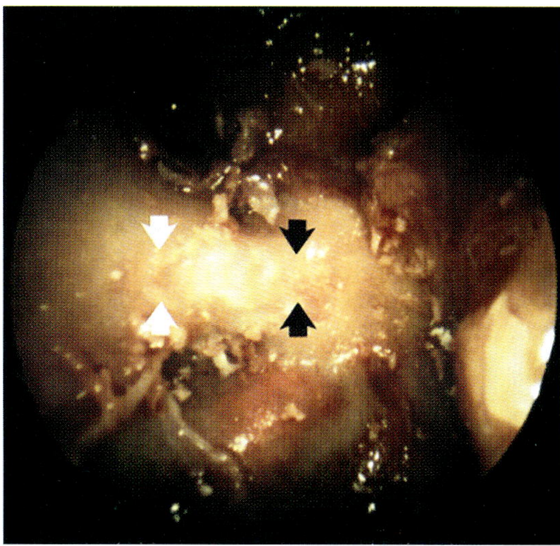

Fig. 14–5. Appearance of right optic nerve following endoscopic decompression. Bone at proximal portion (white arrows) is thicker and more dense than at distal aspect of decompression (black arrows).

Controversy exists as to whether or not the vaginal sheath needs to be incised. If incised, a sharp sickle knife or angled myringotomy knife should be used. A light nonadherent pack coated with antibiotic ointment is placed in the nose to control bleeding and is removed within 24 hours. The patient is placed on cefazolin sodium for 3 days perioperatively.

Postoperative Care

The patient is followed carefully for changes in ocular or visual status, with particular attention to observation for retroorbital hematoma or worsening visual acuity. Cerebrospinal fluid rhinorrhea may occur but should resolve spontaneously without sequelae.[16] Ophthalmology consultation is performed within the first 24 hours postoperatively and throughout the hospitalization to document any change in the examination. Thereafter, the patient should undergo routine follow-up with an ophthalmologist at regular intervals for the first 6 months. The administration of systemic corticosteroids may be performed at the discretion of the treating physician.

Summary

Endoscopic optic nerve decompression that follows the principles of previously described transethmoid procedures is a new approach to the treatment of traumatic optic neuropathy. Adequate exposure of the intracanalicular portion of the optic nerve is gained, and decompression can be performed at the segment where injury to the nerve is believed to have occurred. The endoscopic approach avoids external incisions or a craniotomy. This is especially suited for patients who are medically unstable or have no associated intracranial pathology. Careful patient selection, appropriate preoperative work-up, and extensive familiarity with the extracranial course of the optic nerve, internal carotid artery, and structural variations of ethmoid and sphenoid sinuses are essential to optimizing the surgical management of these patients.

REFERENCES

1. Hughes B. Indirect injury of the optic nerves and chiasma. *Bull Johns Hopkins Hosp.* 1962; 111:98–126.
2. Walsh F, Lindbergh. Pathological clinical correlates: indirect trauma to the optic nerves and chiasm. *Inv Ophthalmol.* 1966; 5:433–449.
3. Francois J. Vascularization of the optic nerve (letter). *Arch Ophthal.* 1977; 95:520.
4. Radius R, Anderson D. Reversibility of optic nerve damage in primate eyes subjected to intraocular pressure above systolic blood pressure. *Br J Ophthal.* 1981; 65:661–672.
5. Lam B, Weingeist T. Corticosteroid responsive traumatic optic neuropathy. *Am J Ophthal.* 1990; 109:99–100.
6. Mahaptra A. Delayed recovery from indirect optic nerve injury. *J Neurosurg Sci.* 1992; 36:151–153.
7. Seiff S. High dose corticosteroids for treatment of vision loss due to indirect injury to the optic nerve. *Ophthal Surg.* 1990; 21:389–395.
8. Call N. Decompression of the optic nerve in the optic canal. *Ophthalmic Plast Reconstr Surg.* 1986; 2:133–137.
9. Messerli J, Vuillemin Th, Raveh J. Primare Opticusdekmopressionbei Mittelgesichtsfrakturen. *Klin Mbl Augenheilk.* 1990; 196:398–401.
10. Nayak S, Kirtam M, Ingle M. Transethmoid decompression of the optic nerve in head injuries: an update. *J Laryngol Otol.* 1991; 105:205–206.
11. Mauriello J, Deluca J, Krieger A, et al. Management of traumatic optic neuropathy—a study of 23 patients. *Br J Ophthalmol.* 1992; 76:349–352.
12. Soudant J, Lamas G, Senechala G, Girard B. Decompression du nerf optique par voie trans ethmoido-sphenoidale dans les traumatismes orbitaires. *Ann Chir Plast Esthet.* 1989; 34:417–420.
13. Jorissen M, Feenstra L. Optic nerve decompression for indirect posterior optic nerve trauma. *Acta Oto-rhinolaryngologica Belg.* 1992; 46:311–324.
14. Bracken M, et al. A randomized, controlled trial of methylprednisolone or naloxone in the treatment of acute spinal-cord injury. *NEJM* 1990; 322:1405–1411.
15. Sewall EC. External operation on the ethmosphenoid frontal group of sinuses under local anesthesia. *Arch Oto.* 1926; 4:378–411.
16. Niho S, Yasuda K, Sato T, et al. Decompression of the optic canal by the transethmoid route. *Am J Opthalmol.* 1961; 51:659–665.
17. Imachi J, Inoue K, Takahashi T. Clinical and histopathological investigations of optic nerve lesions in cases of head injuries. *Jpn J Ophthalmol.* 1962; 12:98–126.
18. Fukado Y. Results in 400 cases of surgical decompression of the optic nerve. *Mod Probl Ophthal.* 1975; 14:474–481.
19. Fujitani T, Inoue K, Takahashi T, et al. Indirect traumatic optic neuropathy—visual outcome of operative and nonoperative cases. *Jpn J Ophthalmol.* 1986; 30:125–134.
20. Takahashi M, Itoh M, Ishii J, Yoshida A. Microscopic endonasal decompression of the optic nerve. *Arch Otorhinolaryngol.* 1989; 246:113–116.
21. Aurbach G, Reck R, Mihm B. Die endonasale, endoskopisch-mikroskopisch kontrollierte Dekompression des N. Opticus. *HNO.* 1991; 39:302–306.
22. Habal M, Maniscalco J, Rhoton A. Microsurgical anatomy of the optic canal: correlates to optic nerve exposure. *J Surg Res.* 1977; 22:527–533.
23. Lang J. *Clinical Anatomy of the Nose, Nasal Cavity and Paranasal Sinuses.* New York, Thieme, 1989, p 89.
24. Fujii K, Chambers S, Rhoton A. Neurovascular relationships of the sphenoid sinus. *J Neurosurg.* 1979; 50:31–39.
25. Walsh F. Pathological clinical correlates: indirect trauma to the optic nerves and chiasm. *Inv Ophthalmol.* 1966; 5:433–439.
26. Silberman S, Chow J, Stankiewicz J. Personal observation.
27. Aurbach G, Ullrich D, Mihm B. Chirurgische Anatomie des Nervus opticus und der Arteria carotis interna in der lateralen Keilbeinhohlenwand. *HNO.* 1991; 39:467–475.
28. Panje W, Gross C, Anderson R. Sudden blindness following facial trauma. *Otolaryngol Head Neck Surg.* 1981; 89:941–948.

15

Evaluation of Rhinologic Headaches

James M. Chow

Headaches or facial pains are common symptoms encountered by the otolaryngologist. Many of the patients that present to the otolaryngologist with a headache do not do so with their headache as the only symptom but rather with a constellation of symptoms such as a headache, nasal congestion, and nasal drainage which directs one towards the nasal cavity or paranasal sinuses. This triad of symptoms is frequently seen in patients with acute or chronic sinusitis. In a study of 100 consecutive patients with a diagnosis of acute or chronic sinusitis, a severe headache was the fourth most commonly encountered symptom, occurring in 48 patients. Nasal congestion, nasal secretion, and fullness or pressure were more frequently experienced.[1] In another study of 400 consecutive patients undergoing endoscopic sinus surgery, 63% complained of having headaches, the third most commonly encountered symptom after nasal congestion and nasal drainage.[2] Although a headache may not be the most commonly encountered symptom in patients with acute or chronic sinusitis, in some instances, it is the major complaint for which the patient seeks relief.

Although the cause of the headache can be attributed to the nasal cavities or the paranasal sinuses in many instances, especially in those patients in whom nasal congestion and nasal drainage are also presenting symptoms, in other patients the cause is not as clear. These individuals need to be evaluated carefully with a thorough history and physical examination to exclude a non-sinus origin of the headache. Diagnostic possibilities include tension headaches, migraine headaches, neuralgias, cervical spine disorders, temporomandibular joint disorders, vascular abnormalities, ophthalmologic disorders, and various intracranial pathologies.[1] Evaluating these patients is complex and compounded by the occasional triggering of tension or migraine headaches or neuralgias by sinus pathology.

Another category of patients is even more difficult to evaluate. These patients present with a headache as their only major symptom. However, no obvious sinus disease can be identified, nor can a non-sinus etiology be positively diagnosed. Prior to a discussion of this group of patients, a discussion of the neural innervation of the nasal cavity and paranasal sinuses is necessary.

Neural Innervation

The lateral nasal wall is innervated by the first and second divisions of the trigeminal nerve (Fig. 15–1). The anterior ethmoidal nerve, which is the terminal branch of the nasociliary nerve of the first division of the trigeminal nerve, provides sensory innervation to the anterosuperior portion of the lateral nasal wall. This nerve supplies a variable portion of the anterior portion of the superior, middle, and inferior turbinates, as well as their respective meati. The inferoposterior portion of the lateral nasal wall is innervated by the posterior nasal branches of the second division of the trigeminal nerve. These nerves supply a greater portion of the inferior, middle, and superior turbinates, as well as their respective meati than the anterior ethmoidal nerve. The anteroinferior portion of the lateral nasal wall is innervated by a small branch of the anterior superior alveolar nerve of the second division of the trigeminal nerve, the nasodental nerve.[3]

The anterosuperior aspect of the septum is innervated by the anterior ethmoidal nerve, a branch of the first division of the trigeminal nerve. Most of the septum is innervated by the nasopalatine nerve and the posterior superior nasal nerves, which are branches of the sphenopalatine nerve of the second division of the trigeminal nerve. A small portion of the anteroinferior nasal septum is innervated by the nasodental nerve of the anterior

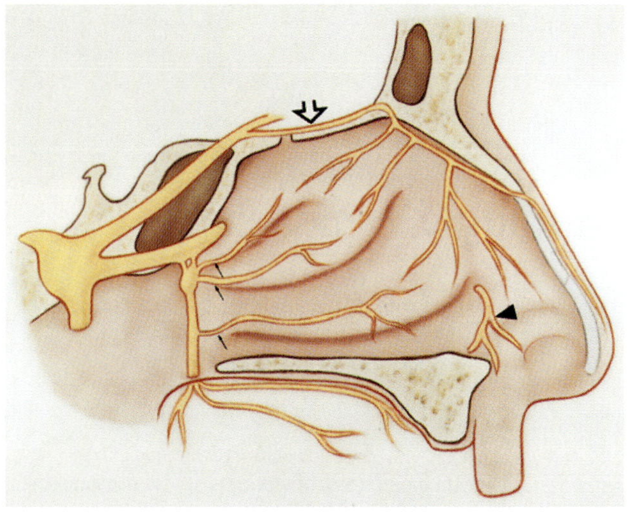

Fig. 15–1. Sensory innervation of the lateral nasal wall. The distributions of the anterior ethmoidal nerve (open arrow), posterior nasal branches of the second division of the trigeminal nerve (small arrows), and a branch of the anterosuperior alveolar nerve (arrowhead) are illustrated.

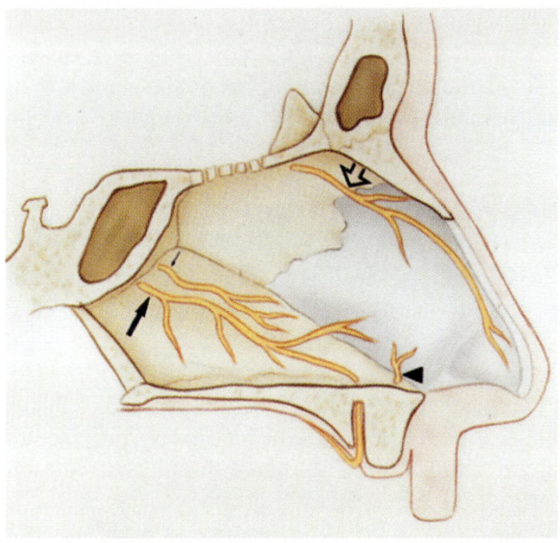

Fig. 15–2. Sensory innervation of the septum. The anterior ethmoidal nerve (open arrow), the nasopalatine nerve (large arrow), the posterior superior nasal nerves (small arrow), and the nasodental nerves (arrowhead) are illustrated.

superior alveolar nerve of the second division of the trigeminal nerve (Fig. 15–2).[3]

The frontal sinus is innervated by the supratrochlear and supraorbital nerves, which are terminal branches of the frontal nerve of the first division of the trigeminal nerve. The anterior ethmoid sinuses are innervated by the anterior ethmoidal nerve. The posterior ethmoid sinuses are dually innervated by some of the posterior nasal branches of the sphenopalatine nerve, which is a branch of the second division of the trigeminal nerve, and the posterior ethmoidal nerve, which is a branch of the first division of the trigeminal nerve. The maxillary sinus is innervated by the superior alveolar nerves, which are branches of the second division of the trigeminal nerve. The sphenoid sinus is also dually innervated by the posterior ethmoidal nerve of the first division of the trigeminal nerve and the posterior nasal branches of the sphenopalatine nerve of the second division of the trigeminal nerve. The posterior ethmoidal nerve supplies the superior portion of the sphenoid sinus, while the posterior nasal branches of the sphenopalatine nerve supply the floor of the sphenoid sinus.[4]

Although some patients with sinus pathology present to the otolaryngologist with complaints of localized headaches, in many instances, the headache or facial pain is not present in the region of pathology. In a report published in 1943, McAuliffe and associates[5] described the results of a study in which they stimulated various areas of the nasal cavity and paranasal sinuses using a variety of noxious stimuli and then recorded the area to which the pain was localized. They determined that the mucosa around the sinus ostia were most sensitive to noxious stimuli, whereas the mucosa of the turbinates were less sensitive, and the mucosa within the sinuses were least sensitive. More importantly, they found that the pain was rarely localized to the sites stimulated but frequently referred to other regions of the head. This can be physiologically understood through the concept of referred pain (Fig. 15–3). This concept is based on an afferent sensory neuron with its receptor in the nasal mucosa and an afferent sensory neuron with its receptor in the skin synapsing on the same sensory neuron of the spinal nucleus of the trigeminal nerve. Because the sen-

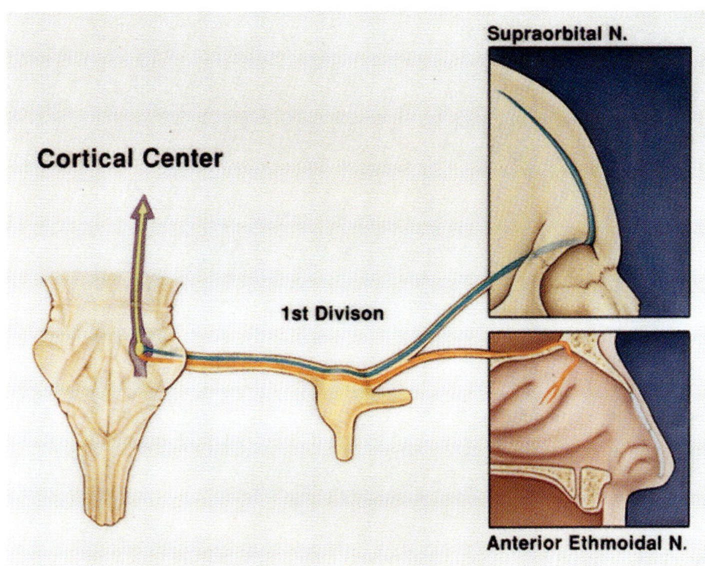

Fig. 15–3. Schematic illustration depicting an afferent sensory neuron from the nasal mucosa and an afferent sensory neuron from the skin synapsing on the same sensory neuron of the spinal nucleus of the trigeminal nerve.

sory neuron of the spinal nucleus of the trigeminal nerve proceeds to a higher cortical center and because the cortical center cannot distinguish the original peripheral source of the impulse, it assigns the pain as coming from the cutaneous skin, based on previous experience.[6,7] To determine the area to which the pain is referred, it is important to review the sensory innervation of the face. The cutaneous distribution of the first division of the trigeminal nerve is to the forehead through the supraorbital and supratrochlear nerves, the medial canthal region through the infratrochlear nerve, the lateral canthal region through the lacrimal nerve, and the lateral aspect of the nose through the external nasal branch of the nasociliary nerve (Fig. 15–4). Thus, stimulation of the anterior aspect of the middle turbinate may be reported as pain in the forehead region, the medial or lateral aspect of the eye, or the lateral aspect of the nose. The cutaneous distribution of the second division of the trigeminal nerve is to the cheek through the palpebral, labial, and nasal branches of the infraorbital nerve and to the temple or zygoma through the zygomaticotemporal and zygomaticofacial nerves, respectively (see Fig. 15–4). Stimulation of the posterior aspect of the middle turbinate may thus be reported as pain in the cheek, temple, or region of the zygoma.

Further investigations into this area have been elucidated through the study of various neuropeptides, one of which is substance P. Stimulation of polymodal nociceptors through infection, chemicals, or pressure leads to an orthodromic pulse that is carried to the central nervous system through unmyelinated C-fibers, resulting in the perception

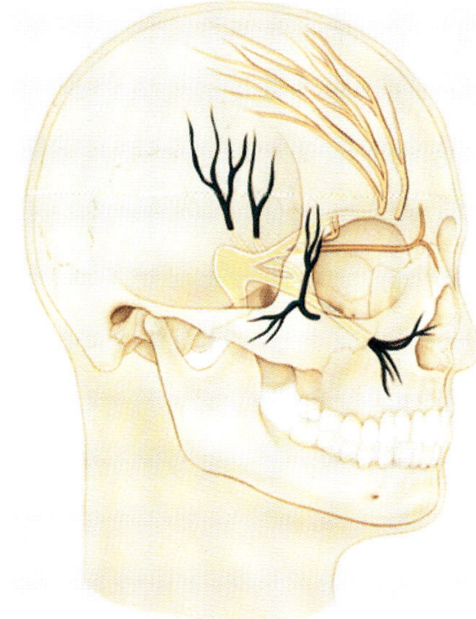

Fig. 15–4. Schematic illustration showing the cutaneous distributions of the first (yellow) and second (black) divisions of the trigeminal nerve.

of pain. Stimulation of polymodal nociceptors also results in the generation of an antidromic impulse leading to the release of substance P at the mucosal site. This causes plasma extravasation, vasodilation, smooth muscle contraction, and hypersecretion. This axon reflex, along with the concept of referred pain, explains how chemical irritants, mechanical pressure, or infection can result in localized or referred pain, mucosal swelling, and increased nasal secretion.[1]

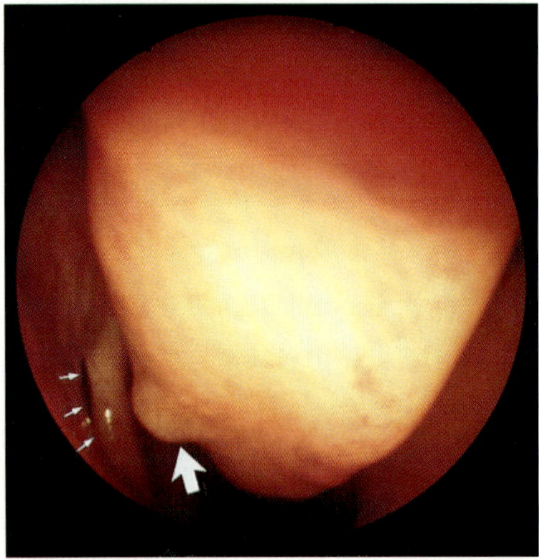

Fig. 15–5. Endoscopic view of the right middle meatus showing a papular area (large arrow) on the lateral aspect of the right middle turbinate opposite an accessory ostium (small arrows).

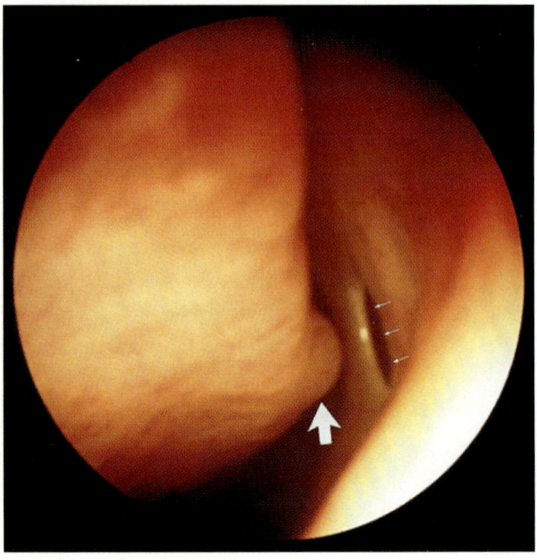

Fig. 15–6. Endoscopic view of the left middle meatus showing a papular area (large arrow) on the lateral aspect of the left middle turbinate opposite an accessory ostium (small arrows).

These concepts are illustrated by the following patient who presented with a complaint of having forehead headaches every time the patient bent over, strained, or lifted heavy objects. Endoscopic examination of this patient showed a localized, papular area on the lateral aspect of each middle turbinate opposite an accessory ostium (Figs. 15–5 and 15–6). On bending over, this patient was noted to have an area of mucosal contact at the margins of the papular area on the lateral aspect of the middle turbinate with the margins of the accessory ostium. This contact point presumably resulted in the stimulation of polymodal nociceptors on the middle turbinate or at the margins of the accessory ostium which resulted in the perception of pain that was subsequently referred to the forehead. Initiation of an antidromic impulse led to the development of localized vasodilation and plasma extravasation, accounting for the edematous papular area located on the lateral aspect of the middle turbinate opposite the accessory ostium. A 3-month course of nasal steroids resulted in subsequent resolution of the pain and papular edematous areas observed on both middle turbinates. The patient has been asymptomatic for 2 years.

As mentioned earlier, there are patients who present with headaches in which a definite pathologic process within the nasal cavity or paranasal sinuses—such as acute or chronic sinusitis, nasal polyps, barotrauma, mucoceles, tumor, etc.—is not readily apparent, nor can a non-sinus origin of the headache be elucidated. These patients present a challenge to the otolaryngologist who must determine the site of origin of the headache.

Use of anesthetic blocks can be a powerful diagnostic tool in evaluating a potential nasal or sinus origin of headache. Relief of a headache or facial pain following administration of a local anesthetic block, within the period of the anesthetic's action, provides strong evidence that the site of origin of the pain is localized to the area where the anesthetic agent was administered or to a location peripheral to where the nerve block was administered. Redevelopment of the headache after the action of the anesthetic agent has elapsed provides even more evidence identifying the site of origin of the headache.

It has been well documented in the literature that septal spurs can cause headaches,[8–13] providing further evidence that areas of mucosal contact are sufficient to initiate headaches. Direct palpation of the mucosa in the areas of contact would be expected to initiate a headache at the site of referred pain if the septal spur was truly the cause of the headache. Application to the area of either a topically applied anesthetic agent or an injectable anesthetic agent resulting in headache relief provides further evidence of localization of the site of origin of the headache. Redevelopment of the headache after the action of the anesthetic agent ceases provides more evidence of identification of the site of the headache's origin.

In some patients presenting with headaches, the site of mucosal contact may not be readily identifiable. Endoscopic examination may show septal spurs that do not seem pathologic. However, in certain circumstances where significant mucosal edema may occur, such as in allergic or irritant states, this may lead to a significant amount of edema, resulting in impaction of the septal spur on the lateral nasal wall and causing the development of a headache. Areas of localized mucosal edema may also exist, indicating potential areas of mucosal contact which could result in headache. Direct palpation of these potential areas of mucosal contact should elicit a headache that is referred to the same area of complaint, providing evidence of identification of the site of origin. Again, achieving relief after application of either a topically applied anesthetic agent or an injectable anesthetic agent into the area supports identification of the site of origin. Redevelopment of headaches after the anesthetic has worn off confirms localization of the site.

In other instances, endoscopic examination may not show any obvious source for the headache. Attention must then be directed towards determining if the site of origin of the headache is the paranasal sinuses. In these instances, direct palpation of the suspected site is obviously much more difficult. Once again, administration of selective anesthetic blocks can be very useful. Application of an anesthetic block to the second division of the trigeminal nerve through the greater palatine foramen will help determine if the site of origin of the headache can be localized to this nerve. If relief of the headache occurs, this directs one's attention to the site of application of the anesthetic block or to an area more peripheral to the nerve block. Careful radiologic evaluation may elucidate the site of origin, such as a dehiscent infraorbital nerve,[14] a retention cyst, or a neuroma. Again, relief from the headache while the anesthetic agent is active and redevelopment of the headache after the anesthetic agent has worn off helps isolate the source of the headache to the site of the nerve block or to a peripheral site. This is illustrated by a patient who presented with right cheek pain resulting from a retention cyst. Application of an anesthetic block to the second division of the trigeminal nerve through the greater palatine foramen using 1% lidocaine with 1:100,000 epinephrine resulted in relief of the sinus headache within 2 minutes. The headache gradually returned a few hours later. A CT scan showed only a retention cyst in the right maxillary sinus (Fig. 15–7). On endoscopic examination of the maxillary sinus, the right anterosuperior alveolar nerve was found to be stretched over the cyst, presumably accounting for the headache (Fig. 15–8). Marsupialization of the cyst resulted in resolution of the headaches.

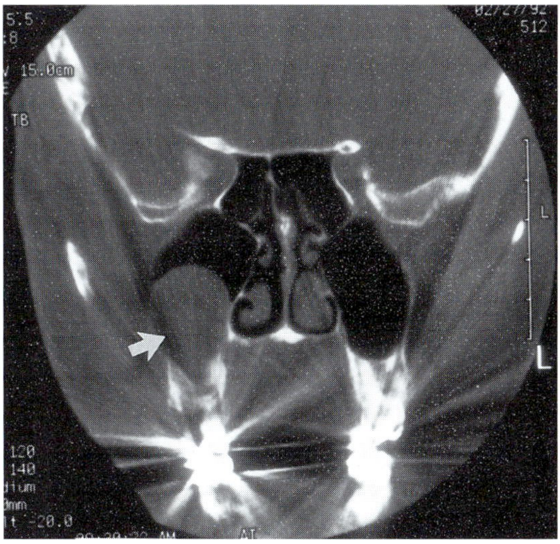

Fig. 15–7. Coronal section CT scan showing a right maxillary sinus retention cyst (arrow).

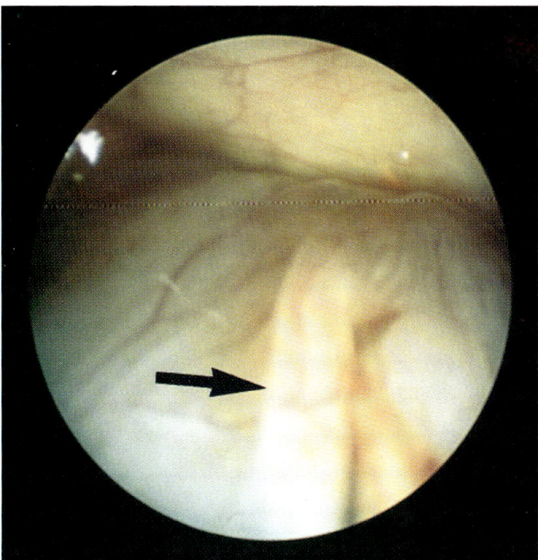

Fig. 15–8. Endoscopic view of the right maxillary sinus showing the anterosuperior alveolar nerve (arrow) stretched over a retention cyst.

REFERENCES

1. Stammberger H, Wolf G. Headaches and sinus disease: The endoscopic approach. *Ann Otol Rhinol Laryngol.* 1988; 97(suppl 134):3–23.
2. May M, Mester SJ, Levine HL. Office evaluation of nasosinus disorders: Patient selection for endoscopic sinus

surgery. In: Levine HL, May M, eds. *Endoscopic Sinus Surgery.* 1st ed. New York, NY: 1993:62.
3. Williams PL, Warwick R, Dyson M, Bannister L, eds. *Gray's Anatomy.* 37th ed. New York, NY: Churchill Livingstone; 1989:1102.
4. Friedman WH, Rosenblum BN. Paranasal sinus etiology of headaches and facial pain. *Otolaryngol Clin No Am.* 1989; 22:1217–1228.
5. McAuliffe GW, Goodell H, Wolff HG. Experimental studies on headache pain from the nasal and paranasal structures. *Am Res Nerve Ment Dis Proc.* 1942;23:185–208.
6. Greenfield H. A study of referred cephalgia secondary to noxious stimulation of specific regions of the nasal mucosa and sinus ostia. Doctors Harold Wolff and Donald Dalessio revisited. Presented as a scientific exhibition at the meeting of the American Academy of Otolaryngology, San Antonio, Texas, Sept. 14–18, 1986.
7. Ballantyne J, Groves J, eds. *Scott-Brown's Diseases of the Ear, Nose and Throat.* 4th ed. London: Butterworths; 1979.
8. Hansen RM. Pain of nasal origin. *Laryngoscope.* 1968:78:1164–1171.
9. Masing H. Functional aspects in septal plasty. *Rhinology.* 1977:15:167–172.
10. Ryan, RE Sr, Ryan RE Jr. Headache of nasal origin. *Headache.* 1979:19:173–179.
11. Koch-Henriksen N, Gammelgaard N, Hvidegaard T, Stoksted P. Chronic headache: the role of deformity of the nasal septum. *Brit Med J.* 1984:288:434–435.
12. Gerbe RW, Fry TL, Fischer ND. Headache of nasal spur origin: an easily diagnosed and surgical correctable cause of facial pain. *Headache.* 1984:24:329–330.
13. Schonsted Madsen U, Stoksted P, Christensen PH, Koch-Henriksen N. Chronic headache related to nasal obstruction. *J Laryngol Otol.* 1986:100:165–170.
14. Whittet HB. Infraorbital nerve dehiscence: the anatomic cause of maxillary sinus "vacuum headache?" *Otolaryngol Head Neck Surg.* 1992:107:21–28.

16

Endoscopic Dacryocystorhinostomy: Primary and Revision

Ralph B. Metson

Endoscopic instrumentation provides the surgeon with a safe and effective technique for opening an obstructed lacrimal sac without the need for an external incision. Although intranasal dacryocystorhinostomy (DCR) was described by West[1] almost a century ago, it never gained widespread popularity because of problems with limited visibility and poor exposure of the lacrimal sac within the narrow confines of the superior nasal cavity. These problems have been overcome by the introduction of nasal endoscopes which provide excellent visualization for surgical manipulation within the depths of the nasal cavity. Surgeons who have developed expertise with endoscopic treatment of sinus disease are applying similar skills for endoscopic treatment of lacrimal obstruction.

Preoperative Evaluation

Patients with obstruction of the lacrimal drainage system usually present with epiphora. They complain of excessive tearing of the affected eye which interferes with vision and can be socially unacceptable. Continued blockage of the sac leads to chronic dacryocystitis with drainage of purulent material from the canaliculi at the corner of the eye. Inflammation of the skin in the region of the medial canthus overlying the obstructed sac may occur, particularly during acute infections.

Preoperative evaluation for endoscopic DCR should include a complete ophthalmologic examination with measurement of visual acuity and visual fields, as well as slit lamp examination of the surface of the eye. The patency of the lacrimal drainage system is accessed by probing the canaliculi for any signs of obstruction or stenosis. The puncta are irrigated with fluorescein dye to access the ease of flow into the nose or the presence of any reflux. The presence of fluorescein in the nose can be verified with a nasal endoscope or by the presence of dye on a strip of gauze placed in the inferior meatus.

Otolaryngologic evaluation and examination should include nasal endoscopy to look for signs of sinusitis or anatomic abnormalities which could contribute to lacrimal obstruction. After installation of a topical decongestant and anesthetic (such as 0.5% phenylephrine HCl and 4% lidocaine HCl), an endoscope is introduced into the nasal cavity. The author prefers a nasal endoscope of 2.7 mm diameter with a 30 degree angle of view for patient examination in the office. This scope provides good visualization with a maximum of patient comfort. The inferior meatus is inspected for any masses which could cause obstruction in the nasolacrimal duct orifice. The middle meatus is examined for the presence of polyps or mucopurulent drainage. A septal deviation or enlarged middle turbinate which may need to be addressed at time of DCR should also be noted.

Computerized tomography (CT) of the paranasal sinus should be performed prior to endoscopic DCR to delineate sinus anatomy and identify any disease not recognized on physical examination. Both axial and coronal scans are preferred. Anterior ethmoid air cells which overlie the lacrimal sac and need to be opened at the time of surgery are found in over 90% of patients.[2] Magnetic resonance scans are not generally obtained because they are unable to image the thin bony sinus partitions.

While many surgeons do not routinely obtain a dacryocystogram prior to DCR, others feel it is essential for identifying and documenting the location and degree of lacrimal obstruction. Radiopaque contrast media is injected into the canaliculi while an x-ray is taken. Normally, the media should be seen flowing freely into the inferior meatus. When obstruction is present, dye will flow only to the site of obstruction and not reach the nasal cavity. The most common site of obstruction is just distal to the lacrimal sac, which may be dilated. Filling defects representing lacrimal stones may also be seen.

Endoscopic Primary DCR

Endoscopic DCR may be performed under either local or general anesthesia, depending upon the condition of the patient and preference of the surgeon. The operation is performed with a video camera attached to the endoscope, so the assistant surgeon can observe the entire procedure on a video monitor.

The patient is placed in a supine position with the head slightly elevated to decrease venous pressure at the operative site. Nasal packing soaked in a 4% cocaine solution is placed along the lateral nasal wall to initiate mucosal decongestion. The nose and affected eye are draped in the operative field. A 4-mm diameter 0 degree nasal endoscope is used for visualization, as submucosal injections of 1% lidocaine HCl with epinephrine 1:100,000 are placed in the middle turbinate and the lateral nasal wall just anterior to the attachment of the turbinate (Fig. 16–1).

The assistant surgeon passes a 20 gauge fiberoptic light probe (Endo-illuminator—Storz Instruments, St. Louis, Mo.) through a canaliculus into the lacrimal sac. The probe transilluminates the lateral nasal wall, providing information about the

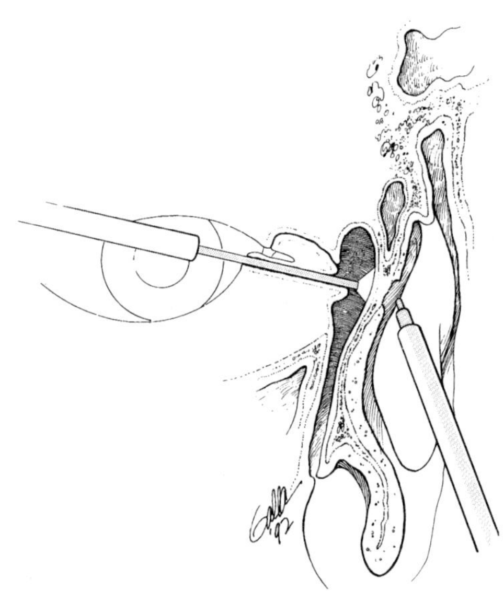

Fig. 16–2. Endoscopic approach to the lacrimal sac for primary DCR is shown in this frontal section through the right nasal cavity. A fiberoptic light probe is passed through a canaliculus into the lacrimal sac. Transillumination of the lateral nasal wall guides laser removal of mucosa and bone overlying the lacrimal sac. From Metson R: Endoscopic Laser DCR. *Laryngoscope.* 104:269-274, 1994. By permission.

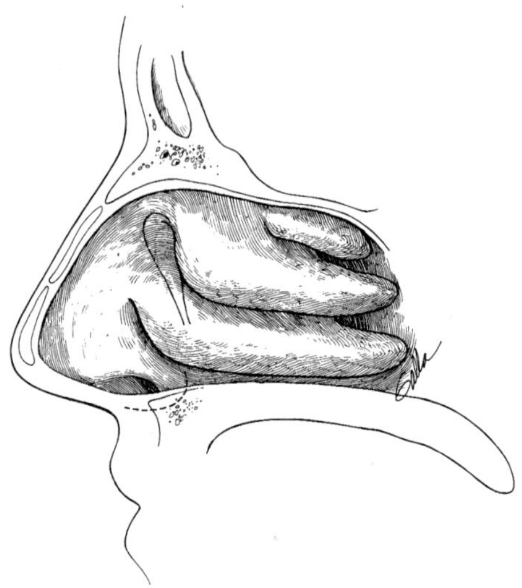

Fig. 16–1. View of the right lateral nasal wall demonstrates the relationship of the lacrimal sac and nasolacrimal duct to the turbinates. Note how a portion of the sac may extend beneath the middle turbinate, requiring turbinate resection for adequate exposure. From Metson R: Endoscopic Surgery for Lacrimal Obstruction. *Otolaryngology-Head and Neck Surgery* 104:473-479, 1991. By permission.

location of the lacrimal sac (Fig. 16–2). The area of maximal brightness corresponds with the posterior end of the lacrimal sac where the overlying bone is thinnest, not the center of the sac (Fig. 16–3).

Surgical dissection is begun with removal of an approximately 1-cm diameter circle of mucosa and underlying bone at the area of transillumination along the lateral nasal wall (Fig. 16–4). Initial tissue removal usually includes a portion of the uncinate process located posterior to the maxillary line. An air space is often entered which corresponds to the infundibulum or an anterior ethmoid air cell overlying the lacrimal sac. As dissection is carried more anteriorly, the lacrimal bone is opened and the underlying medial wall of the sac will be exposed. Movement of the light probe will confirm the location of the sac wall.

The maxillary bone which forms the anterior aspect of the lacrimal fossa must then be removed. Removal of this relatively thick bone is technically the most difficult step in the surgery. Bone removal may be accomplished with a drill, curette, or back-biting forceps. Because of limitations with conventional instrumentation, the surgical laser has become a popular tool for primary endoscopic DCR to facilitate bone removal and hemostasis. Although the argon,[3] carbon dioxide, and potassium titanyl phosphate (KTP)[4] lasers have all been used

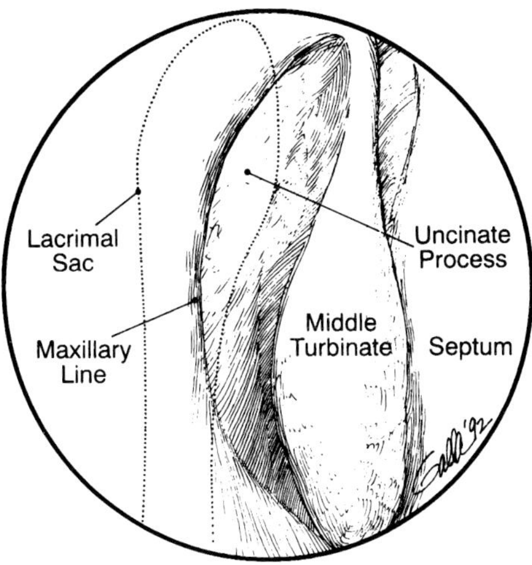

Fig. 16–3. Endoscopic view of right nasal cavity demonstrates location of the lacrimal sac (dotted outline) underlying the lateral nasal wall. The light probe transilluminates the thin lacrimal bone and uncinate process which usually overlie the posterior aspect of the lacrimal sac. The maxillary line, a bony eminence which originates at the middle turbinate attachment, is a reliable anatomic landmark for location of the sac. From Metson R: Endoscopic Laser DCR. *Laryngoscope* 104:269-274, 1994. By permission.

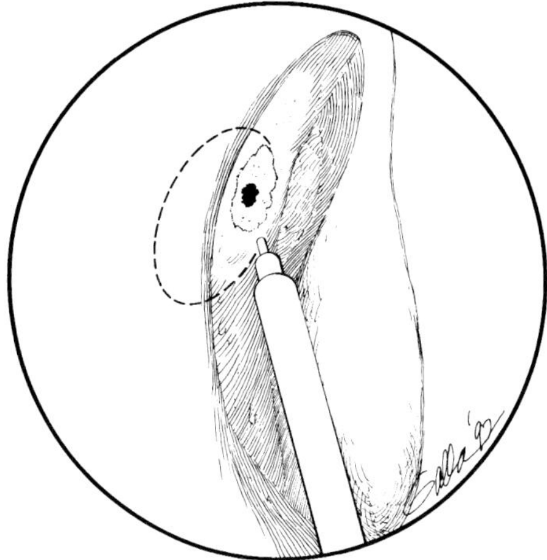

Fig. 16–4. A small bony opening in the lateral nasal wall is seen as the laser is used to ablate mucosa and bone overlying the lacrimal sac. Surgical dissection begins at the area illuminated by the light probe within the sac. The final bony opening (dashed line) will extend anteriorly past the maxillary line and inferiorly to the sac-duct junction. From Metson R: Endoscopic Laser DCR. *Laryngoscope* 104:269-274, 1994. By permission.

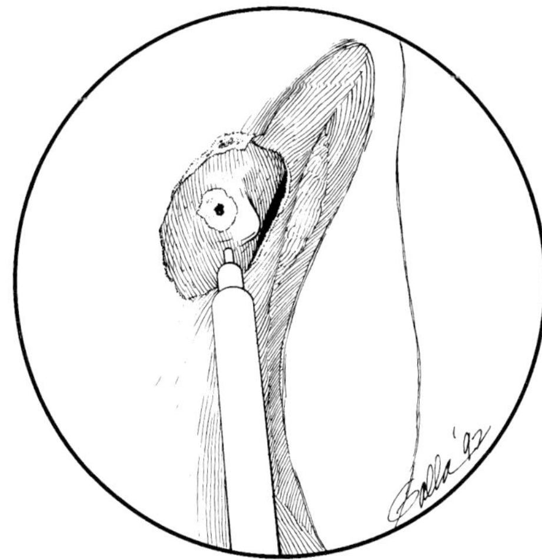

Fig. 16–5. Once the bony opening has been enlarged, the laser is used to open the lacrimal sac. This step is facilitated by tenting up the medial sac wall with the light probe. From Metson R: Endoscopic Laser DCR. *Laryngoscope* 104:269-274, 1994. By permission.

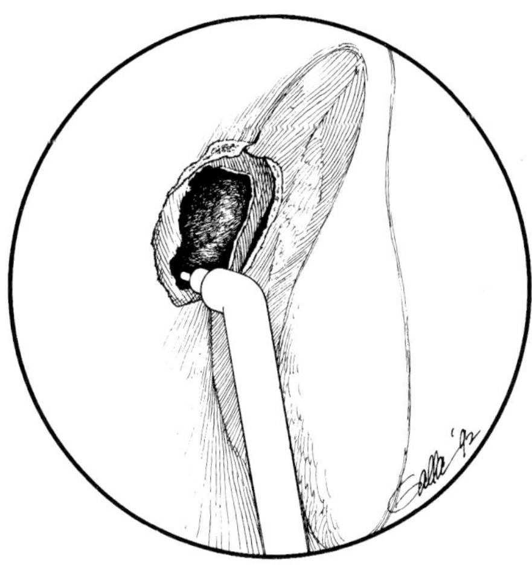

Fig. 16–6. The opening into the lacrimal sac is enlarged with an angled laser probe. From Metson R: Endoscopic Laser DCR. *Laryngoscope* 104:269-274, 1994. By permission.

for transnasal endoscopic DCR, the holmium:YAG laser is particularly well suited for this procedure because of its effective bone-cutting capabilities.[5]

After the medial sac wall has been exposed, it is entered with either the laser or an angled Blakesley forceps. The laser provides for a more hemostatic sac opening, whereas the forceps allows for a tissue specimen to be obtained for pathologic examination. It is often helpful to use the light probe or a lacrimal probe within the sac to tent up the medial sac wall as it is opened (Fig. 16–5). This maneuver serves to isolate the medial wall and prevent inadvertent injury to the underlying structures. Once the sac is entered, the probe will be visible.

The sac opening is enlarged to a diameter of 5 to 10 mm (Fig. 16–6). Its inferior edge should

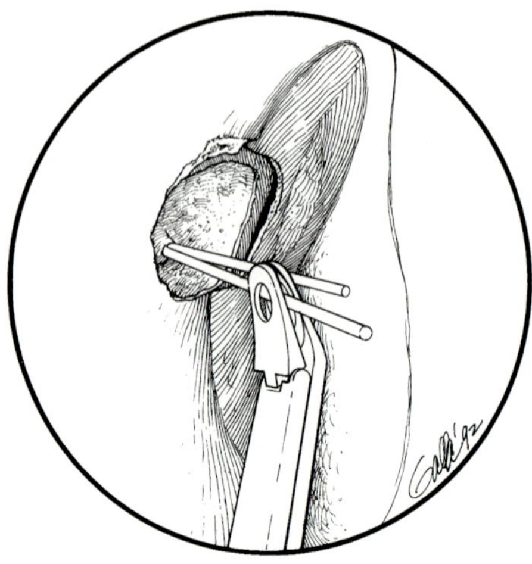

Fig. 16–7. Lacrimal probes threaded with Silastic tubing are passed through the canaliculi, grasped with forceps, directed out of the nasal cavity, trimmed, and tied. Note the location of the internal common punctum where the catheters enter the sac interior. From Metson R: Endoscopic Laser DCR. *Laryngoscope* 104:269-272, 1994. By permission.

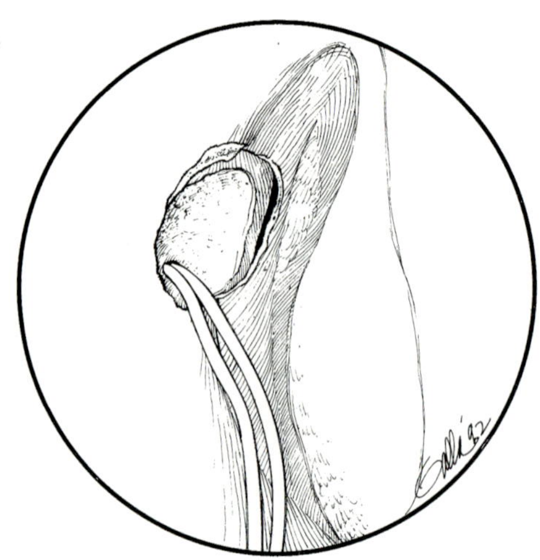

Fig. 16–8. View of the tubing that stents the intranasal opening into the lacrimal sac during the healing period. From Metson R: Endoscopic Laser DCR. *Laryngoscope* 104:269-272, 1994. By permission.

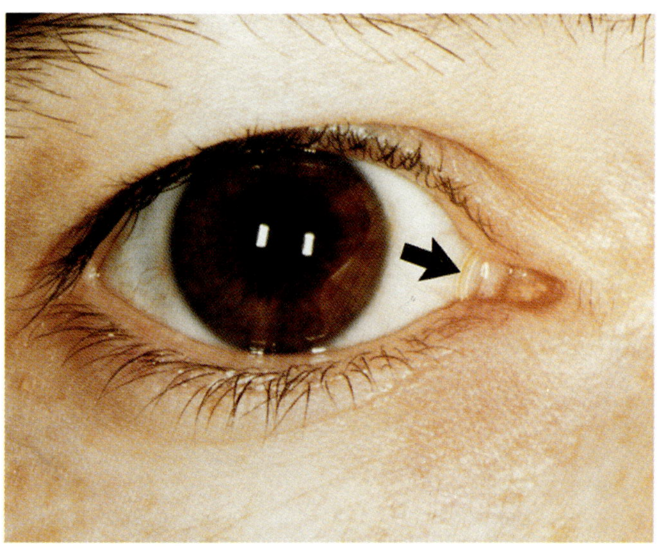

Fig. 16–9. Silastic tubing (arrow) which serves as a stent during the healing period is seen at the medial canthus in this patient who underwent endoscopic primary laser DCR. This tubing passes from the canaliculi through the lacrimal sac and into nasal cavity where it is tied to form a continuous loop. From Metson R: Endoscopic Laser DCR. *Laryngoscope* 104:269-272, 1994. By permission.

extend to the level of the sac-duct junction. No attempt is made to create mucosal flaps.

The location of the common punctum is verified by passing stents attached to a Silastic tubing (Guibor Canaliculus Intubation Set—Concept Inc., Largo, Fl) through the superior and inferior canaliculi. The stents are grasped with a Blakesley forceps (Fig. 16–7), withdrawn from the nasal cavity, and cut from the tubing. The ends of the tubing are then tied and trimmed within the nasal cavity to form a continuous loop around the canaliculi (Figs. 16–8 and 16–9). This tubing serves to stent the surgical ostium during the postoperative healing period (Figs. 16–10, 16–11, 16–12).

Endoscopic Revision DCR

Because bone along the lateral nasal wall has already been removed during prior surgery, endoscopic revision DCR is technically easier than

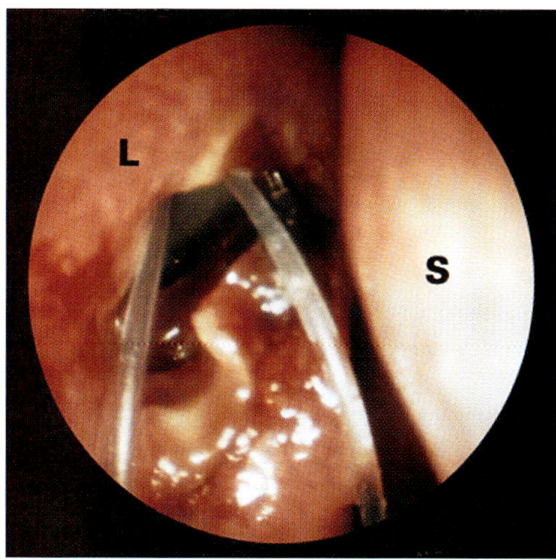

Fig. 16–10. Endoscopic view of same patient shown in Figure 16-9 demonstrates the Silastic catheters entering the lacrimal sac through the surgically-created ostium in the lateral nasal wall (L). Inflammation at the surgical site is evident one week following laser DCR. Nasal septum (S). From Metson R: Endoscopic Laser DCR. *Laryngoscope* 104:269-272, 1994. By permission.

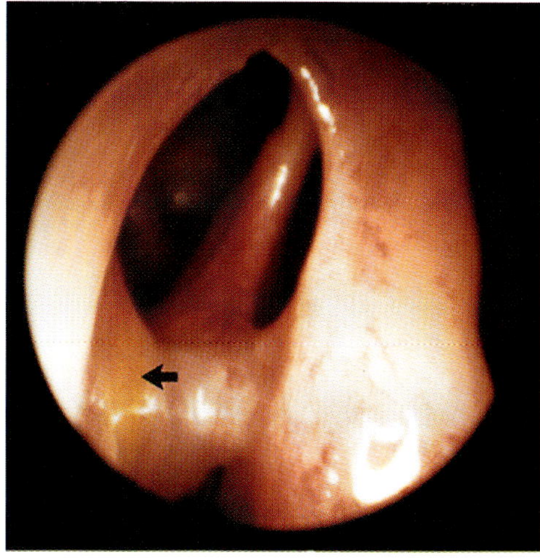

Fig. 16–12. Endoscopic view of same patient shown in Figures 16-9 to 16-11 once the Silastic catheters have been removed. Yellow color along lateral nasal wall (arrow) demonstrates free-flow of fluorescein dye from the right eye into the nasal cavity through the patent surgical ostium. From Metson R: Endoscopic Laser DCR. *Laryngoscope* 104:269-272, 1994. By permission.

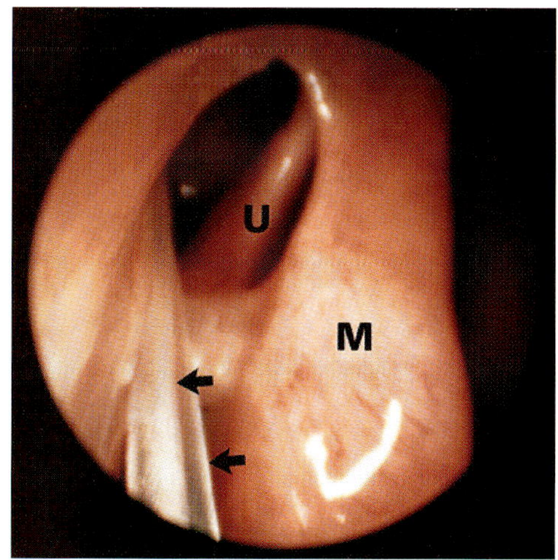

Fig. 16–11. Healed surgical site two months following surgery. Pair of catheters (arrows) is seen passing lateral to the middle turbinate (M) and edge of partially resected uncinate process (U) into the lacrimal sac. From Metson R: Endoscopic Laser DCR. *Laryngoscope* 104:269-272, 1994. By permission.

primary endoscopic DCR and more suitable for the surgeon who is learning the endoscopic DCR technique.

Once the patient has been anesthetized and the nasal cavity prepared in the manner described above for primary DCR, the assistant surgeon passes a lacrimal probe through a canaliculi into the obstructed lacrimal sac. The tip of the probe can be observed with the endoscope as it tents the mucosa of the lateral nasal wall (Fig. 16–13). The endoscopist then uses a sickle knife to make a curvilinear incision in the nasal mucosa approximately 1 cm anterior to the underlying probe tip. If there is extensive submucosal fibrosis from prior surgery, the mucosa posterior to this incision may have to be elevated sharply with the sickle knife. The posterior mucosal flap is grasped with straight Blakesley forceps and removed with a twisting motion (Fig. 16–14). Similar bites of adjacent mucosa may be necessary to enlarge this intranasal opening to a diameter of at least 10 mm.

If the lacrimal sac has already been entered, the tip of the lacrimal probe will be exposed. Frequently, however, there is additional scar tissue which needs to be removed to enter the sac interior. The intranasal opening is deepened with an angled Blakesley forceps directed laterally towards the sac (Fig. 16–15). Since scarring from previous surgery may obscure sac anatomy, it is important to use the probe which lies within the sac as a guide for tissue removal. Care must be taken to remove only tissue directly surrounding the probe to avoid inadvertent exposure of periorbital fat. The assistant who is directing the lacrimal probe can alert the endoscopist if it appears to be

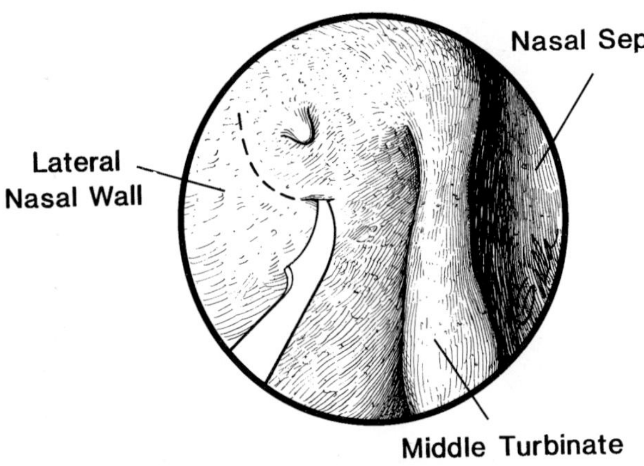

Fig. 16–13. Revision endoscopic DCR. Lacrimal probe passed through a canaliculus is seen tenting the nasal mucosa just anterior to the attachment of the middle turbinate. This probe indicates the location of lacrimal sac. Nasal mucosa overlying anterior edge of sac is incised with a sickle knife. From Metson R: The Endoscopic Approach for Revision DCR. *Laryngoscope* 100:1344-1347, 1990. By permission.

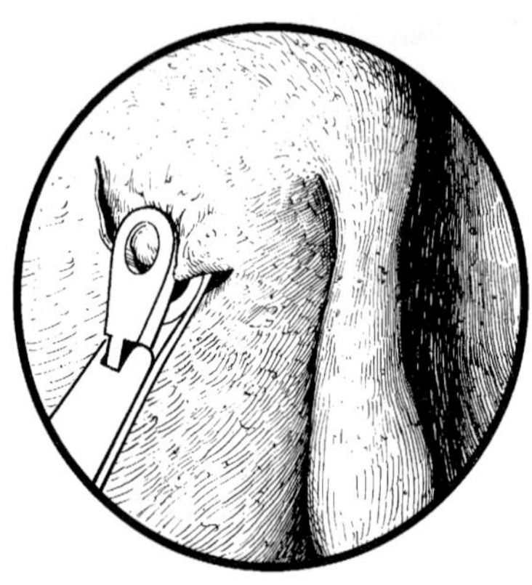

Fig. 16–14. Posterior flap of nasal mucosa covering lacrimal sac is grasped with biting forceps and removed. Mucosal opening is enlarged to a diameter of approximately 10 mm. From Metson R: The Endoscopic Approach for Revision DCR. *Laryngoscope* 100:1344-1347, 1990. By permission.

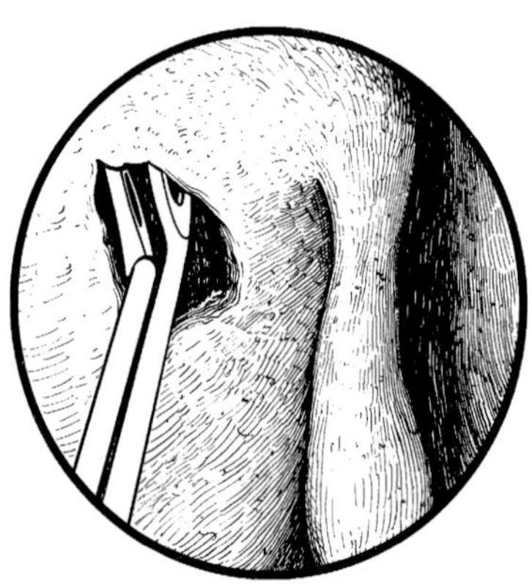

Fig. 16–15. Angled biting forceps is directed laterally to enlarge opening into lacrimal sac. Exposed lacrimal probe is used as a guide for tissue removal. After the opening into the lacrimal sac has been adequately enlarged, probes should pass freely into the nose from both the superior and inferior canaliculi. From Metson R: The Endoscopic Approach for Revision DCR. *Laryngoscope* 100:1344-1347, 1990. By permission.

approaching too close to the medial canthus, which could injure the canaliculi. Once the intranasal opening has been sufficiently enlarged, the sac interior and internal common punctum are usually visible with a 30 degree endoscope. Lacrimal probes should pass freely into the nose from both the superior and inferior canaliculi.

The lacrimal probe is then replaced by silastic tubing that has its ends threaded over a rigid wire (Guibor Canaliculus Intubation Set). This tubing may be used instead of a lacrimal probe from the start of the case. The rigid ends of tubing are passed through the superior and inferior canaliculi into the nose via the newly created opening into the lacrimal sac. These ends are grasped with the Blakesley forceps (Fig. 16–16) and guided out of the nose. The silastic tubing is trimmed and tied within the nasal cavity. The tubing thus forms a continuous loop which passes through the intranasal ostium and around the canaliculi, and is unlikely to become dislodged (Fig. 16–17). Unless bleeding is a problem or a septoplasty has been performed, no nasal packing is used.

Postoperative Care

If nasal packing is placed at the conclusion of surgery, it is removed the following morning. Patients are discharged with instructions to begin twice-a-day nasal saline irrigations with a bulb syringe. Any remaining intranasal debris is removed from the operative site at the first postoperative visit 1 week following surgery.

The Silastic tubing used to stent the surgical ostium is typically removed 2 months after surgery by cutting the exposed tubing at the medial canthus and withdrawing it through the nose. It may be removed sooner if excessive granulation tissue formation is seen to occur around the tube at the ostium. In revision cases in which postoperative

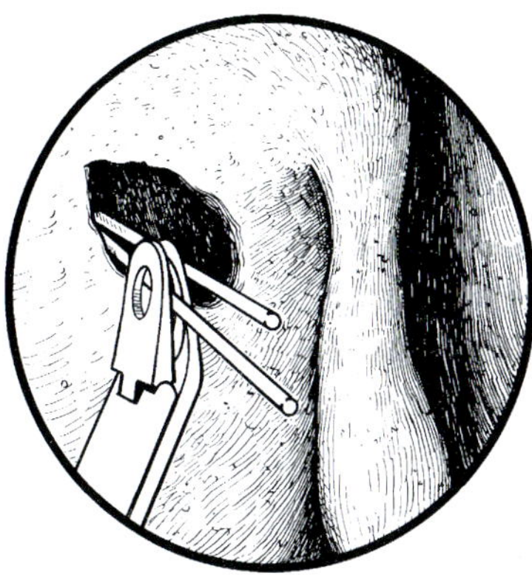

Fig. 16–16. The rigid ends of Silastic intubation catheters passed through the canaliculi are grasped with forceps, directed out of the nose, trimmed, and tied. From Metson R: The Endoscopic Approach for Revision DCR. *Laryngoscope* 100:1344-1347, 1990. By permission.

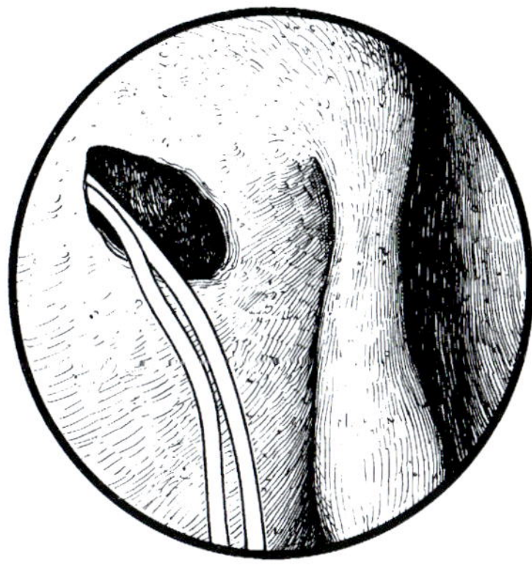

Fig. 16–17. View of Silastic catheters which stent the intranasal opening into the lacrimal sac during the healing period. From Metson R: The Endoscopic Approach for Revision DCR. *Laryngoscope* 100:1344-1347, 1990. By permission.

scarring has been a problem, stents may be left in place for 6 months or longer. Patency of the lacrimal drainage system is verified by irrigation of the canaliculi, as well as endoscopic observation of fluorescein dye flowing from the eye through the surgical ostium into the nose (Fig. 16–18).

Complications

The performance of safe and effective endoscopic lacrimal surgery requires specialized instrumentation and training. This surgery should be performed only by those who are experienced in endoscopic intranasal techniques. If excessive bleeding occurs during endoscopic DCR, the procedure should be terminated or converted to an open DCR. Occasionally, orbital fat is exposed while removing bone to uncover the lacrimal sac. Care must be taken not to disturb this fat to prevent injury to underlying orbital structures. Damage to the adjacent medial rectus and superior oblique muscles can lead to diplopia. Blindness can result from laceration of intraorbital vessels with subsequent hemorrhage or by direct injury to the optic nerve itself.

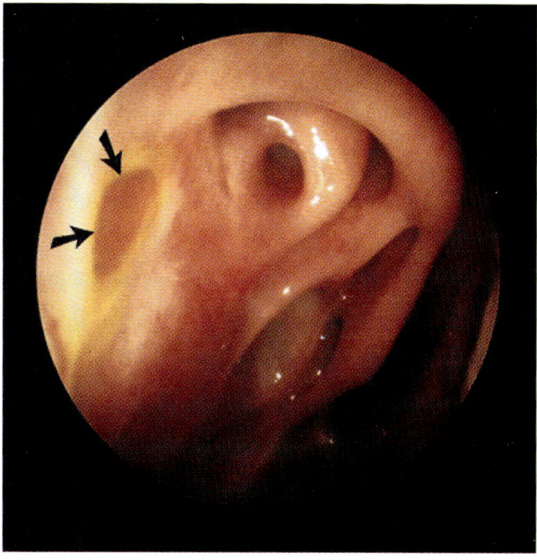

Fig. 16–18. Endoscopic view of right lateral nasal wall following revision endoscopic DCR shows flow of fluorescein dye through the surgical ostium (arrows) into the nose. Prominent structures seen in the center of the figure are openings into the ethmoid sinuses in this patient who has undergone an ethmoidectomy and middle turbinate resection. From Metson R: Endoscopic Surgery for Lacrimal Obstruction. *Otolaryngology–Head and Neck Surgery* 104:473-479, 1991. By permission.

Postoperative epistaxis severe enough to require nasal packing occurs in less than 5% of cases. Bleeding usually occurs within 1 week after surgery and is caused by a branch of the sphenopalatine artery supplying the remnant of a partially resected middle turbinate. Postoperative infection involving the nose or orbit following DCR is rare. Perioperative antibiotics are administered in an attempt to avoid this complication.

Postoperative adhesions are one of the most common causes of surgical failure for both external[6,7] and endoscopic[8] DCR. These adhesions usually span the lateral nasal wall and middle turbinate or septum, causing obstruction of the surgically created ostium. The incidence of this complication can be reduced by avoiding surgical trauma to the turbinate mucosa or resecting the anterior half of the turbinate so that it is not in the proximity of the ostium. Correction of a deviated septum also reduces the likelihood of postoperative adhesion formation, as does meticulous cleaning of debris from the intranasal operative during the postoperative period.

Surgical Results

The reported success rate for primary endoscopic DCR ranges from 82% to 86%. Although these results have not reached the 90% to 97% efficacy typically described for external DCR,[9] it is likely that the success of this relatively new technique will increase with greater clinical experience.

In a series of transnasal endoscopic DCR cases followed for 4 to 26 months, McDonogh[10] reported successful relief of lacrimal obstruction in 20 of 23 cases (86%). Gonnering[4] and Massaro[3] described a total of 16 laser-assisted endoscopic DCRs with no failures, although 7 patients still had lacrimal stents in place at time of publication. Woog[11] reported a long-term ostial patency rate of 82% for 40 laser-assisted DCR procedures performed on 37 patients. Follow-up ranged from 6 to 91 weeks. If it occurred, surgical failure, defined as the inability to perform lacrimal irrigation through the DCR ostium, was evident within 14 weeks of surgery in all cases.

Metson[5] described 46 endoscopic laser DCRs performed on 40 patients who were followed for more than 1 year and found that surgery relieved nasolacrimal duct obstruction in 85% of cases. Most surgical failures were the result of gradual closure of the surgical ostium. In one case, a subsequent external DCR revealed an inadequately drained diverticulum of the lacrimal sac as a cause of recurrent dacryocystitis. Revision laser DCR in patients who had already failed a primary laser DCR was not found to be beneficial.

Mannor and Millman[12] suggested that lacrimal sac anatomy on preoperative dacryocystogram is an important prognostic factor for successful endoscopic DCR. In a series of 18 non-laser endoscopic DCRs, they found that those patients with a normal or dilated lacrimal sac had a success rate of 82%, whereas those with a scarred sac had only a 29% likelihood of success.

Revision endoscopic DCR[13,14] with or without a laser has been found to be a worthwhile surgical endeavor for those patients who have failed a primary conventional DCR. Metson[8] reported a 75% success rate for those patients who had persistent epiphora or dacryocystitis following external DCR. Common causes of DCR failure, such as intranasal adhesions, concurrent ethmoiditis, and an enlarged middle turbinate, can be readily identified and corrected with endoscopic instrumentation. In the case of patients who fail repeated DCR attempts, consideration must be given to missed causes of lacrimal obstruction, such as canalicular scarring, which would require a conjunctivodacryocystorhinostomy (CDCR) for successful treatment.

Comments

The current role of endoscopic DCR is not to replace external DCR, but to serve as an alternative approach for the treatment of lacrimal obstruction in selected patients. For the younger patient with epiphora who wishes to avoid a surgical scar on the face, endoscopic DCR offers an excellent alternative to conventional techniques.

Endoscopic DCR also appears to have a place for revision surgery in the patient who has already failed an external DCR. Endoscopic instrumentation provides excellent visualization within the nasal cavity for the identification and removal of adhesions which are a common cause of DCR failure. Other intranasal factors that contribute to DCR failure, such as middle turbinate hypertrophy, septal deviation, and ethmoid sinusitis, also lend themselves to endoscopic correction.

Endoscopic DCR has the potential to reduce patient morbidity through improved intraoperative hemostasis, greater utilization of local anesthesia, and shorter hospitalization as compared to conventional techniques. Alternatively, the issues of increased operative time and cost associated with a new surgical procedure, particularly if a laser is used, must also be considered. As clinical expertise with endoscopic DCR techniques increases, these considerations become less of a factor.

REFERENCES

1. West JM. Eine Fensterresektion des Ductus naso-lacrimalis in Fallen von Stenose. *Archiv fur Laryngologie und Rhinologie.* 1910; 24:62–64.
2. Blaylock WK, Moore CA, Linberg JV. Anterior ethmoid anatomy facilitates dacryocystorhinostomy. *Arch Ophthalmol.* 1990; 108:1774–1777.
3. Massaro BM, Gonnering RS, Harris GJ. Endonasal laser dacryocystorhinostomy: a new approach to nasolacrimal duct obstruction. *Arch Ophthalmol.* 1990; 108:1172–1176.
4. Gonnering RS, Lyon DB, Fisher JC. Endoscopic laser-assisted lacrimal surgery. *Am J Ophthalmol.* 1991; 111:152–157.
5. Metson R, Woog JJ, Puliafito CA. Endoscopic laser dacryocystorhinostomy. *Laryngoscope.* 1994; 104:269-274.
6. Welham RAN, Henderson PH. Results of dacryocystorhinostomy: analysis of causes for failure. *Trans Ophthalmol Soc U K.* 1973; 93:601–609.
7. Allen KM, Berlin AJ, Levine HL. Intranasal endoscopic analysis of dacryocystorhinostomy failure. *Opthal Plastic Recon Surg.* 1988; 4:143–145.
8. Metson R. Endoscopic surgery for lacrimal obstruction. *Otolaryngol Head Neck Surg.* 1991; 104:473–479.

9. McLachlan DL, Shannon GM, Flanagan JC. Results of dacryocystorhinostomy: analysis of reoperations. *Ophthalmic Surg.* 1980; 11:427–430.
10. McDonogh M. Endoscopic transnasal dacryocystorhinostomy—results in 21 patients. *S Afr J Surg.* 1992; 30:107–110.
11. Woog JJ, Metson R, Puliafito CA. Holmium:YAG endonasal laser dacryocystorhinostomy. *Am J Opthalmol.* 1993; 116:1–10.
12. Mannor GE, Millman AL. The prognostic value of preoperative dacryocystography in endoscopic intranasal dacryocystorhinostomy. *Am J Opthalmol.* 1992; 113:134–137.
13. Metson R. The endoscopic approach for revision dacryocystorhinostomy. *Laryngoscope.* 1990; 100:1344–1347.
14. Orcutt JC, Hillel A, Weymuller EA. Endoscopic repair of failed dacryocystorhinostomy. *Opthal Plastic Recon Surg.* 1990; 6:197–202.

17

Endoscopic Treatment of Epistaxis

Leonard H. Wurman

The treatment of epistaxis, especially posterior epistaxis, must be considered one of the more vexing problems for the otolaryngologist. Anterior epistaxis, except in unusual cases such as trauma or hereditary hemorrhagic telangiectasia, is usually located to the anterior septal blood vessel complex known as Kiesselbach's area. This bleeding is usually seen directly and can be cauterized quite readily. Posterior epistaxis, however, tends to be a more vigorous bleed, is more difficulty to identify, and more troublesome to control. Superior or ethmoid artery epistaxis seems to be septal in origin, but high and anterior.

A number of different treatments are used to control posterior epistaxis. For years, probably the only effective treatment was the placement of a posterior nasal pack. While this method is usually effective over time, there is significant morbidity and even mortality. Indeed, the placement of a posterior pack is difficult for the physician and most uncomfortable for the patient, the latter requiring sedation and pain control medications not only during the pack insertion, but also during maintenance of the pack itself. There is frequent residual oozing of blood with a posterior pack in position, and the pack is usually left in for 3 to 5 days after the oozing has finally stopped. Transfusions are occasionally necessary during this oozing period, increasing the risk of a transmittable disease. The hypoxia and hypoventilation associated with posterior packing increase the rate of myocardial infarction and cerebrovascular accident.[1] Packing has been postulated to stimulate a nasovagal reflex that causes bradycardia, a decrease in cardiac output, hypotension, and inhibition of respiration in dogs.[2] More recently, posterior packing was documented to produce sleep apnea.[3] It would appear that posterior packing should not be the treatment of choice for posterior epistaxis.

Nasal balloon tamponade is a variant of posterior packing. It does not work as well, but certainly has the advantage of being easy to insert for both the patient and the physician. Maintenance of the balloon is also less uncomfortable for the patient than is a posterior pack, and when bleeding restarts, adding more water to the balloon may stop the bleeding. There are, however, disadvantages with the balloons as well. The balloons leak, so pressure decreases over time. They are uncomfortable to maintain, and certain balloons risk pressure necrosis of the lateral nare skin which, if not prevented, may lead to skin erosion, subsequent scar formation, and air flow obstruction.

The most effective treatment for posterior epistaxis appears to be ligation of the internal maxillary (IM) or anterior ethmoid (AE) artery.[4] Once experience has been gained with this procedure, and the proper instruments are used (Weck Hemaclip Applicator—Edward Weck & Company, Inc., Research Triangle Park, NC; Wurman Internal Maxillary Artery Ligation Speculum—Richards Medical Company, Memphis, Tn; and the Schuknecht Speculum Holder—Richards Medical Company, Memphis, Tn), it is not a difficult procedure. Most patients are discharged within 24 hours. Its two disadvantages are that it is costly and it does require a general anesthetic. The risks are those associated with general anesthetia, the possibility of numb or devitalized teeth, and, as with any canine fossa (Caldwell-Luc) approach, intraoperative bleeding and postoperative sinusitis. The risk of infraorbital hypesthesia seems to have been eliminated with the use of the ligation speculum.

Nasal Blood Supply

The nasal blood supply has three sources with multiple anastomoses. The sphenopalatine artery must be considered the primary source supplying much of the turbinates and meati laterally and the posterior and inferior septum medially. The anterior and posterior ethmoidal arteries, both branches of the ophthalmic artery of the internal carotid system, provide blood to both the lateral and medial nasal mucosa superiorly. The anterior septum and the lateral anterior nasal mucosa are supplied by the superior labial branch of the facial artery.

Ethmoidal artery bleeding is only an occasional occurrence, but can be identified endoscopically. Ethmoidal bleeding loci are usually on the septum superior to the middle turbinate and can be identified endoscopically only after the middle turbinate has been vasoconstricted and fractured laterally. The author is not aware of the lateral wall as the cause of superior epistaxis. Ethmoidal artery bleeding can be controlled with the same posterior endoscopic cautery technique described later for posterior epistaxis.

Until recently, the actual bleeding site of posterior epistaxis was not well identified. In the 1940s, Woodruff published his triologic thesis on posterior epistaxis,[5] then called cardiovascular epistaxis because of its suspected association with hypertension. Using the old style nasopharyngoscope, with the bulb located at the distal end, he identified what he believed was a venous plexus located posteriorly. Harrah named this area Woodruff's nasopharyngeal plexus.[6]

Although Woodruff discussed a venous plexus, posterior epistaxis may be venous or arterial, as evidenced by the occasional pulsatile nature of the flow. As the sphenopalatine artery penetrates through the sphenopalatine foramen it breaks into a number of vessels (Fig. 17–1), the primary branches being the source of posterior epistaxis. The eponymous Woodruff's plexus will be used to describe the blood vessels in the following areas: the posterior 1 cm of the nasal floor, inferior meatus, inferior turbinate, and the middle meatus; the vertical strip of mucosa anterior to the eustachian tube cartilage; and the mucosa lateral and superior to the posterior choana covering the adjacent sphenoid rostrum (Figs. 17–2, 17–3, 17–4, 17–5). True posterior epistaxis almost always arises from these sites; it is unusual to find bleeding coming from the posterior septum, but this has occurred. If one visualizes bleeding as coming from within the inferior or middle meatus or from the lateral surface of the inferior turbinate, it is easy to see that neither gauze packing nor balloon tamponade can effectively exert pressure directly onto the bleeding site.

Posterior Endoscopic Cautery

ADVANTAGES, DISADVANTAGES, AND RISKS

Essentially, the control of posterior epistaxis with the endoscope and cautery combines the new sinus endoscopes with the old standard nasal suction

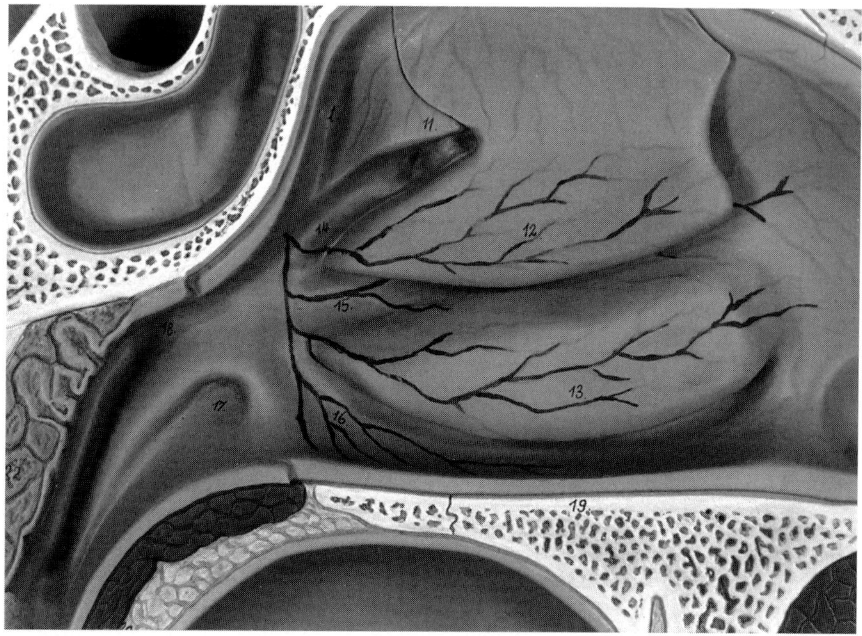

Fig. 17–1. Branching of the left sphenopalatine artery on a model of the left lateral nasal wall. 12, middle turbinate; 13, inferior turbinate; 14, sphenopalatine artery; 17, eustachian tube orifice. From Wurman LH, et al: The treatment of posterior epistaxis by internal maxillary artery ligation and posterior endoscopic cautery, in Johnson JT (ed): *American Academy of Otolaryngology/Head and Neck Surgery*, v3, 1990.

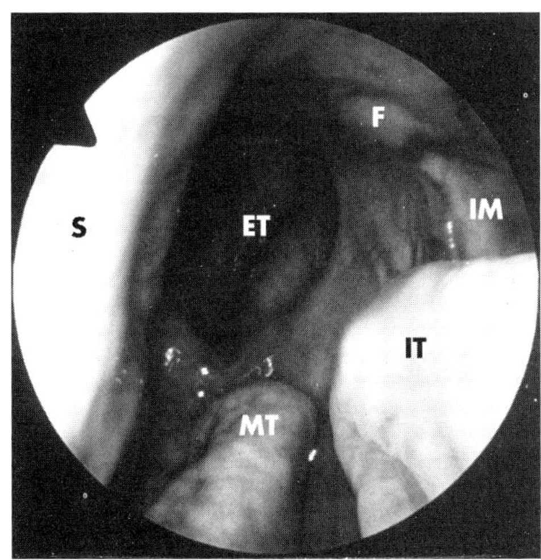

Fig. 17–2. Prominent vessels on the right inferior meatus and posterior to the inferior turbinate. S, septum; F, floor; IT, inferior turbinate; ET, eustachian tube orifice; IM, inferior meatus; MT, middle turbinate. From Wurman LH, et al: The treatment of posterior epistaxis by internal maxillary artery ligation and posterior endoscopic cautery, in Johnson JT (ed): *American Academy of Otolaryngology/Head and Neck Surgery*, v3, 1990.

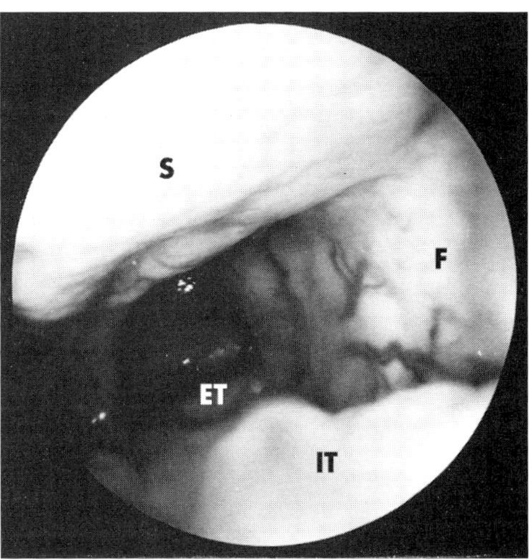

Fig. 17–3. Prominent vessels on the posterior right nasal floor. S, septum; F, floor; IT, inferior turbinate; ET, eustachian tube orifice. From Wurman LH, et al: The treatment of posterior epistaxis by internal maxillary artery ligation and posterior endoscopic cautery, in Johnson JT (ed): *American Academy of Otolaryngology/Head and Neck Surgery*, v3, 1990.

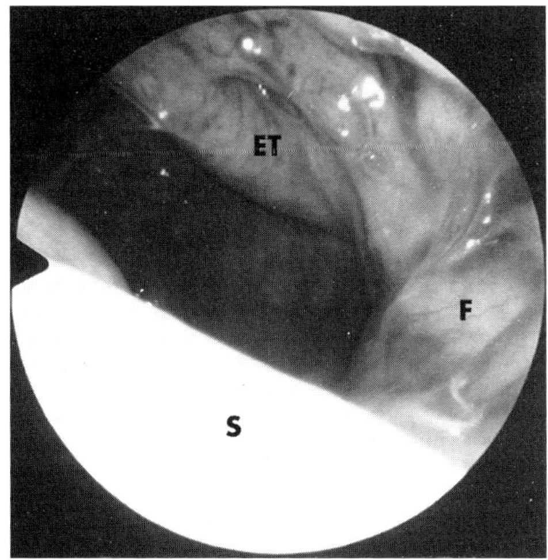

Fig. 17–4. Prominent vessels anterior to the left eustachian tube orifice. S, septum; F, floor; ET, eustachian tube orifice. From Wurman LH, et al: The treatment of posterior epistaxis by internal maxillary artery ligation and posterior endoscopic cautery, in Johnson JT (ed): *American Academy of Otolaryngology/Head and Neck Surgery*, v3, 1990.

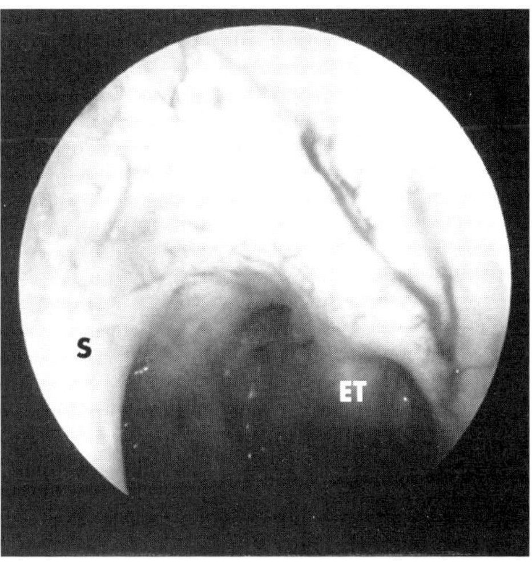

Fig. 17–5. Prominent vessel on the lateral left sphenoid wall. ET, eustachian tube orifice.

cautery unit. Every patient with posterior epistaxis is a candidate for posterior endoscopic cautery (PEC) (this is the treatment of choice in our office). We rarely, if ever, use posterior packing. We may occasionally use the balloon tamponade, although that technique is probably more commonly used by the referring doctors in the smaller towns in northern Wisconsin.

There are significant advantages to PEC. First, the success rate approaches 90%. When our office first started using this method, we were not this effective, but as our experience grew, so did our effectiveness. We initially took some patients to the operating room for the procedure, but now perform PEC in the office or emergency room. If possible, an intramuscular narcotic or sedative is administered. Most patients are treated as outpatients, especially if they live locally, but some may be admitted overnight, especially if they reside outside of town, are elderly, or if blood loss has been significant. PEC's further advantages include considerable cost savings compared with the AE or IM ligation and posterior packing, no long-term effects on nasal function, and no occurrence of sinusitis or postoperative pain. The disadvantages of PEC are that electrocautery to the posterior lateral nose may be painful. We initially thought this mucosa was difficult to reach with anesthetic. We now feel that some of the pain is due to the electric current or the heat affecting the greater palatine nerve. This discomfort has been overcome by administering local anesthetic directly into the posterolateral nasal mucosa with, occasionally, a transoral greater palatine nerve block. For years, we did not use the greater palatine nerve block, so we cannot credit the success of PEC with the temporary positive effect of stopping posterior epistaxis by the nerve block itself.

There are several risks with PEC. Perhaps 25% of patients will have palate numbness, although none have had a permanent problem. Most patients recover completely, while a few believe that numbness is still present but is not bothersome. Having become aware of this possibility, we are now careful to cauterize only the mucosa to avoid damaging the underlying bone.

One initial concern was that the cautery would disrupt nasal function by causing scarring and synechiae. This has not occurred. The coagulum that occurs (Fig. 17–6) when Woodruff's plexus is coagulated heals with time if care is used to avoid cauterizing closely opposed mucosal surfaces. Patients who undergo cautery of the posterior tip of the inferior turbinate may indeed lose that portion of the turbinate (Fig. 17–7) without any loss of nasal function. One of our concerns, though one we have not seen, is permanent serous otitis media secondary to eustachian tube damage. The mucosa on the anterior lip of the nasopharyngeal opening of the eustachian tube must be identified and cautery avoided.

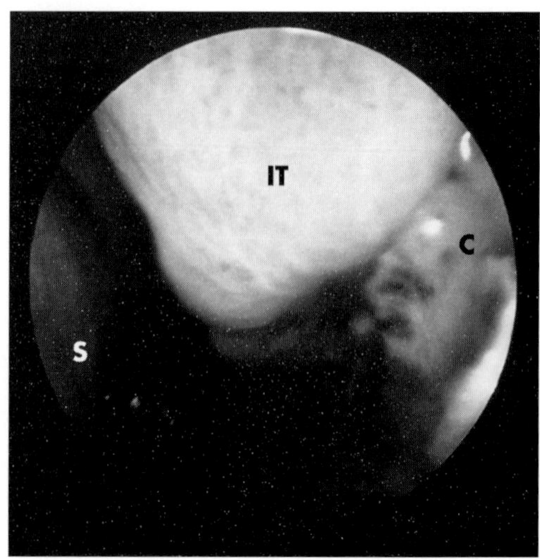

Fig. 17–6. Coagulum in left inferior meatus 2 weeks after cautery.

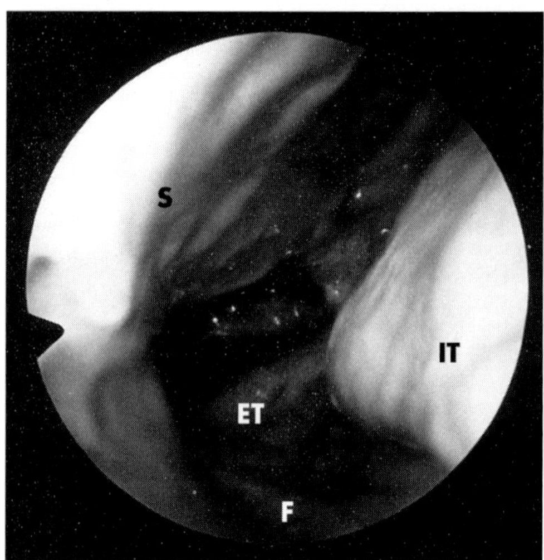

Fig. 17–7. Absent posterior tip of left inferior turbinate. IT, inferior turbinate; S, septum; F, floor; ET, eustachian tube orifice.

TECHNIQUE

The PEC technique is relatively straightforward. To the standard nasal cautery armamentarium are added 0.5- × 1.5-inch neurosurgical cottonoids, oxymethazoline (Afrin®), 4% topical xylocaine, the 4-mm straight or slightly angled nasal endoscope (the 2.7 is used quite well too in our office), a 10-cc syringe of xylocaine with epinephrine, and a 22 gauge 3.5-inch spinal needle (Fig. 17–8). A tonsil needle can be used instead of a spinal needle. If there are no contraindications, a narcotic is usually administered for intramuscular sedation. This may be ordered by phone to the emergency room nurse so that it has taken effect by the time the otolaryngologist arrives.

The posterior nature of bleeding is ascertained through patient history and anterior rhinoscopy. Because topical vasoconstriction may stop the bleeding, it is worthwhile to attempt to examine the bleeding site endoscopically before applying intranasal medications. The patient is essentially "talked through" this part of the procedure since both the endoscope and suction are inserted intranasally without any anesthetic. Having the patient's head tilted back encourages the posterior flow of the blood and increases the chance of identifying the bleeding locus. Oxymethazoline

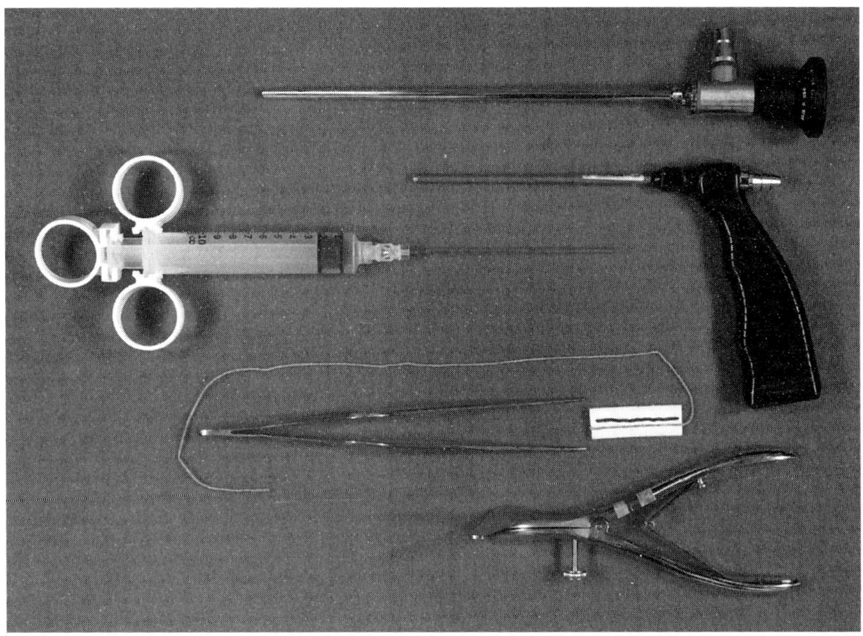

Fig. 17–8. PEC instruments. Top to bottom, 4 mm, 25-degree endoscope, standard nasal suction cautery unit, 10 cc syringe with 3.5 inch 22 gauge spinal needle, a 0.5 by 1.5 inch neurosurgical cottonoid, bayonets, and a nasal speculum.

(Afrin®) and 4% topical xylocaine are mixed half and half and applied to cotton pledgets or cottonoids, and then applied intranasally, first anteriorly and then further posteriorly. This frequently stops or slows bleeding. The nurse now grounds the standard suction cautery unit to the patient. As soon as the mucosa have become anesthetized, the endoscope and nasal suction are again inserted to identify the bleeding site if bleeding is continuing.

If the site cannot be identified, then all of Woodruff's plexus requires cautery. Unfortunately, the vasoconstriction and anesthesia needed to comfortably slip the scope into the posterior nose will often not just slow but stop the bleeding. If further anesthesia is necessary at this point, it is obtained by directly injecting the septum, nasal floor, and inferior turbinate (Fig. 17–9) with a local anesthetic with epinephrine using the spinal or tonsil needle. The surgeon, when concentrating on the posterior cautery, may not realize the extent of anterior nasal pressure, so liberal injections of the local anesthetic are helpful. If bleeding is still present, but is yet unidentified, the scope is again used to identify the site of the bleeding. The local anesthetic-vasoconstriction mix is now injected under endoscopic control using the spinal needle bent 30 degrees at the hub and slightly angled at the tip. If the bleeding site is known, anesthesia is injected in this location only; if not, then it should be injected into all planned cautery locations.

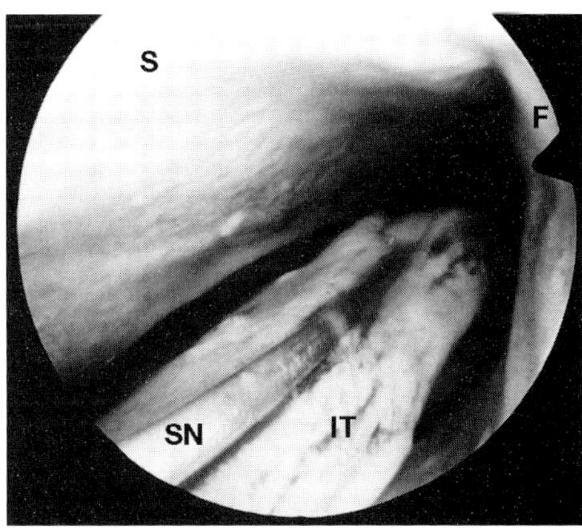

Fig. 17–9. Infiltration of local anesthetic—vasoconstrictor into posterior portion of right inferior turbinate with a spinal needle. S, septum; F, floor; IT, inferior turbinate; SN, spinal needle. From Wurman LH, et al: The treatment of posterior epistaxis by internal maxillary artery ligation and posterior endoscopic cautery, in Johnson JT (ed): *American Academy of Otolaryngology/Head and Neck Surgery*, v3, 1990.

Under endoscopic control, the suction cautery is now used to coagulate the mucosa at the bleeding site (Fig. 17–10). If no bleeding site is found, all of Woodruff's plexus can be cauterized. If the patient were to still feel the cautery current, a

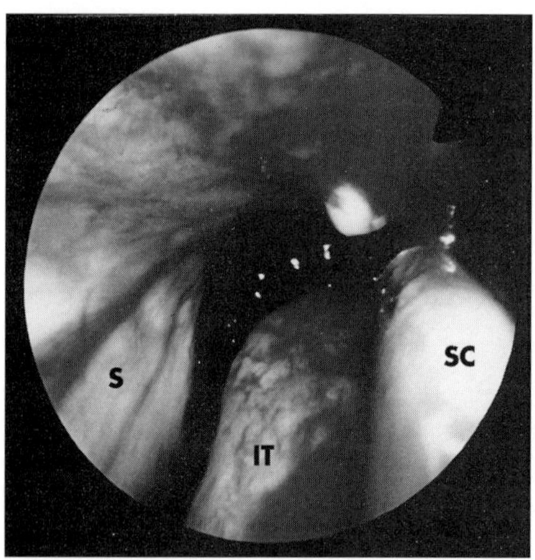

Fig. 17–10. Cautery of a right posterior inferior meatus bleeding site. IT, inferior turbinate; S, septum; SC, suction cautery. From Wurman LH, et al: The treatment of posterior epistaxis by internal maxillary artery ligation and posterior endoscopic cautery, in Johnson JT (ed): *American Academy of Otolaryngology/Head and Neck Surgery*, v3, 1990.

greater palatine nerve block transorally is required. It sometimes helps to mobilize the inferior turbinate medially for adequate vision and to allow room to work in the inferior meatus. Likewise, if one must approach the posterior portion of the middle meatus, the inferior turbinate is fractured laterally and the middle turbinate medially. Most bleeding sites seem to be located high in the very posterior portion of the lateral wall of the inferior meatus, tucked beneath the overhanging inferior turbinate. If the inferior turbinate is still obstructing, cautery directly on it will cause it to shrivel up visibly. This technique vastly improves posterior nasal visibility. In addition, by pushing the middle turbinate medially, access to the basal lamella is possible. The sphenopalatine artery and its branches can be cauterized inferiorally on the basal lamella as the vessels cross from the pterygomaxillary space to the middle turbinate and septum. We have noted bleeding coming from the posterior 1 cm of the nasal floor, inferior meatus, inferior turbinate, and the middle meatus; from the strip of mucosa posterior to the turbinates and anterior to the eustachian tube cartilage; and even from the mucosa of the adjacent face of the sphenoid. If no bleeding is identified, the mucosa in all of these potential bleeding locations must be cauterized. Aside from the loss of the posterior tip of the inferior turbinate, no other postcautery anatomic abnormalities have been identified, and the only clinical symptom patients have noted has been transient palate hypesthesia.

No packing is used postoperatively. Most patients are discharged or perhaps kept several hours in a holding bed if there is a question of the effectiveness of the cautery technique itself. Saline nasal sprays may help postoperatively to lessen the likelihood of crusting or to allow crusts that do form to detach without tearing the mucosa. Failure of what appears to be well-performed PEC usually leads to an internal maxillary artery or anterior ethmoid ligation, but if a coagulation profile is obtained first there should be no undiagnosed bleeding tendency.

REFERENCES

1. Cassisi NJ, et al. Changes in arterial oxygen tension and pulmonary mechanics with the care of posterior packing in epistaxis: a preliminary report. *Laryngoscope.* 1971; 81:1261.
2. Angell JE. Nasal reflexes. *Proc R Soc Med* 1969; 62:1287.
3. Wetmore SJ, et al. Sleep apnea in epistaxis patients treated with nasal pack. *Otol Head Neck Surg.* 1988; 98:596.
4. Wurman LH, et al. In: Johnson J, ed. *Instructional Courses,* Vol 3. Mosby; 1990:129–140.
5. Woodruff GH: Cardiovascular epistaxis and the nasopharyngeal plexus. *Laryngoscope.* 1949; 59:1238.
6. Hara HJ: Severe epistaxis. *Arch Otolaryngol.* 1962; 75:258.

18

Computer-Assisted Endoscopic Sinus Surgery

Jack B. Anon and S. James Zinreich

Use of computer imaging technology to increase the accuracy of stereotactic localization dates back to the mid 1970s when authors such as Brown[1] published reports on the use of computed tomography in conjunction with a marked, head-mounted stereotactic frame for targeting brain lesions in neurosurgery. Over the next decade, a series of technologic modifications gradually led to replacement of the original, cumbersome device with a variety of frameless systems.[2,3] In addition to increased maneuverability and greater access to the surgical field, the most important advantage of the newer frameless technology was the capability for real-time use of previously obtained information, imaging which is not possible with the framed devices.

Due to the position of bony anatomy within the paranasal sinuses, endoscopic surgery is extremely well suited to application of computer assisted visualization techniques. Computer assisted localization technology was first applied directly to the field of otolaryngology in 1987, when Schlondorff and colleagues[4] reported their development of and experience with a jointed, intraoperative probe correlated to a three-dimensional model created from a preoperative computed tomography (CT) scan. Continued refinement of CT technology has culminated in development of the ISG Intraoperative Viewing Wand, introduced in the United States in 1990 by Zinreich[5] and further detailed by Legget and associates[6] in 1991. Prior to the introduction of this device, surgeons depended on their direct visualization of the actual operative field, their previous surgical experience, and their ability to mentally translate data from a two-dimensional CT scan to the operating field. Clearly, there was a need to improve the accuracy of this "transferral" process. The device discussed in this chapter brings this improvement.

The Intraoperative Navigational Device

The "Wand" we currently use for our endoscopic surgeries is based on stereotactic software created by ISG Technologies (Mississauga, Ontario, Canada) and is currently implemented with a Hewlett Packard 715 workstation.

The workstation is interfaced with the Surgicom (Faro Technologies, Lake Mary, Fl), a passive mechanical arm with 2 degrees of freedom at each of the joints. A metallic probe is attached to the arm at the last joint. Sensors at each of the six rotational axes pass information about the relative angles of the arm segments to the computer by means of an analog-to-digital conversion board. These data are used in conjunction with known geometric information about the arm and the probe to trigonometrically solve for the spatial position and orientation of the device.

The device is fully extendable into the operating field or may be locked into a neutral position when not in use. It is attached either to a mount connected to the T-rail of the operating table, or directly to a Mayfield headrest system, which obviously secures the arm and prevents intraoperative motion.

A high-resolution computer monitor is used to display four images simultaneously: the triplanar image, which includes axial, sagittal, and coronal views; and the three-dimensional reconstructed image.

Preoperative Requirements for Computer Assisted Surgery

If the physical examination, patient history, lack of response to medical management, and baseline

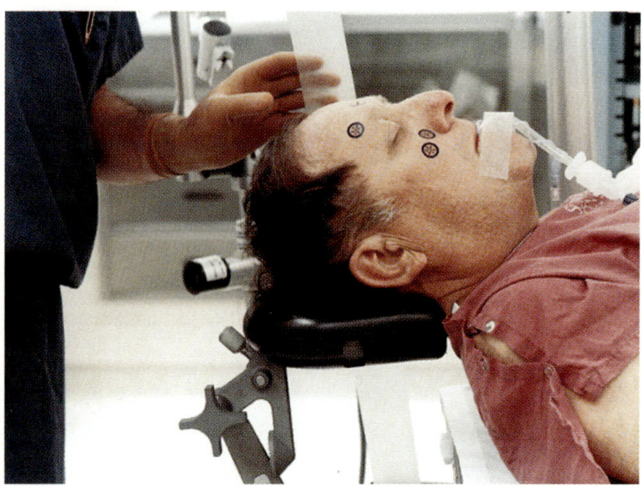

Fig. 18–1. Patient's head resting on padded horseshoe headrest. Plastic tape is used to secure the head in position.

coronal CT scan confirm the need for sinus surgery, and computer assisted surgery is planned, a new axial CT scan is required. The scanner should be set to a 3-mm slice thickness with a 3-mm table incrementation and targeted to include the area from the top of the frontal sinus to the upper incisors, including all soft tissue of the head between these areas. Fiducial markers are placed on the face for landmark identification and registration.

The acquired digitized CT data are transferred to the ISG-Allegro workstation via a nine-track magnetic archive tape, optical disc, or Ethernet, for reconstruction of the patient's face and underlying bony structures into a three-dimensional model. The original images and the three-dimensional (3-D) reconstructions are then stored on cartridge tape and transferred to the Viewing Wand system, located in the operating room.

Intraoperative Procedure

With the patient supine on the operating table, general anesthesia is induced and endotracheal intubation performed. The patient's head is then supported and the head of the operating table replaced by a padded horseshoe headrest. In our initial series, a Mayfield vertical horseshoe headrest was used.[7] Currently, the headrest has been replaced by a flat, padded U-shaped headrest, which supports a larger surface of the skull. The head is then secured by 3-inch plastic tape, which is secured to the lower aspect of the headrest, as shown in Figure 18–1.

The computer screen is then placed directly opposite the surgeon, the patient is draped in the usual fashion, and a plastic drape is used to cover the exposed articulated arm (which in turn is connected to the computer). Once the surgical team is scrubbed and gowned, a sterile probe is attached to the articulated arm of the Viewing Wand via a small hole in the drape, subsequently sealed with a sterile rubber band. At this point, previously placed cocaine pledgets are removed, the nose is examined endoscopically, and the lateral nasal wall is injected with 1% lidocaine with 1:100,000 epinephrine.

Registration Sequence

Registration may be performed in either of two ways: using fiducials (registration numbers) or anatomic landmarks. The registration process conveys to the computer (containing the 3-D reconstruction of the anatomic region to be evaluated) the precise location and orientation of the anatomic object, such that the image of the probe tip on the computer screen shows the actual position of the probe tip on, or in, the object. As each registration marker on the patient is touched with the tip of the probe, the corresponding marker's representation on the computer image is identified by a mouse-driven cursor on the screen (Figs. 18–2 and 18–3). This results in a point pair file that contains the real space and image space locations of each of the markers or anatomic landmarks. The computer then processes this point pair file to register the real space to the image space (that is, it registers the patient's anatomy to the imaged anatomy). A visual check of the registration is made by touching widely separated anatomic points on the surface of the patient's head and confirming the indicated locations on the computer screen.

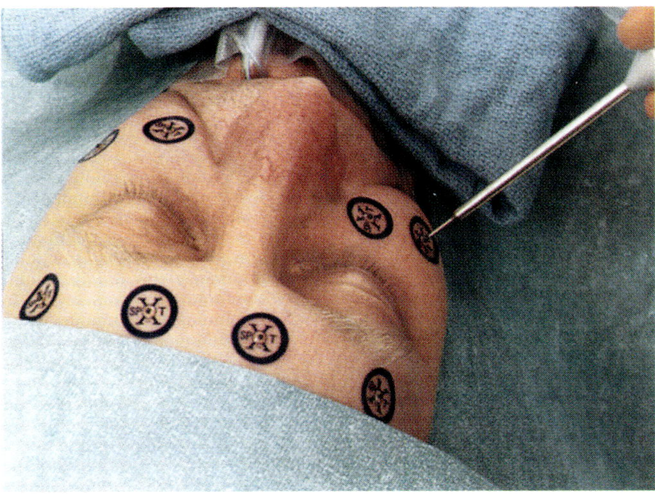

Fig. 18–2. Fiducial marker registration: Viewing Wand probe placed on center of fiducial marker.

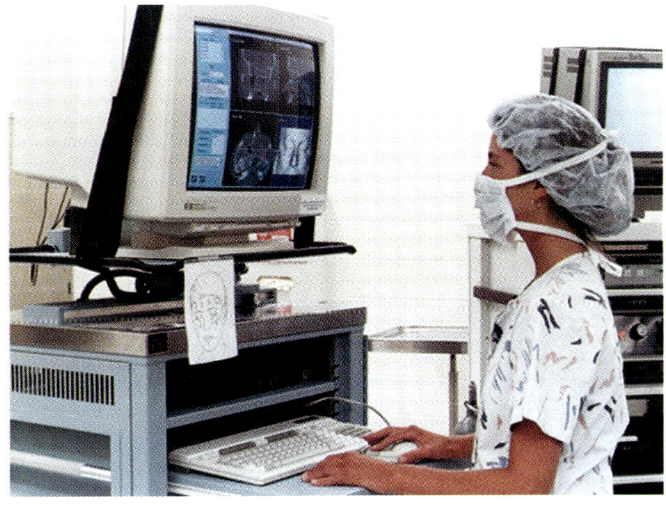

Fig. 18–3. Simultaneous to Viewing Wand probe being placed on fiducial marker, the operating assistant uses the computer mouse to position the cursor over the corresponding point on the three-dimensional virtual image.

The second method of registration uses the patient's facial, physical features as landmarks and as surface contours. For example, the Viewing Wand probe is placed on the lateral canthal area of the right eye; simultaneously, the mouse is used to place the cross-hairs over the same landmark on the three-dimensional computer generated image, and the location of the cross-hair is registered into the computer (Figs. 18–4 and 18–5). The contralateral lateral canthal and both left and right nasal alar regions are similarly entered. The probe is then placed along approximately 40 additional positions on the patient's face. The computer actually matches the patient's facial surface contour to the identical contour pattern of the three-dimensional reconstructed object, thereby allowing a precise correlation of each point in the CT scanned volume with its corresponding x-y-z coordinate within the reconstructed information on the computer screen.

Following the registration process, the computer displays the root mean square (RMS) value, which represents an expression of the deviation for each individual point of the registration set as compared to the whole. Clinical observations indicate lower RMS values correspond with a more accurate registration. The registration accuracy is subsequently corroborated by placing the probe tip on the center of one of the markers on the patient's face and visually checking its corresponding position on the computer screen, shown by the position of the cross-hair. Also, the distance between the actual fiducial and the imaged fiducial can be obtained by placing the cursor on the imaged fiducial and the probe on the actual fiducial. The difference between the imaged and actual fiducials

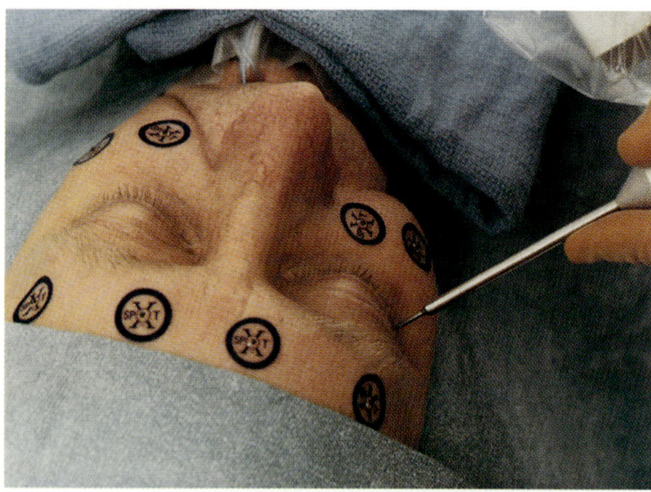

Fig. 18–4. Anatomic registration: the probe is positioned on the lateral canthal region of the right eye.

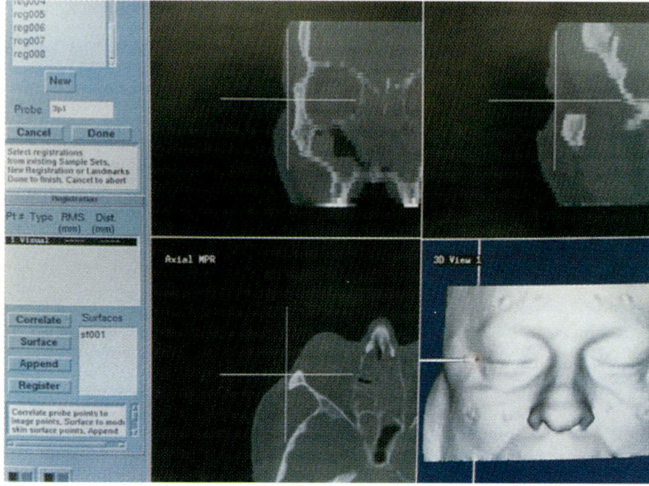

Fig. 18–5. Anatomic registration: the cross-hairs demonstrate the lateral canthal region on the two-dimensional triplanar views as well as the 3-D virtual image.

reveals the true accuracy of the registration. Using this technique, we have found our accuracy to range from 1 to 3 mm.

The combination of general anesthesia and the tightly fixed head position of our patients has prevented any problems with motion; however, with any motion, registration must be recalibrated. Instead of repeating the entire registration sequence, an abbreviated process can be used that involves marking four points on the patient's skin with a fine point marking pen and establishing those points in the computer system. If the patient's head moves, those four points alone can be used to reestablish registration. If fiducial registration is used, the fiducial markers can be established as landmarks in a similar manner.

Once preparatory procedures are completed, the actual surgery proceeds as usual, with the Viewing Wand used to define the operative field at various stages (Fig. 18–6). We initially use the "probe" to identify the bulla ethmoidalis and confirm our position medial to the lamina papyracea. Throughout the procedure the probe is used to identify position and landmarks. Once the anterior ethmoid cells are entered and disease eradicated, the probe identifies the entry point into the posterior ethmoid cells. The fovea ethmoidalis can easily be identified with the probe and, if disease is present in the sphenoid sinus, such pathology is also accessible using the probe to identify the entry point (Figs. 18–7, 18–8, 18–9). The probe has also proven to be very useful in identifying the exact point of penetration into the maxillary sinus and to avoid damaging the orbit. Initially, the frontal recess and frontal sinus were difficult areas to approach, as the trajectory of the straight probe could not be rotated easily back into this area. A newly designed curved probe is expected to resolve this problem.

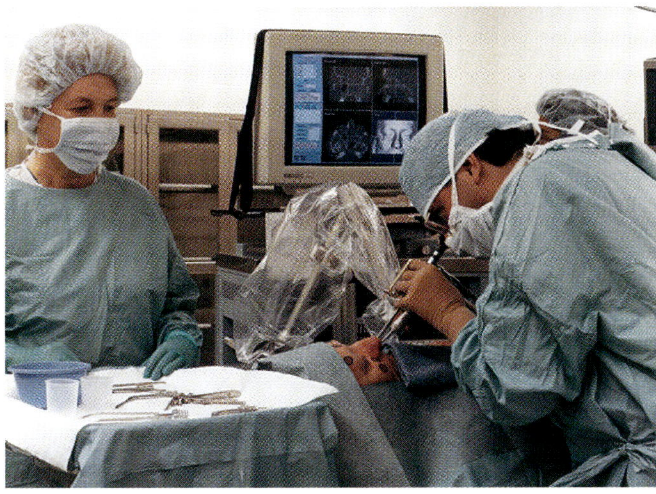

Fig. 18–6. Operation in progress: overall view demonstrating computer position relative to the surgeon. Note, the draped multijointed Viewing Wand arm attached to the operating table.

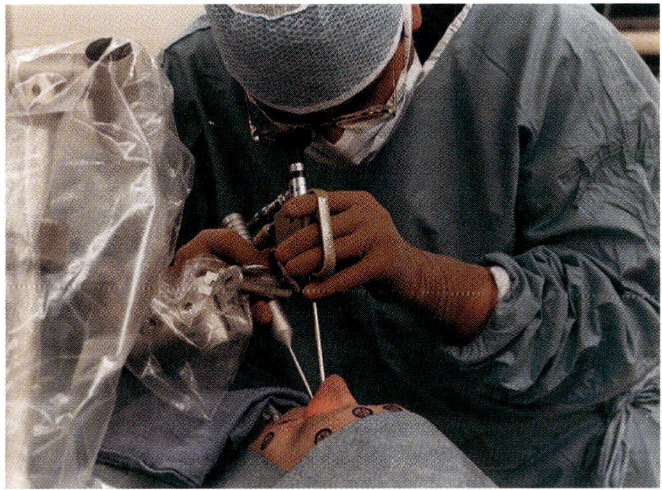

Fig. 18–7. The probe is used *para*endoscopically.

Discussion

The ISG Viewing Wand system offers a significant improvement over previously used radiographic technology. Compared with the fluoroscopic C-arm, for example, the Viewing Wand is more manageable, allows for easy visualization of all anatomic planes, and, since it does not involve radiation exposure, avoids the need for cumbersome radiation protection with the use of the C-arm.[8]

Disadvantages of the Viewing Wand are essentially minor. For example, we feel that the need for a second axial CT scan is a minor point, since the radiation exposure associated with this type of scan is far below the 50% cataract dose. The margin of safety imparted by use of the Viewing Wand during surgery far outweighs the minor drawback of an additional radiation dosage.

One important consideration in weighing the benefits of the Viewing Wand system is the increased cost of instrumentation. In addition to the obvious costs of the computer system itself, a technician is needed to produce the three-dimensional image from the initial CT scan data.

Specific indications for use of this device include revision surgery, massive disease or disease within the sphenoid sinus, the presence of Onodi cells or potentially complicating factors, and frontal recess disease. It also has been used for optic nerve decompression and sinonasal carcinoma.[9] With continued research it becomes clear that computer assistance may play an important role in procedures for other conditions of the head and neck as well, including drainage of orbital or epidural abscesses secondary to complications of acute sinusitis and decompression of orbital contents for Graves' disease.[10] In a review of other

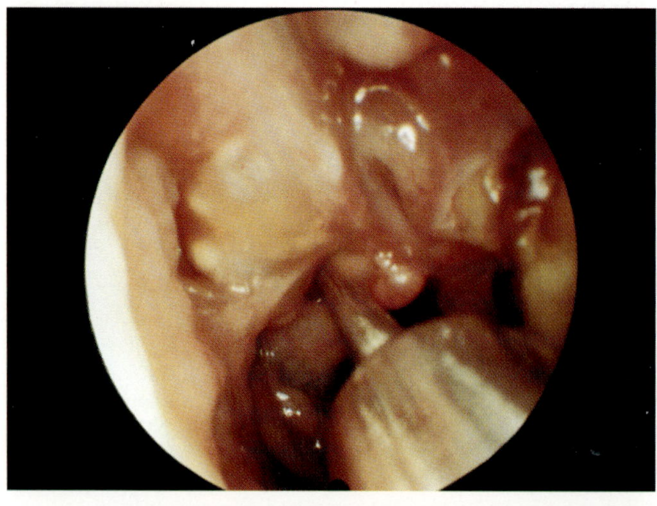

Fig. 18–8. Endoscopic view of probe tip in sphenoethmoidal recess region.

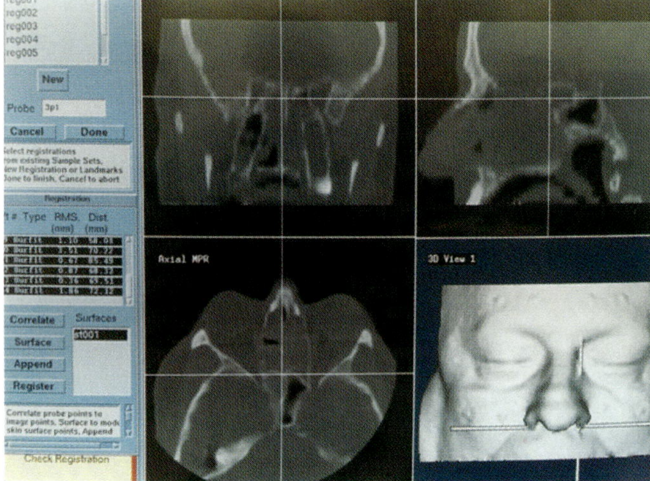

Fig. 18–9. Corresponding computer image with cross-hairs demonstrating exact position of Viewing Wand probe.

indications, an investigative group in Germany[11] reported that a device similar to the Viewing Wand had been used in ENT cases including procedures involving the paranasal sinuses and nasopharynx, cochlear implants, and head and neck tumors. They also listed indications such as endonasal and open approaches to the skull base, and translabyrinthine approaches for acoustic neuromas. The "Wand" had been used successfully for neurosurgical procedures at the Johns Hopkins Medical Institute since 1990.[12]

Computer assistance allows the surgical field to be more clearly defined, thus safer sinus surgery is performed. In addition, this allows more thorough dissection, as "hidden" cells can be better identified.

Computer assisted guidance is no substitute for a carefully trained, experienced surgeon with a thorough understanding of surgical anatomy, but in such hands it can be valuable in assuring and improving accuracy.

REFERENCES

1. Brown RA. A computerized tomography—computer graphics approach to stereotaxis localization. *J Neurosurg.* 1979;50:715–720.
2. Roberts DW, Strohbehn JW, Hatch GF, et al. Frameless stereotaxis interpretation of computerized tomographic imaging and the operating microscope. *J Neurosurg.* 1986:65:545–549.
3. Watanabe E, Watanabe T, Manaka S, et al. Three-dimensional digitizer (neuronavigator): new equipment for computed tomography-guided stereotaxic surgery. *Surg Neurol.* 1987; 27:543–547.
4. Schlondorff, G, Meyer-Ebrecht D, Mosges R, et al. CAS—computer assisted surgery in der kopf-und hals-chirurgie. *Arch Oto-Rhino-Laryng.* 1987;11(5):45.
5. Zinreich SJ. Intraoperative computer imaging for endoscopic sinus surgery. Presented at the First International Symposium on Contemporary Sinus Surgery, Pittsburgh, PA, Nov. 4–6, 1990.

6. Leggett WB, Greenberg M, Gannon W, et al. The viewing wand—a new system for three-dimensional computed tomography-correlated intraoperative localization. *Curr Surg.* 1991;48(10):674–678.
7. Anon JB, Lipman SP, Oppenheim D, Halt RA. Computer-assisted endoscopic sinus surgery. *Laryngoscope.* 1994; 104(7):901-905.
8. Anon JB, Lipman SP, Guelcher RT. Intraoperative use of the fluoroscopic C-arm during endoscopic intranasal sinus surgery. *Oper Techn Otolaryngol Head Neck Surg.* 1991;2(4):266–268.
9. Loury M, Cummings C, Zinreich SJ. Intraoperative use of an interactional three-dimensional imaging system. Presented at the Southern Section Triological Society, Sea Pines, GA, Jan. 1992.
10. Synderman C, Hopson S. Computer assisted orbital decompression for graves' disease. Presented at the First Computer Assisted Sinus Endoscopic Surgery Course, Pittsburgh, PA, May 7–8, 1993.
11. Klimek L, Mosges R, Bartsch M. Indications for CAS (Computer Assisted Surgery) systems as navigational aid in ENT surgery. In: Lembke HU et al, eds. (*HRSG*): *Computer-Assisted Radiology '91.* Springer Verlag; New York, NY; 1991.
12. Zinreich SJ, Tebo S, Long DL, et al. Frameless stereotactic integration of CT imaging data: accuracy and initial applications. In press.

19

Complications of Endoscopic Sinus Surgery and Malpractice

James A. Stankiewicz

The complications of endoscopic sinus surgery are the same whether for revision or primary surgery. In the first part of this chapter, complication avoidance will be stressed with an eye toward avoiding malpractice. The second part of the chapter will discuss management of specific complications.

Complication Avoidance

The greatest advantage of endoscopic diagnosis and surgery is the ability to put all patient information together in a workable database. Sifting through all available information helps the surgeon anticipate problems and greatly reduces the risk of complications.

Preoperative assessment is important, from the history to the informed consent and decision to operate. The history should be screened carefully for all potential problem areas. A questionnaire addressing all areas of history is important and should be comprehensive. It can be reviewed with the patient and will provide an excellent record and much valuable information. The patient's medication history is also very important. The patient's previous treatment history has to be reviewed for intensity and duration of antibiotic therapy. If antibiotics have been used ineffectively or inappropriately to treat acute or chronic sinusitis, this problem has to be addressed before deciding upon surgery. The first thing a lawyer will look at in the case of a complication is whether the surgery was necessary, if proper antibiotic therapy was given, and if the patient is a treatment failure. Antibiotics need to be given for at least 3 to 4 weeks before a decision for surgery is considered. Most often, patients will have been treated for 7 to 10 days with single or repeated doses of an antibiotic that is clearly inappropriate for chronic sinusitis. Recommendations for appropriate medical treatment are available and should be followed.[1] Medications that can cause bleeding problems should be noted to prevent complications. As a rule, aspirin and nonsteroidal anti-inflammatory medications should be stopped 10 days prior to surgery. Specific questions regarding the intake of aspirin need to be asked because patients frequently will not mention these over-the-counter medications. Surgical and medical history should be noted. The presence of previous sinus surgeries is important due to loss of landmarks and, in extensive cases, increased risks.[2] Patients who have had previous complications are obviously at high risk and should be evaluated very carefully to diminish the chances of a repeat complication as much as possible. It should be obvious to these patients that they are at great risk. If they are unaware of this, they should be told frankly. Asthmatics usually have sinus disease that is the most difficult to treat medically and surgically, and preoperative planning is important.

The physical exam should be complete and well documented. A graphic chart report is helpful. However, there are times when the examination appears relatively normal and symptoms require further evaluation. Endoscopic examination and radiographic evaluation are most important. Similarly, there are times when obvious disease is present on examination, but a computerized tomography (CT) scan shows only nasal swelling with normal sinuses indicating rhinitis. Most importantly, especially for revision cases, is the documentation of scarring, landmark changes, and extent of disease.

The radiographic study of choice is the coronal CT scan, which can delineate the bony anatomy and extent of disease. In cases where previous complications have occurred or in extensive disease where there is concern for bony erosion, the coronal and axial CT scans work well. In cases of orbital or skull base infection, it is necessary to rule out periorbital or dural invasion, and an MRI scan can provide this information. These studies allow selection of proper surgical procedures and afford better preparation to diminish the risk of complication.

Informed consent is one of the key factors in avoiding litigation. Along with establishing a reason for surgery, complicated sinusitis or failure of medical therapy, actual surgery, and postoperative care, informed consent is one of the keys to defending a lawsuit. It is my experience that patients should be told about the recommended surgery as well as how it is done and why it should be done. Risks and alternatives to surgery, with their risks, should be covered. Sinus surgery is hazardous, and all risks should be discussed. A handout elucidating the risks of sinus surgery is helpful. Blindness, double vision, and brain complications unfortunately do occur. The experienced surgeon can summarize these risks by discussing with the patient his/her personal experience with complications. In my practice, patients have not been lost due to aggressive informed consent.

Operative Avoidance of Complications

Upon entering the surgical suite, the surgeon should have the CT scan on the light box. Both the CT scan and office records should be reviewed. Adequate time for topical vasoconstriction (and local anesthesia if it is used) is paramount to avoid bleeding and visualization problems. Patients under general anesthesia should be prepared topically and parenterally in the same fashion as the patient under local anesthesia. Patients under general anesthesia are more prone to complications due to lack of patient response to inadvertent entrance into the orbit or skull base. The eyes must not be obstructed by anything (for example, tape, goggles, and towels) so the surgeon can observe eye movement or swelling during surgery. Instrumentation should be checked by the nurse and the physician to make sure the instruments are familiar and functional. During the surgery, the endoscope should be clean, and fogging should be prevented with Ultrastop™, a suitable alternative such as Fred™, or the scope scrubber. Suction irrigation may be helpful, especially when the middle turbinate is not present. Correct location is paramount. If the surgeon is

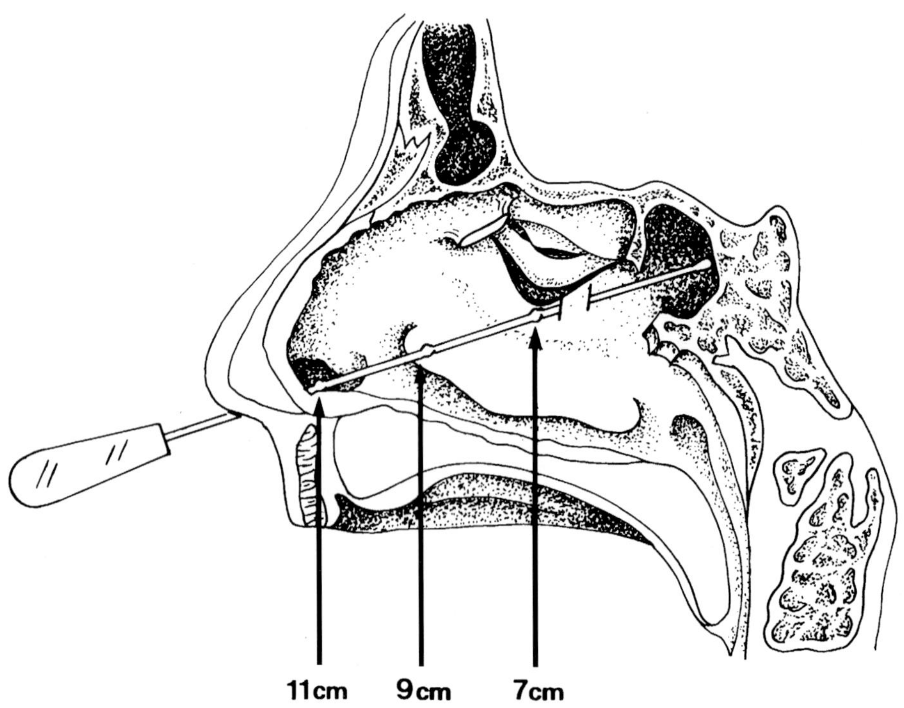

Fig. 19–1. Beaded probe measurements to important anatomical sites.

unsure of instrument location or anatomy, he or she should remove the endoscope and look with a headlight or use the endoscope as a light. Remember that the endoscope is not binocular, and depth of field may occasionally become a problem. The use of a cross table plain film or fluoroscopy can help to identify anatomic location and prevent entrance into the base of the skull, cribriform plate, lamina papyracea, or fovea ethmoidalis.[3] A beaded probe (Skillern-Storz, St. Louis, MO) or other measuring device can identify distances to the basal lamella of the middle turbinate, sphenoid sinus, posterior nasopharynx, base of the skull, and fovea ethmoidalis (Fig. 19–1). Anatomy should be respected and used advantageously. Techniques such as watching the eye or palpating the medial canthal ligament and lacrimal bone to feel vibration, indicating the lamina papyracea has been reached, are helpful. Palpation of the eye while examining the lamina papyracea intranasally with the endoscope to de-

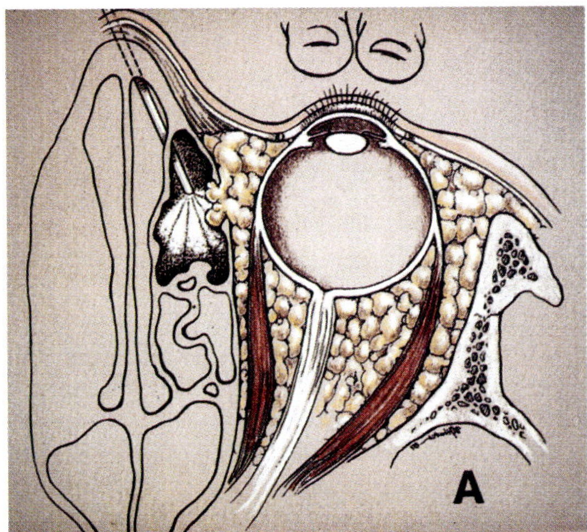

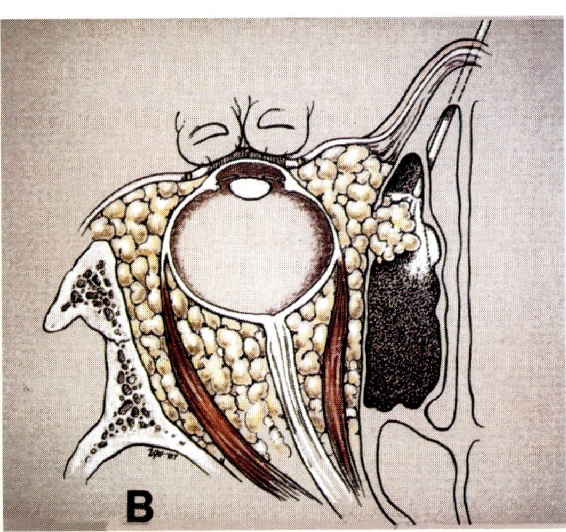

Fig. 19–2. Technique of simultaneous eye palpation and intranasal endoscopic examination. **A**, Endoscope in place examining lateral nasal wall lamina papyracea. Note hole in lamina papyracea with mild fat exposure. **B**, Simultaneous eye palpation and endoscopic observation. If hole in lamina papyracea is apparent with periorbita or orbital fat exposed, early visualization of defect is possible. (From Stankiewicz JA: Blindness in intranasal endoscopic ethmoidectomy: Prevention and management. Otolaryngol Head Neck Surg, 101:320-329, 1989. By permission.)

ANATOMY RELATIONSHIPS TO PREVENT COMPLICATIONS

1. The lamina papyracea lies superior to and not any more lateral to the natural ostia.
2. Operate lateral to the middle turbinate, never medial.
3. The antrostomy should be placed just above inferior turbinate with the surgical instrument lying on top of the inferior turbinate.
4. The antrostomy should not be made more anterior than the anterior end of the middle turbinate.
5. The nasofrontal duct lies at 6.0 to 6.5 cm from the nasal opening.
6. The anterior ethmoid artery and base of the skull (posterior-superior fovea ethmoidalis) is 7 cm from the nasal opening.
7. The sphenoid sinus anterior wall is 7 cm from the nasal opening.
8. The basal lamella of the middle turbinate is 6 cm from the nasal opening (posterior ethmoids lie behind this).
9. The nasopharyngeal wall approximates the posterior sphenoid wall to within 1 cm.
10. Identify and cannulate the sphenoid ostia if possible. The posterior middle turbinate may need to be removed to do this because the ostia lies one-third of the way up the anterior wall from the choana just next to the septum.
11. The anterior wall of the sphenoid sinus lies at a plane between the superior inferior turbinate and bottom of the middle turbinate.
12. The antrostomy is at the level of the inferior orbital rim.
13. If the middle turbinate has to be removed, remove only the inferior part of the turbinate with scissors; preserve the superior part as an anatomic landmark.
14. The bone of the skull base is yellow, not white like the ethmoid.
15. The skull base/ethmoid is thinnest at the medial part of the fovea ethmoidalis in the ethmoid at the level of the anterior ethmoid artery adjacent to the middle turbinate.
16. The skull base slants downward as the surgeon moves posteriorly and is not straight back, putting the posterior ethmoid/sphenoid area at risk.
17. The fovea ethmoidalis anteriorly at the level of the ethmoid artery and frontal recess is higher than the cribriform plate, whereas posteriorly the skull base flattens out.

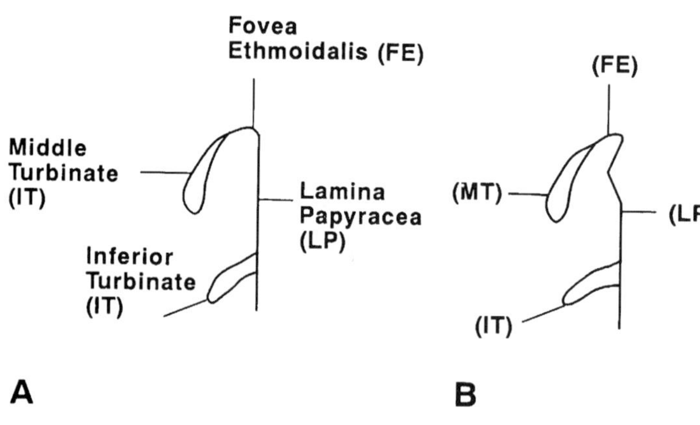

Fig. 19–3. Anatomical differences on the left side of nasal cavity concerning portion of lamina papyracea. **A**, To right-handed surgeon, left side apparent anatomy. **B**, Anatomy in reality with orbit pushing into ethmoid superiorly and laterally. (Otolaryngol Head Neck Surg 101:320-329, 1989. By permission.)

termine presence of the lamina papyracea or entrance into the orbit is very important and should be repeatedly employed (Fig. 19–2).[4,5] Right-handed surgeons should begin on the right side because there is some evidence the anatomic direction is more conducive to complications. Endoscopic surgeons should be wary, however, about anatomy on the left side, which brings the lamina papyracea more in a direct line for injury (Fig. 19–3).[4] Precise identification of landmarks intraoperatively is essential. If a sphenoidotomy and antrostomy have to be done first to establish landmarks, so be it. In extensive surgery, a "blueprint" plan for surgical technique and approach should be prepared ahead of time (see box on previous page).

Avoidance technique, as noted above, with the inclusion of intraoperative radiology to find location and define landmarks is very important. Traditional surgery should be combined with endoscopic surgeries or used alone if it is the safest way for a surgeon to proceed. In addition, each surgeon should have a "game plan" of what to do if an operative complication should occur.

Specific Complications

HEMORRHAGE

Significant hemorrhage can occur intraoperatively. Patients can lose two units of blood or more in a given procedure, but this is rare. This extent of blood loss can mean that an intracranial complication has occurred, or it is a signal to stop surgery and reevaluate. In my experience, patients who have had multiple polypectomies and sinus surgeries are at greater risk of hemorrhage. Usually their disease is extensive and requires sphenoethmoidectomy and polypectomy to control. Major bleeding points are the anterior ethmoid and posterior septal arteries. The anterior ethmoid artery usually will retract into its bony canal unless avulsed.[6] On occasion, severe bleeding can occur nasally or intraorbitally, requiring cautery and packing (see discussion under *Blindness*). The posterior septal artery, which provides blood to the posterior middle turbinate and the septum, can bleed vigorously and is controlled with cautery or packing. Usually this hemorrhage is related to removal, totally or partially, of the middle turbinate. Cautery of all turbinate remnants is the best way to control this and prevent postoperative bleeding. While blood can ooze from several sites during surgery, the amount of blood loss is often not realized until the end of surgery. Once all of the pathology has been removed, bleeding, unless arterial, will slow. Bleeding can become brisk enough that vision is impaired. In this circumstance, it is better to pack the nose and either go to the other side or terminate the surgery. To proceed with surgery (and possibly get into trouble) is hazardous. Patients understand the need for stopping surgery under this circumstance. Although they may not be happy that the procedure could not be finished, patients are usually willing to come back another day. Interestingly, for whatever reason, bleeding seems to be much reduced the next time around. In my experience, patients who undergo general anesthesia average about 75 to 100 cc more blood loss than patients getting local anesthesia. In cases in which bleeding is anticipated, autologous transfusion may be extremely useful. Chapter 4 discusses major carotid artery hemorrhage and should be reviewed.

CEREBROSPINAL LEAK (SEE CHAPTER 10)

BLINDNESS

Blindness can occur temporarily or permanently. Permanent blindness occurs as a result of direct optic nerve injury or prolonged intraocular pressure that causes neural injury.[8] Direct injury to the optic nerve is irreversible. Increased intraocular pressure can be reversed. Major orbital injury occurs as a result of entrance through the lamina papyracea and, in most cases, the periorbita.

Prevention of blindness begins preoperatively when evaluating the patient for the first time and carries over to operative and postoperative considerations. Patients who have extensive disease and have had previous surgeries warrant caution and careful evaluation. Operatively, the patient's eyes are not covered and are closely observed. Eye movement during surgery, ecchymosis, proptosis, or pupillary change are all signs that indicate the orbit has been entered. The finding of the natural antrostomy defines the lamina papyracea as a landmark, which is superior and slightly lateral to the antrostomy, especially in revision surgery. Palpation of the eye while viewing the ethmoid complex and lamina papyracea intranasally will, very early on, indicate dehiscence of the lamina papyracea, periorbita, or orbital fat, and keep the surgeon out of trouble (see Fig. 19–8).[8] Orbital fat should not be tampered with, and the patient should be observed closely for signs of orbital hematoma. Patients who develop signs consistent with entrance into the orbital cavity (for example, ecchymosis, lid edema) should be admitted for close observation. Usually ecchymosis first appears in the medial upper lid. Minimal nonexpanding lid discoloration can be observed on an outpatient basis, but specific instructions must be provided to the patient and family about the risks and how to contact the surgeon if problems develop.

Blindness secondary to increased orbital pressure is of two types: 1) Slow small vessel hemorrhage secondary to periorbital/lamina papyracea injury with slowly expanding hemorrhage and proptosis, and 2) sudden, large postvessel (arterial) hemorrhage with immediate onset vision loss, proptosis, and chemosis. Treatment differs according to cause. Slow vessel injury is gradual, with a better chance of responding to medical treatment as outlined below. Fast vessel injury needs to be acted upon immediately. While pressures may be such with slow vessel injury that danger to the vascular supply to the optic nerve is not a problem

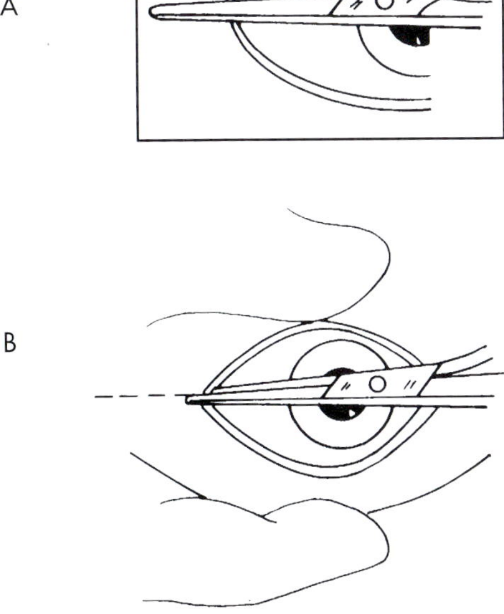

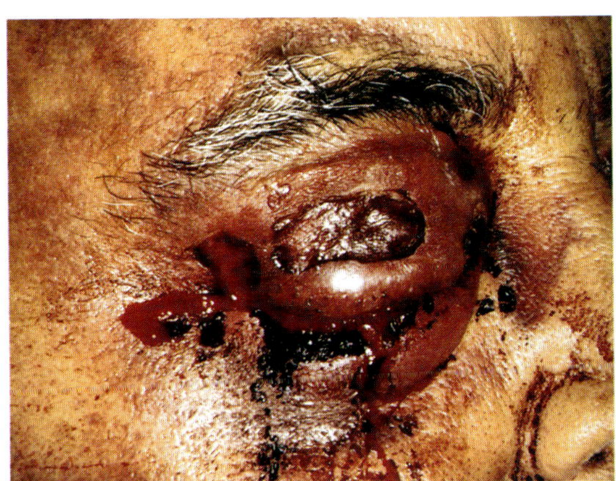

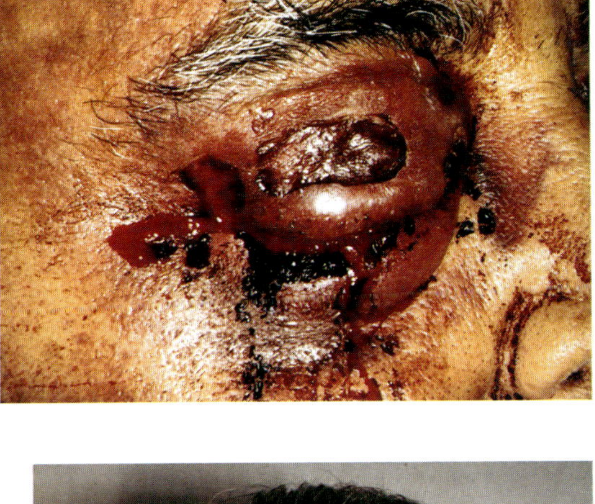

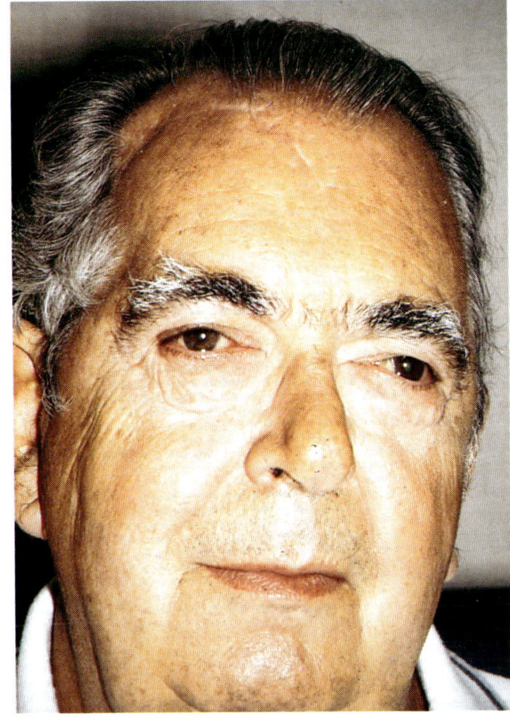

Fig. 19–4. **A** and **B,** Lateral canthotomy technique. **C,** Preoperative view; marked proptosis with orbital pressure 50 mm Hg. Note lid ischemia. **D,** Postoperative healing with resolution of pressures and no vision loss with lateral canthotomy.

for 60 to 90 minutes, acute pressure changes with fast vessel injury may compromise the optic nerve in as little as 10 to 15 minutes. The typical scenario for fast vessel injury is avulsion of the anterior ethmoid artery with direct intraorbital hemorrhage, with proptosis occurring in minutes. The lamina papyracea may be intact. Treatment requires less medical management and more aggressive decompression. Other than orbital massage there is no medical treatment that will reduce pressures in 10 to 15 minutes. If the eye remains firm and proptotic, an immediate lateral canthotomy is necessary (Fig. 19–4). If no change occurs, then medial orbital decompression via (Lynch) external ethmoidectomy with control of ethmoid area hemorrhage is necessary. The lamina papyracea needs to be decompressed, as well, to control pressures. High dose prednisone, for optic nerve trauma, may prove helpful intraoperatively and postoperatively. The patient needs close observation postoperatively by ophthalmologists, with medical therapy geared towards keeping pressures down.

A patient who develops slow vessel blindness should be treated immediately with mannitol 1 to 2 gm/kg, intravenously, infused over 30 to 60 minutes. Eye consultation is obtained and orbital massage is begun immediately (Fig. 19–5).[8] If blindness does not resolve and the optic nerve is not injured directly (Marcus Gunn pupil), then lateral canthotomy or Lynch incision with external ethmoidectomy is performed. The periorbita should be incised to help provide drainage and decompression.

There is no evidence that steroids do or do not benefit these slow vessel patients; thus, they are not necessary. Gradual proptosis and increased orbital pressure can also occur over several days, and patients should be aware of this and return for immediate treatment.

Postoperatively, it is important that the patient, nurses, and family be told of possible complications and what to look for. Any problem occurring during surgery should be discussed with them. Their immediate response, based on good postoperative teaching, may make the difference.

ORBITAL HEMATOMA

Orbital hematoma occurs as a result of entrance into the lamina papyracea or periorbita. Close observation for signs of increased intraocular pressure is necessary as noted above. Ecchymosis occurs and usually resolves within 1 to 2 weeks (Fig. 19–6).[4,5]

DIPLOPIA (DOUBLE VISION)

Diplopia (double vision) is related to direct or indirect injury to the medial rectus muscle or its nerve or vascular supply. Entrance through the lamina papyracea and periorbita is usually the

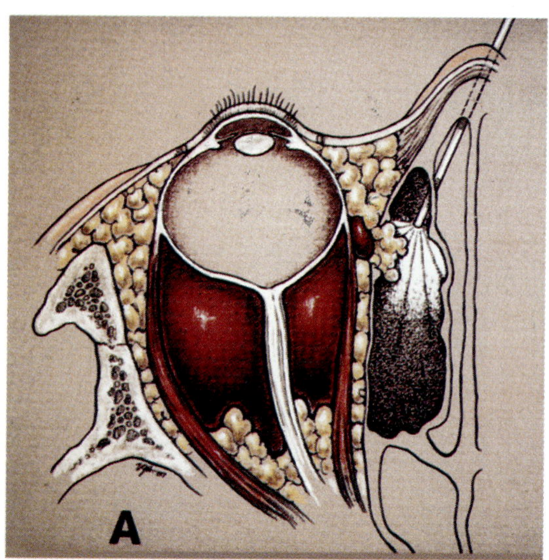

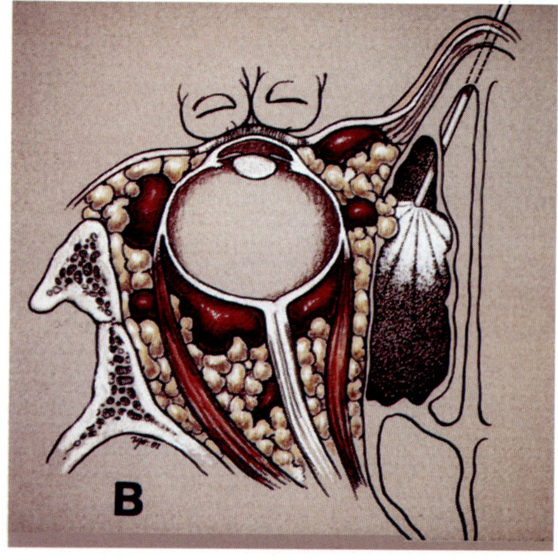

Fig. 19–5. Orbital massage technique and how it affects intraocular pressure. **A**, Retrobulbar hemorrhage after entrance into lamina papyracea and injury to periorbita. **B**, Redistribution of orbital hemorrhage utilizing orbital massage, resulting in decreased orbital pressure. (From Stankiewicz, JA: Blindness and intranasal endoscopic ethmoidectomy: Prevention and management. Otolaryngol Head Neck Surg 101:320-329, 1989. By permission.)

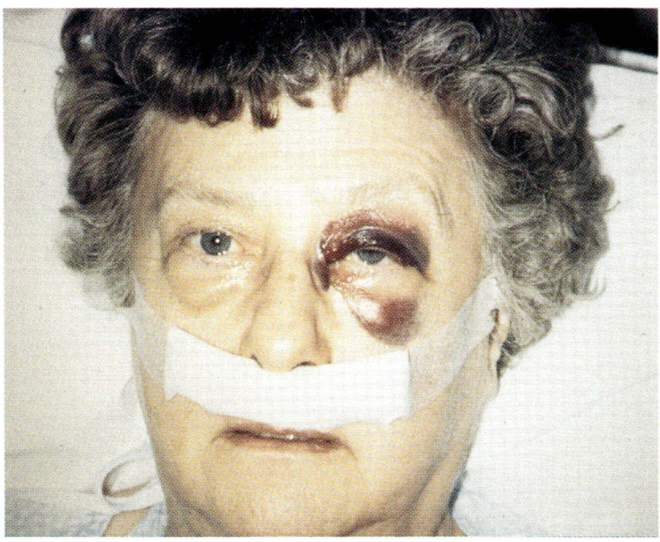

Fig. 19–6. Patient with orbital hematoma caused by entrance into lamina papyracea.

main cause. Radiologic and anatomic studies show the medial rectus to be within a few millimeters of the lamina papyracea (Figs. 19–7 and 19–8). However, cautery or laser surgery on or through the periorbita is a potential cause. Some diplopia is related to edema, and is temporary. This may be due to intraorbital injection of xylocaine. If persistent diplopia develops, the treatment is ophthalmologic surgery, which may not result in relief.[9]

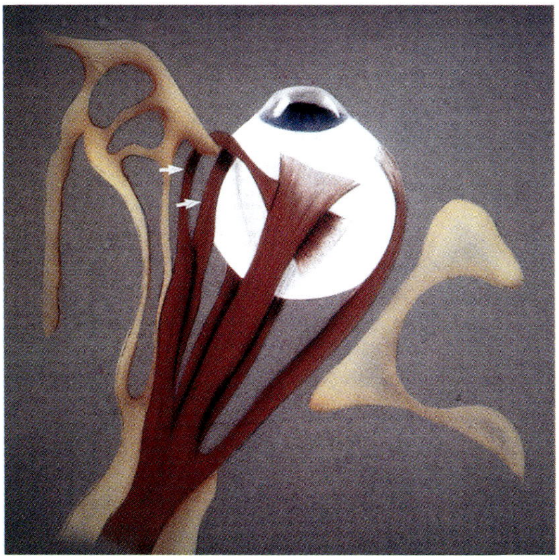

Fig. 19–7. Illustration of eye muscle possibly injured during sinus surgery. Most common is medial rectus and then superior oblique (see arrows).

SUBCUTANEOUS ORBITAL EMPHYSEMA

Subcutaneous orbital emphysema results from entrance into the lamina papyracea. Usually, air enters as a result of a Valsalva maneuver, such as

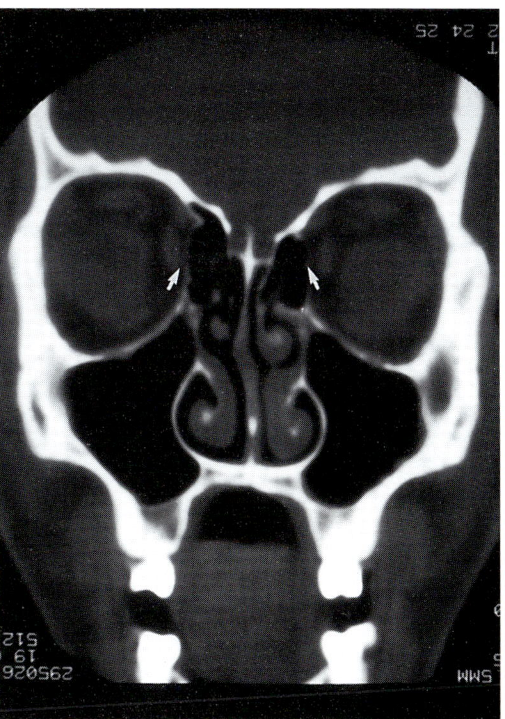

Fig. 19–8. CAT scan coronal view showing close distance (see arrows) of medial rectus to lamina papyracea.

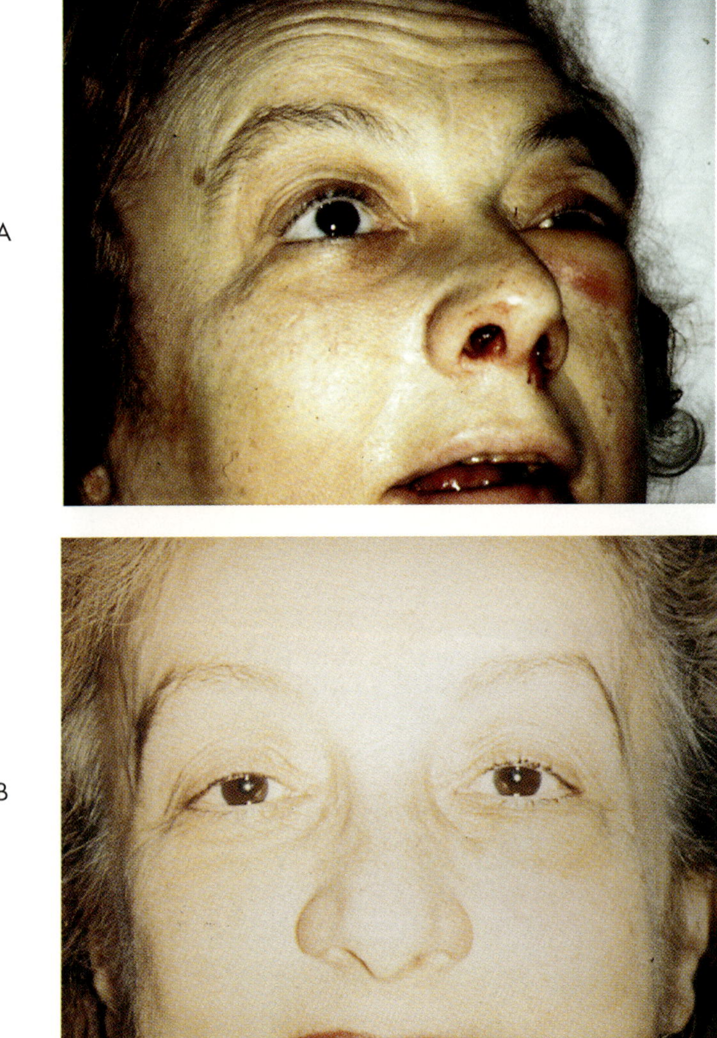

Fig. 19–9. **A**, Operative subcutaneous emphysema. **B**, Resolution at 10 days. Note slight persistent lid puffiness that eventually resolved.

with vomiting, nose blowing, extubation, or anesthesia masking. This will resolve within 1 week (Figs. 19–9A, B).[4,5]

Postoperative Complications

PREVENTION

Postoperative considerations regarding close observation and appropriate order writing are important. Patients who look normal at the end of surgery can look horrendous 1 to 2 hours after surgery. Any patient about whom the surgeon is concerned should be considered for a same-day admissions. Appropriate orders reflecting the surgeon's concern for the eye and/or brain should be written so the surgeon is notified immediately if something is wrong. Nurses unfamiliar with these new procedures should be told what they are and what to expect. Endoscopic sinus surgery patients do not look like Caldwell-Luc patients postoperatively. Family members should be told what to expect and informed about potential complications or about the surgeon's concerns about a possible complication. Strict information about what to call the surgeon for, especially for problems in the eye or brain area, need to be given to the patient's family. A handout that summarizes the above is very helpful. All of this avoids waiting for complications to occur and gives the best chance for treatment. Following the above recommendations reduces litigation risk if a complication should occur.

Specific Postoperative Complications

SYNECHIA

Synechia formation is the most common complication, if it is indeed a complication, occurring with endoscopic sinus surgery. Because of the functional nature of the surgery, the middle turbinate is often preserved. Whenever two raw surfaces oppose one another, as is often the case when the middle turbinate is preserved, scarring can occur. Measures to counteract synechia should be taken. Various types of spacers are available. Some surgeons routinely remove the anterior part of the middle turbinate as an alternative to using a spacer. When the turbinate is preserved, meticulous postoperative care and observation are necessary. The surgeon should lyse all adhesions and place a spacer, if necessary. Adhesions usually occur anteriorly. It should be noted that the middle turbinate has a natural tendency to move laterally, contributing to synechia formation. If synechia occur to the extent that the middle meatus is blocked with return of disease, revision surgery is necessary. If the turbinate is again preserved, a spacer must be placed to avoid readhesion. Partial turbinectomy may be necessary, depending on the extent of disease and synechia formation.[4] The key to avoiding synechia is truly functional surgery causing minimal injury to surrounding tissue.

NASOLACRIMAL DUCT INJURY

The natural antrostomy should not be opened anteriorly to the anterior end of the middle turbinate to avoid injury to the nasolacrimal duct. This is especially important in children. The bone covering the nasolacrimal duct is much harder than that covering the natural ostia and fontanelle area. The best time to find the natural antrostomy is at the beginning of surgery after the uncinate process is removed. The use of a probe to find the antrostomy and dilate the opening is very helpful. If backward biting is restricted anteriorly and the ostia is opened inferiorally and posteriorly, this complication can be eliminated. If injury occurs, patients will complain postoperatively of increased tearing (i.e., with tears running down their face). Dacryocystitis may then occur. Ophthalmology consultation may require probing and dilation. Eventually dacrocystorhinostomy may be necessary.

POSTOPERATIVE HEMORRHAGE

In most cases, postoperative hemorrhage requiring packing, surgery, or possible transfusion is due to arterial hemorrhage from the sphenopalatine artery branches to the middle turbinate and posterior ethmoid area and less so to the anterior ethmoid artery. Patients need to be cautioned about too vigorous activity or travel, postoperatively. Any aspirin or nonsteroidal anti-inflammatory medications are avoided. Hard fixed crusts should be left alone to loosen and soften prior to removal. If removed, the adjacent tissue can be traumatized enough for major arterial bleeding to occur. Because most of these hemorrhages occur in the area of a removed middle turbinate, I have treated these patients with endoscopic cautery, which avoids the morbidity of a posterior pack and allows patients to be discharged the next day.

RARE COMPLICATIONS

The following complications have been reported but are extremely rare: cavernous sinus-internal carotid artery fistula, anterior cranial fossa brain damage, anesthesia-related cardiac arrhythmia and malignant hyperthermia, and dysesthesia cheek.[10,11]

Summary

Complication rates for intranasal sinus surgery range from 2% to 17%. This range identifies the difference between experienced and inexperienced sinus surgeons.[2,4,12] Endoscopic sinus surgeons encounter the same risks as traditional intranasal or external sinus surgeons. New technology demands added training and increased vigilance so that complication rates remain as low as possible. Synechia formation, orbital hematoma, and antrostomy closure are the most common complications. Cerebral spinal fluid leak with meningitis, double vision, and blindness are the most devastating complications. Reducing complications begins with prevention, which is achieved through diligent preparation. Careful surgical technique—based on both old and new principles and combined with compulsive postoperative care—is necessary for safe sinus surgery.

REFERENCES

1. Stankiewicz JA, Osguthorpe JD. Medical treatment sinusitis. *Otolaryngol Head Neck Surg.* 1989; 110:361–362.
2. Freedman HM, Kern EB. Complication of intranasal ethmoidectomy: A review of 1000 consecutive operations. *Laryngoscope.* 1979; 89:421.

3. Greenfield H. A controlled approach to avoid pitfalls and complications of ethmoid and sphenoid surgery. American Academy of Otolaryngology-Head and Neck Surgery. Instruction course, Washington, D.C., September, 1993.
4. Stankiewicz JA. Complications of endoscopic intranasal ethmoidectomy. *Laryngoscope.* 1987; 97:1270.
5. Stankiewicz JA. Complications of endoscopic nasal surgery: Occurrence and treatment. *Am J Rhinol.* 1987; 1:45.
6. Freidman WH. The ethmoid sinus, In: Blitzer A, Lawson W, Friedman W, (eds). *Surgery of the paranasal sinuses,* Philadelphia, 1985; WB Saunders, p 146.
7. Kainz J, Stammberger H. The roof of the anterior ethmoid: A place of least resistance in the skull base. *Am J Rhinol.* 1990; 3:191–199.
8. Stankiewicz JA. Blindness and intranasal endoscopic ethmoidectomy: Prevention and management. *Otolaryngol Head Neck Surg.* 1989;101:320-329.
9. Stammberger H. Endoscopic endonasal surgery. Concepts in treatment of recurring rhinosinusitis. Part I. Anatomic and pathophysiologic considerations. Part II. Surgical technique. *Otolaryngol Head Neck Surg.* 1986; 94:143.
10. Maniglia AJ. Fatal and major complications secondary to nasal and sinus surgery. *Laryngoscope.* 1989; 99:276.
11. Maniglia AJ. Rare complications following ethmoidectomies: A report of eleven cases. *Laryngoscope.* 1981; 91:1234.
12. Friedman WH, Katsantonis GP, Rosenblum BW. Sphenoethmoidectmy: The case for ethmoid marsupialization. *Laryngoscope.* 1986; 96:473.

20

New Concepts and the Use of Powered Instrumentation (the "Hummer") for Functional Endoscopic Sinus Surgery

Reuben C. Setliff, III

The three major issues in functional endoscopic sinus surgery (FESS) are *visualization, instrumentation,* and *the extent of surgery* in a given clinical situation. *Visualization* has become a minor issue as a result of the advent of the endoscope and improved lighting. However, current development of three-dimensional, virtual reality, and other endoscopic displays reflects an ongoing concern for visualization and orientation. Furthermore, the lack of real-time suction during the procedure compromises both visualization and safety.

Instrumentation is the second major issue, undergoing little change since the inception of endoscopic operative intervention for sinus disease. Concepts regarding the surgery are relatively new, especially the functional approach; however, the instruments, although more refined, fall short of enabling the surgeon to deliver a precise technique.

For the most part, available instrumentation influences the decision regarding the third major issue, *the extent of surgery.* Obviously, the functional approach to surgery dictates as limited a procedure as necessary to reestablish mucociliary clearance. Most physicians agree that sinus outflow tracts are small in healthy individuals (Fig. 20–1) and are often measured in millimeters. In many instances, sinus function is surprisingly well maintained, even when the area is diseased or partially obstructed. The ultimate surgical success seems to be a sinus with a small outflow tract that can be returned to health. However, the traditional concept of "large-hole surgery," ie, converting a small ostium to a larger opening, remains alive and well.

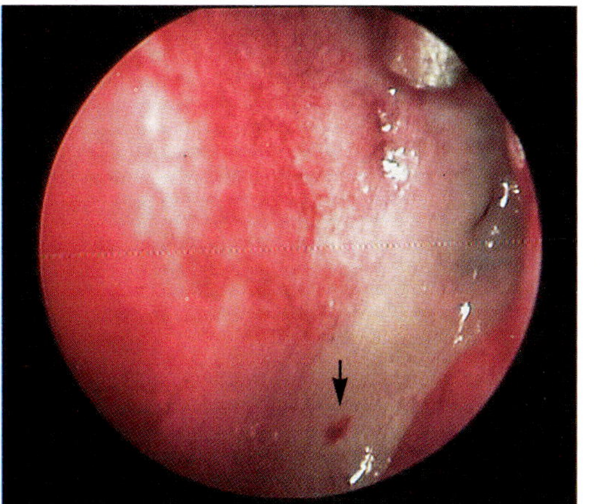
A

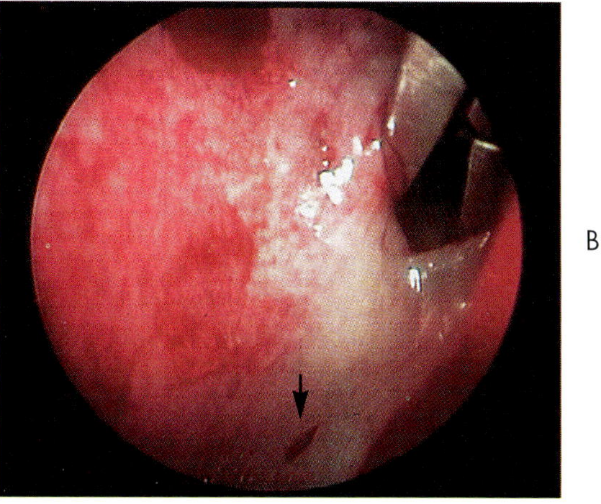
B

Fig. 20–1. **A** and **B,** Healthy sphenoid sinus despite pin-point ostium (see arrows).

The lack of resolution in the above issues relating to visualization, instrumentation, and extent of surgery impacts directly on the pervasive fear that underlines most sinus surgery. The surgeon's remedy for fear is precision—the kind of precision that eliminated the nightmarish outcomes of mastoid surgery before the microscope and powered cutting burr were introduced. Is it possible that another powered instrument could deliver real-time suction, thus improving the physician's visualization and orientation? Might the same instrument also create a precise technique that could reduce the risks to neighboring structures and make the elusive goals of functional surgery a reality? Finally, would it then be possible to explore the "small-hole" limits of functional surgery and answer the questions relating to the extent of surgery necessary to reverse chronic sinus disease?

Searching for answers to the above questions during August of 1992, the genesis of powered instrumentation for sinus surgery occurred at Great Plains Regional Medical Center in North Platte, Nebraska. The unit was an existing off-the-shelf device originally designed for temporomandibular joint (TMJ) surgery. Although the promise of the device was evident in early trials, this experience belied the future. Questions quickly arose regarding tip selection, suction requirements, hook up, prevention of line clogging, clearing of lines when clogging occurred, and sinus surgery possibilities using the device.

Initially utilized as an adjunct to the procedure, (ie, for clean up or touch up following traditional instrumentation) it soon became evident for use with all sinuses but the frontal that the device could replace most of the instrumentation used for sinus surgery. In addition, a more limited and less traumatic procedure could be performed with healing measured in days, rather than weeks or months.

The power instrumentation (the "Hummer") used in these efforts is made by Stryker Endoscopy of San Jose, California. Although there are similar devices, our experience is limited to the Stryker unit (Fig. 20–2).

As of August 1994, the "Hummer" has been used by the author in 261 adult and 64 pediatric patients in primary cases. The patients are drawn from a stable, rural midwest population. Postoperative results are pending and only preliminary observations will be reported in this chapter.

The potential advantages of the instrument became a reality with increasing experience. The benign contours of the relatively small diameter tip (3.5 mm) dramatically reduced inadvertent trauma to nasal mucosa (Fig. 20–3). The blunt end appeared to decrease the risk of violating the lamina papyracea, lateral lamella of the cribiform, or skull base. The closed nonworking side of the

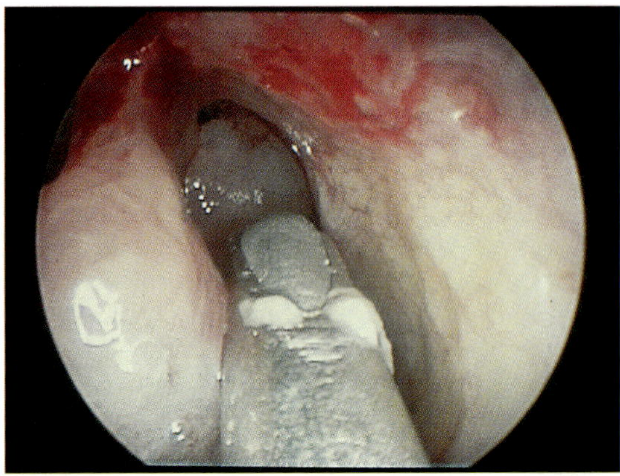

Fig. 20–3. "Hummer" tip with benign contours and window closed.

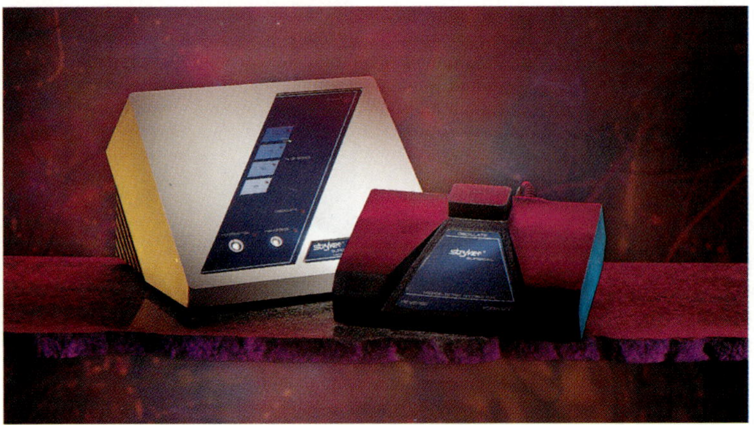

Fig. 20–2. The "Hummer" power unit and footswitch.

tip proved to be advantageous and relatively atraumatic for access in the middle meatus when slight medial retraction was required.

Tip length (8 cm) and the blunt end appeared to dramatically reduce the possibility of optic nerve or carotid artery violation via the sphenoid. The tip also proved sturdy enough to handle most required approaches to bony structures and for repositioning tissue.

The actual mechanism of the tip action in the nose and sinuses, especially with polyps, was both fortuitous and dramatic. The notion of pulling tissue into a small window by suction and then removing it with an internal spinning blade was not a new idea, but attempting this without continuous irrigation in the nose and sinuses was.

It became evident with the first attempt that powered instrumentation for nasal polyps would become the technique of choice. No other approach compares with the precision, speed, and visualization available with this technique. Further, the anatomic structures within the nose and middle meatus can clearly be defined, thereby converting a difficult procedure to a routine one.

Even now, approximately 2 years later, some physicians would recommend the technique for nasal polyps only; nothing could be further from the truth. In fact, the only real limitation to global sinus surgery is the lack of a curved tip to access the frontal recess—although many frontal cases have been performed with the available instrumentation.

What is the mechanism of action, and how is the "Hummer" used in sinus surgery other than polyps? (See *Utilization of a Powered Micro-debrider System in Functional Endoscopic Sinus Surgery.*) The tip has two parts (Fig. 20–4): an outer protecting sheath with a window near the end and a rotating insert with an accompanying window. The rotating insert is the blade, the recessed cutting action providing a measure of safety.

Its effectiveness is dependent upon suction through the hollow core of the blade pulling tissue, bone, blood, and irrigation fluid into the window (Fig. 20–5), resecting or removing the same from the operative field. Any clogging of the suction line is immediately recognized as a reduced efficiency of this action.

After much experimentation, it was determined that the most effective vacuum pressure was 170 to 180 mm Hg. This setting allowed for effective removal of surgical by-products without unwanted stripping of mucous membrane. A simple suction hookup to facilitate irrigation clearing of an occa-

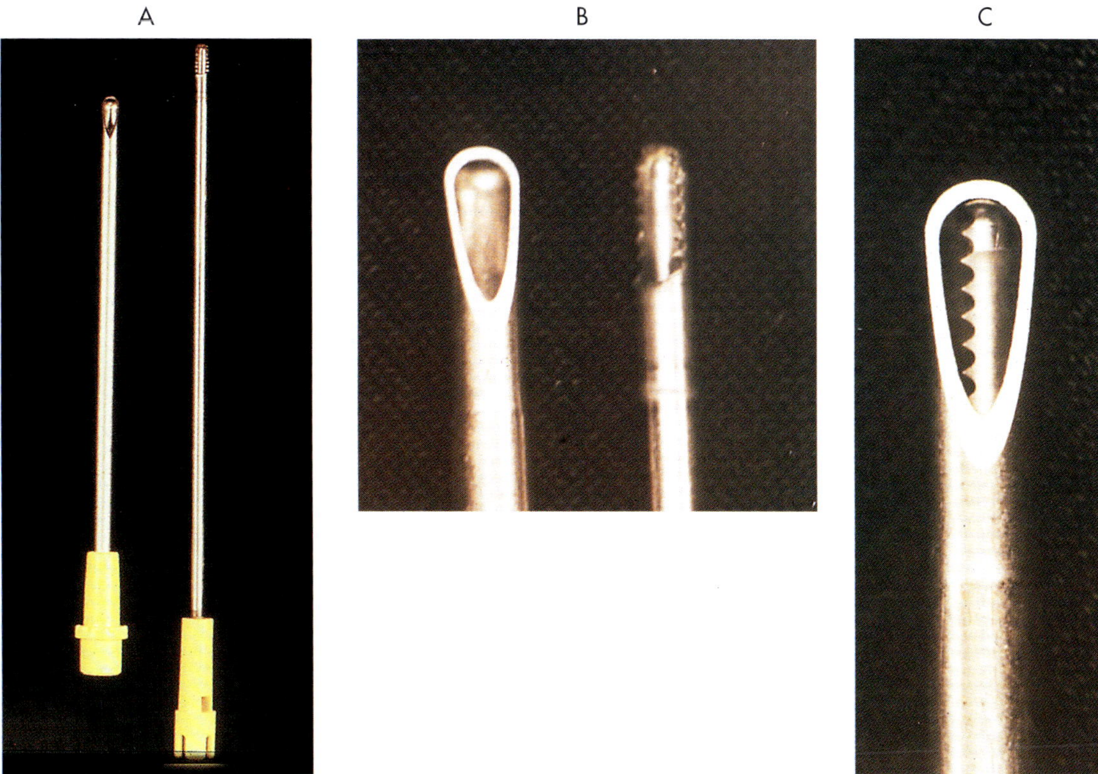

Fig. 20–4. **A,** Unassembled sheath on the left and insert on the right; **B,** unassembled sheath on the left and insert on the right; **C,** assembled window partially opened.

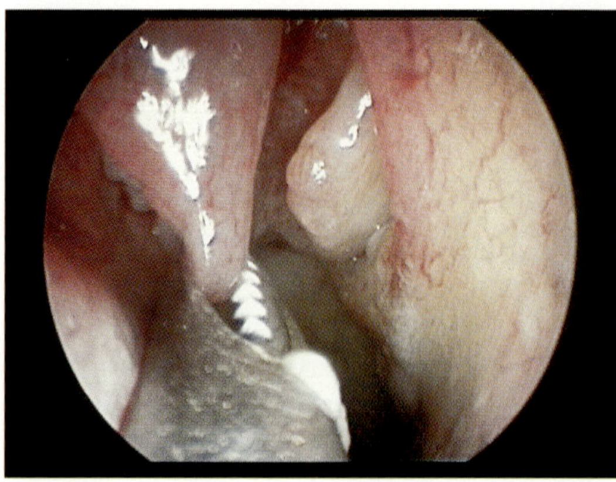

Fig. 20–5. Suction of polyp into window.

sionally clogged line is shown in *Utilization of a Powered Micro-debrider System in Functional Endoscopic Sinus Surgery.* Commercial set-ups designed for this purpose and for collecting specimens for pathology are now available.

The theoretic advantages of real-time continuous suction have long been appreciated. Ingenious modifications of forceps represent attempts to implement the concept for sinus surgery. However, they do fall short of real-time suction operative devices.

The theoretic advantages of real-time suction become a reality with powered instrumentation. Because the resected tissue or bone and blood are removed up the suction line, withdrawing the instrument from the nose to remove tissue or clear the operative field of blood is no longer necessary, reducing the probability of trauma to nasal mucosa or soiling of the endoscope lens. Should the endoscope become soiled, it can be cleared with targeted irrigation down the barrel of the endoscope, immediately removing the irrigation fluid from the field. In the *absence* of line clogging, visualization at the surgery site is unimpaired and real-time with respect to the resection.

As mentioned, the device was originally designed for TMJ surgery. However, the handpiece is remarkably adaptable to sinus surgery, whether working through the scope or off of the monitor (Fig. 20–6). It weighs 5 ounces, is 6 inches long, and is connected to its power source by a 10-foot coaxial cable. A suction port on the handpiece is the proximal end of a tube within the handpiece that runs to a chamber. In this chamber, the tip connects and delivers the evacuated material from the operative field. Tissue and debris then move from the chamber, through the handpiece, and on to the collecting system.

The power unit offers a range of power setting selections up to 1600 RPMs at a 100% setting. Speed can be varied by the degree of the depression on the foot switch. Cutting action is possible in forward, reverse, and oscillation settings. Sinus surgery is most effectively performed with full power—full depression of the foot switch and the oscillation setting. An increased frequency of oscillation further enhances the device's effectiveness and can be a retrofit on existing units.

Although both cutters and burrs are available for insertion into the handpiece by a quick-lock collar; the burrs are mentioned only to point out their limited application in early cases. Cutters are available in many configurations in both 2.5- and 3.5-mm diameters (Fig. 20–7). The aggressive straight cutter in a 3.5-mm diameter has proved to be most effective in both pediatric and adult sinus surgery. Limited experience with prototype curved tips indicates some added advantage for frontal sinus surgery.

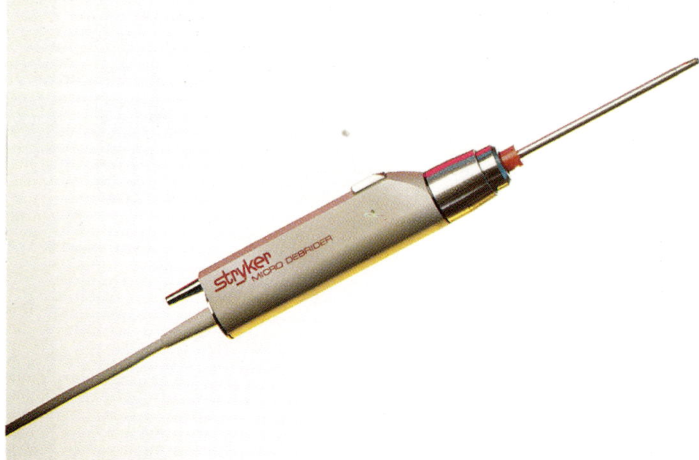

Fig. 20–6. Close-up of handpiece.

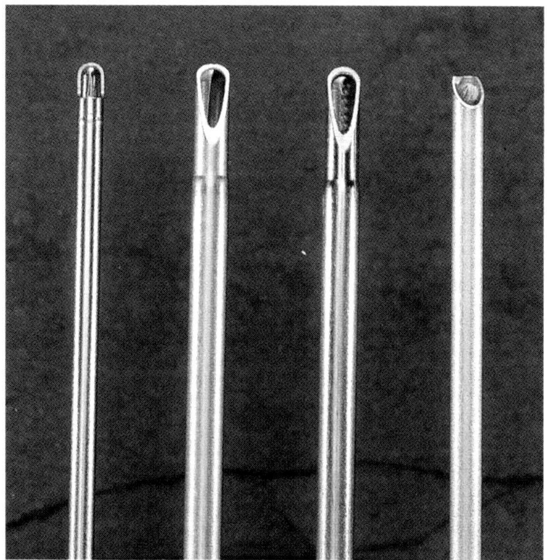

Fig. 20–7. "Hummer" tips; the aggressive cutter is third from the left.

At this time, the early promise of powered instrumentation has become a reality. The use of the device addresses all of the major issues of concern with today's sinus surgeon. Real-time suction makes the visualization potential of the improved endoscope a reality. The increased visualization with the precise and less traumatic surgery afforded by the "Hummer" causes less bleeding and a reduced healing burden for the patient.

Anatomic structures and variations can be appreciated with the "Hummer" as with no other approach. Powered instrumentation FESS can be approached as a dissection, not a "grab and tear" best effort. Preservation of the middle turbinate is possible in all cases and the early recommendations for performing the surgery under local anesthesia are considerably enhanced.

Our experience with the use of powered instrumentation has spawned several surgical techniques that have proved invaluable in standardizing the procedure. Using retrograde resection of the uncinate process as recommended by Parson, we modified the approach, creating a window into the infundibulum. Two new anatomic concepts, the exit and the final common pathway of the infundibulum, can be defined in all cases. Furthermore, a progression anteriorly from the exit along the final common pathway of the infundibulum will invariably track to the natural maxillary sinus ostium, dropping off inferiorly and laterally (Fig. 20–8).

Although the concept of leaving the natural ostium undisturbed is not new, a new procedure for ostium management has also been developed. Powered instrumentation has allowed the resection of the uncinate to the anterior limits of the infundibular window and a submucosal resection of the remaining inferior and tail portions of the uncinate. By trimming the resulting musocal flaps, a mucosal seam is created that allows direct entry of the maxillary sinus ostium into the nasal fossa. No instrumentation is performed to the natural ostium or the surrounding mucosa (Fig. 20–9). This nonmiddle meatal antrostomy approach has been performed on 240 consecutive patients, both pediatric and adult, since February 1993, with no patients returning for maxillary revision at the time of this chapter's completion (August 1994). Formal data collection is underway and will be reported elsewhere.

An additional surgical technique developed with the use of powered instrumentation involves removal of the ethmoid bulla from its medial interface with the middle turbinate, working from medial to lateral (Fig. 20–10). The surgeon can in all cases, then, clearly define the basal lamella or sinus lateralis of the ethmoid.

Powered instrumentation can also be used to resect the residual upper portion of the uncinate. If the frontal recess must be inspected or approached, the surgeon can enter the agger nasi cell inferiorly and with precision approach, the postero-medial wall of the agger nasi cell to evaluate the frontal recess and drainage (Fig. 20–11).

There are many other possible applications for the instrumentation, including transnasal removal of choanal adenoids, selective adenoidectomy, clean up of the delayed epistaxis case, the creation of abrasions resulting in small planned synechia between the middle turbinate and the septum to medialize the turbinate, and in choanal atresia (Fig. 20–12).

Surgery on the sphenoid sinus—an area of much concern to the sinus endoscopist—has been greatly simplified by the use of powered instrumentation. If outflow tract obstruction is indeed the culprit, powered instrumentation by way of a direct approach to the face and natural ostium of the sphenoid has proved to be most effective. The ostium is quite readily cleared or enlarged with the device. More extensive sphenoid surgery, and the accompanying increased risk, has been reserved for use in fungal sinusitis of the sphenoid or other uncommon clinical presentation.

UTILIZATION OF A POWERED MICRODEBRIDER SYSTEM IN FUNCTIONAL ENDOSCOPIC SINUS SURGERY

Basic Set-Up and Technique

The following guidelines are designed to help otolaryngologists obtain maximum effectiveness

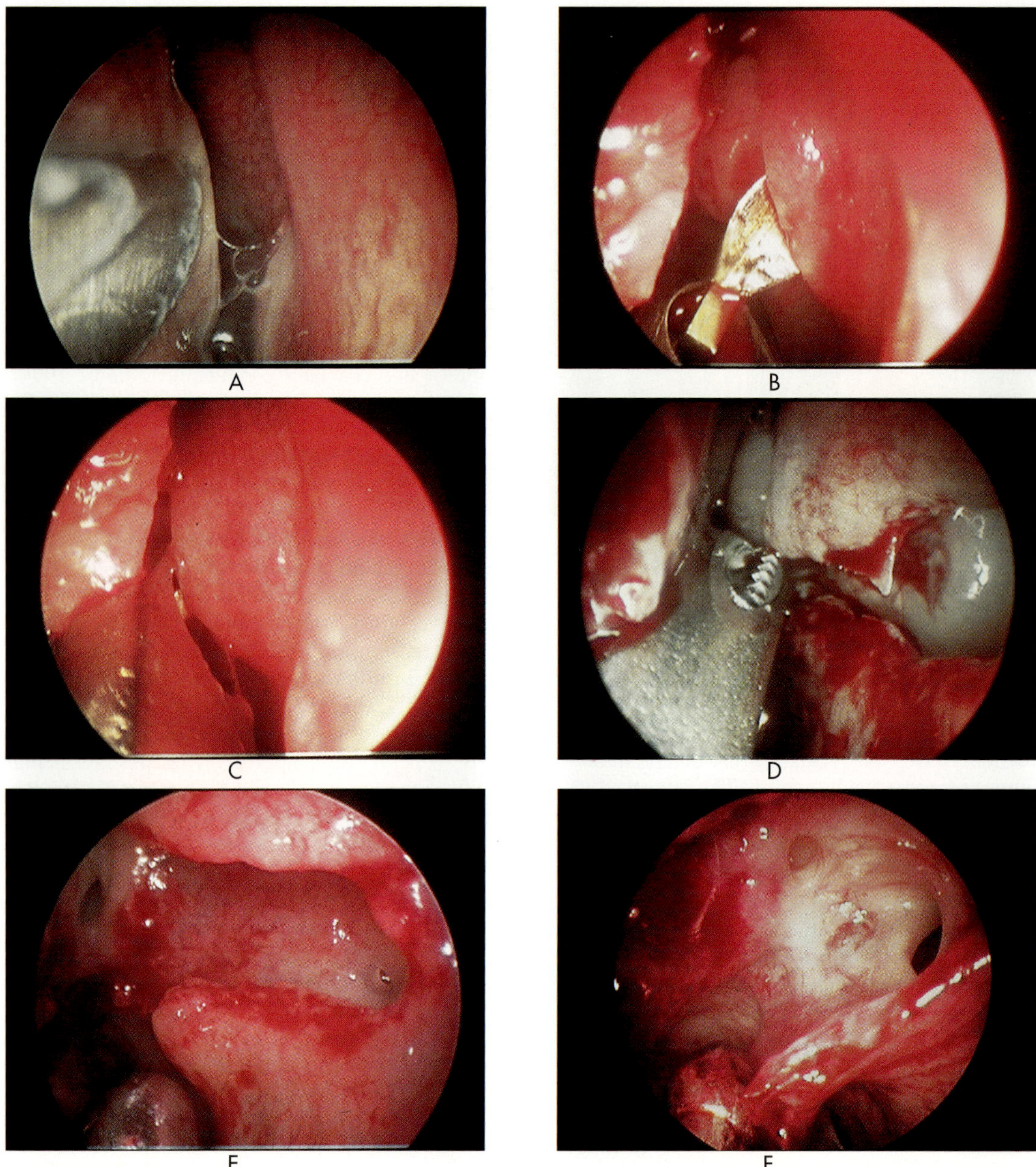

Fig. 20–8. **A,** Pus from exit of infundibulum; **B,** back-biter entering infundibulum; **C,** back-biter prior to first uncinate cut; **D,** window roughly cut; **E,** window after edging; **F,** exit and final common pathway of infundibulum, leading to the natural ostium of the maxillary sinus.

A
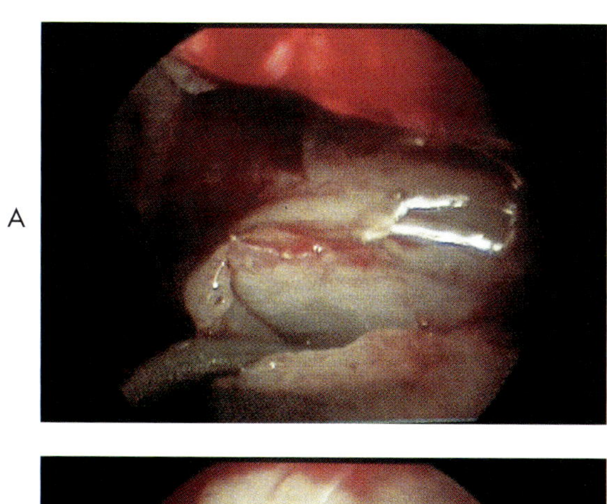

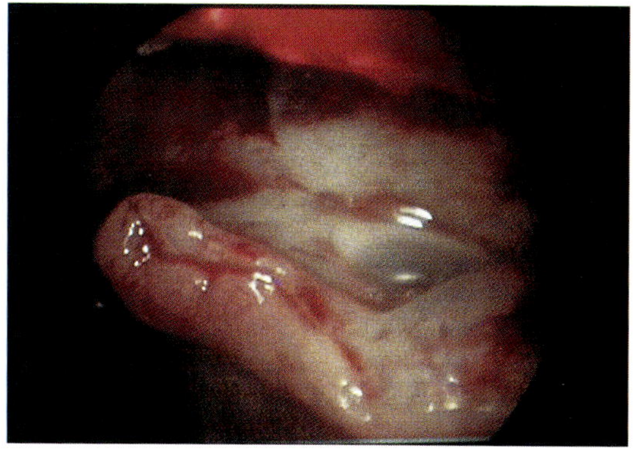
B

C
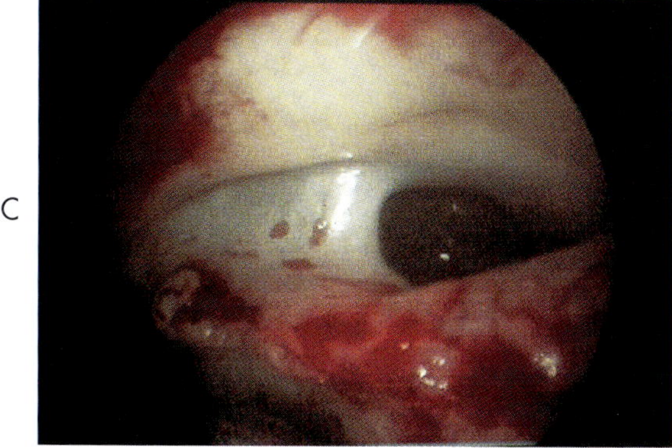

Fig. 20–9. **A,** Submucosal dissection of inferior uncinate; **B,** mucosal seam after uncinate removal; **C,** final appearance of the natural ostium in lieu of the middle meatal antrostomy.

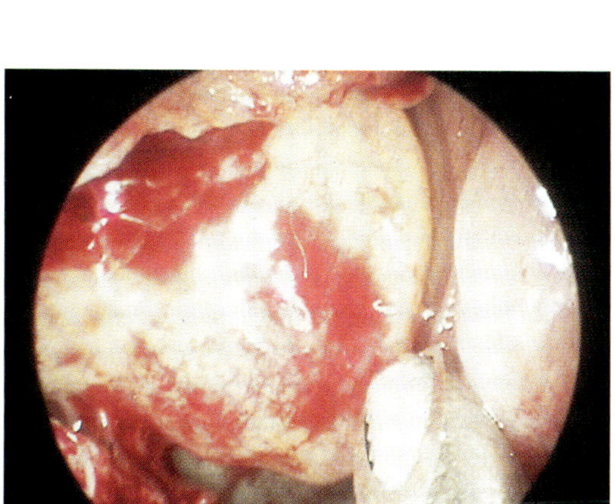

Fig. 20–10. "Hummer" positioned to begin medial to lateral dissection of the ethmoid bulla.

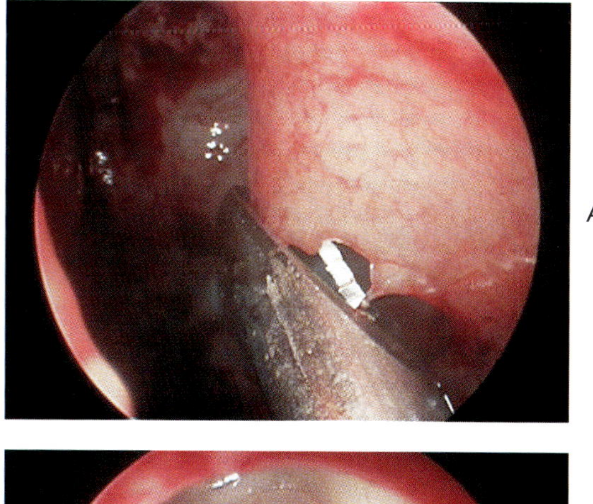
A

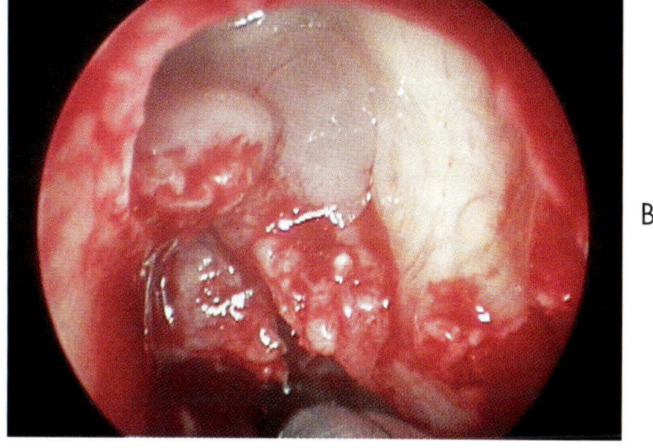
B

Fig. 20–11. Resection of upper uncinate to access agger nasi cell. **A,** "Hummer" positioned to resect upper uncinate; **B,** agger nasi cell.

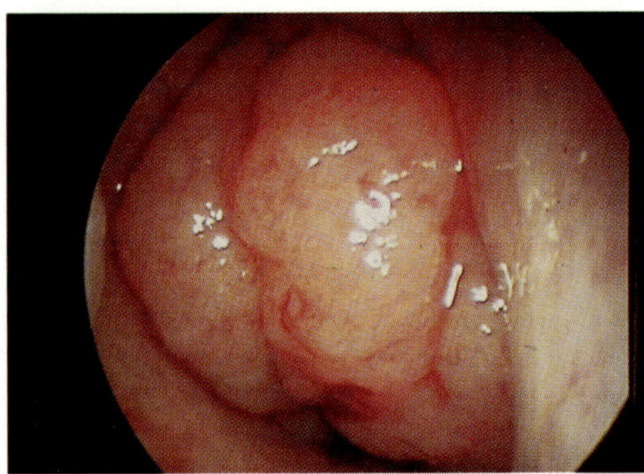

Fig. 20–12. Choanal adnoid.

in the application of a powered rotary shaving device (micro-debrider system) to functional endoscopic sinus surgery (FESS). These guidelines were developed after experience was obtained 250 patients from both with more than a private practice and a university referral center.

Surgeons are advised to begin slowly using the micro-debrider as an adjunct to standard surgical technique. Polypectomy and touch-up, clean up are simple and safe applications that allow the surgeon to get the feel of the instrument and learn the basic techniques of the cutter tip action and suction control that are important for success in more procedures complex. A natural progression to wider application of the instrument will occur as the surgeon gains both experience and confidence.

At this point in our experience, the micro-debrider system has replaced 80% or more of the manual instrumentation normally used for FESS. Its effect on the course of FESS is analogous to the effect of powered drills on mastoid surgery when they were introduced.

Required equipment

Micro-debrider system (1)

2.5-mm and 3.5-mm aggressive cutters (2)

51-cm intravenous extension set (Baxter No. 2c5625 or equivalent)

Three-way stopcock (Baxter No. K75 or equivalent)

30- to 50-mL syringe

Equipment set-up

Attach the handpiece and the footswitch to the console of the micro-debrider system. Refer to the operations manual for instructions on set-up and sterilization.

Insert a cutter into the handpiece.

Attach an intravenous extension set to the suction port at the rear of the micro-debrider handpiece.

Interpose a three-way stopcock between the extension set and the catheter tip adapter.

Attach the adapter to standard suction tubing. Connect suction tubing to the suction canister and the wall suction. Set the wall suction at 180 mm Hg.

Attach the syringe filled with saline to the third port of the stopcock.

See schematic (Fig. 20–13)

Basic technique

Set the micro-debrider to 100% speed level and oscillating mode. The oscillating mode has proved to be the most effective cutting mode for sinus tissues.

Stabilize the cutter shaft against the piriform aperture or some other point to act as a fulcrum for cutter motion if needed.

A useful technique for cutting is that of brief contacts of the tip with tissue or bone during the dissection allowing brief non-contact intervals for evacuation of blood and dissected tissue. However, cutter tip action may vary from a dabbing, curetting, and rolling motion of the tip to a more aggressive technique depending on the consistency of the tissue being resected and the angle of approach of the cutter mouth. Experience will dictate the appropriate technique for various types of tissue.

Utilizing the proper technique, any indication of a lack of dissection progress will most likely be the result of obstruction of the suction path at some point in the system.

Suction Control

Suction is a critical component of the dissection technique. The micro-debrider depends on suction to pull tissue into the cutter window, stabilize it for resection by the oscillating blade, and remove it from the operative field. To minimize the potential for suction line blockage, observe the following:

- Do not share suction with another instrument.
- The micro-debrider should have a discrete suction line.
- Suction should be set at 180 mm Hg. Hospital suction systems vary. Wall-mounted control boxes are not always accurate. Suction may vary throughout the day depending on the number of operating rooms in use. In general, set the suction in the high range. Experience will dictate the appropriate setting for your operating room.
- Whenever the instrument is withdrawn from the nose, insert the tip of the

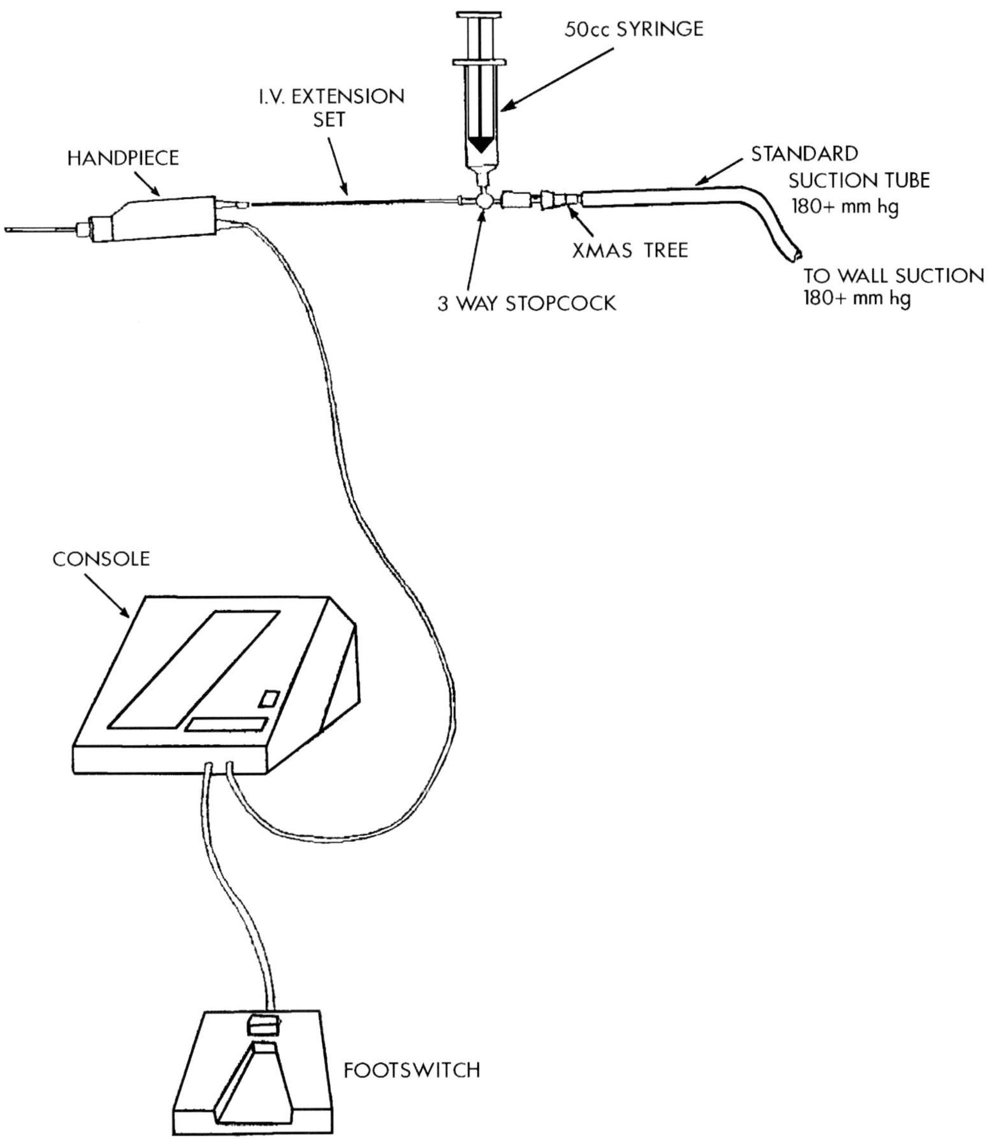

Fig. 20-13. Suction control set-up for micro-debrider system.

cutter into a bowl of saline and run the handpiece with full power to clear the suction line.

If the above does not clear the handpiece and cutter completely, shut off the suction with the three-way stopcock and inject saline through the third port of the stopcock. This will flush the handpiece toward the tip of the cutter. Be sure the cutter window is in the open position and activated.

Occasionally, it may be necessary to flush toward the suction canister or disconnect the intravenous extension set from the suction port and insert a 19-gauge blunt needle into the suction port and flush.

Rarely, it may be necessary to remove the cutter from the handpiece, disassemble it, and clean it manually.

General recommendations

When the patient is under general anesthesia,

it is possible to clean the endoscope with irrigation rather than frequently withdrawing it for cleaning. The irrigation fluid also helps to keep the suction line clear.

When the middle turbinate mechanically limits access to the middle meatus, as in a severe paradoxical curvature, limited removal of its lateral surface (thinning the middle turbinate) may be performed in lieu of more extensive turbinectomy.

A partial uncinectomy or the creation of an uncinate window using a back biter and the micro-debrider instead of a sickle knife approach is possible as the beginning surgical step. Reduced bleeding and an enhanced prospect of precise identification of the natural ostium of the maxillary sinus are advantages of this approach.

The remaining upper uncinate may be removed with the micro-debrider. Submucous removal of uncinate bone with pediatric forceps may facilitate this step.

Following the removal of the superior uncinate (and without the use of tissue forceps) the dome of the agger nasi and frontal recess are usually visible with a 30° scope. The frontal recess may sometimes be enlarged with the micro-debrider by removal of the postero-medial wall agger nasi.

When using the micro-debrider to begin the ethmoid dissection, start at the interface between the medial wall of the ethmoid bulla and the middle turbinate, working from medial to lateral. Remove large or free-floating bone fragments with pediatric forceps as needed to continue the dissection.

Identification of the sinus lateralis and basal lamella is assured if the previous step is carefully done. The micro-debrider is quite effective in dissecting the thinner bony partitions and large cells of the posterior ethmoids with preservation of mucous membrane at the limits of the dissection.

The benign contours of the micro-debrider allow a relatively atraumatic approach to the face of the sphenoid. Cleaning the natural ostium of the sphenoid is readily done with the instrument.

Index

D

E